FREE Study Skills Videos/DVD Offer

Dear Customer,

Thank you for your purchase from Mometrix! We consider it an honor and a privilege that you have purchased our product and we want to ensure your satisfaction.

As part of our ongoing effort to meet the needs of test takers, we have developed a set of Study Skills Videos that we would like to give you for FREE. These videos cover our *best practices* for getting ready for your exam, from how to use our study materials to how to best prepare for the day of the test.

All that we ask is that you email us with feedback that would describe your experience so far with our product. Good, bad, or indifferent, we want to know what you think!

To get your FREE Study Skills Videos, you can use the **QR code** below, or send us an **email** at studyvideos@mometrix.com with *FREE VIDEOS* in the subject line and the following information in the body of the email:

- The name of the product you purchased.
- Your product rating on a scale of 1-5, with 5 being the highest rating.
- Your feedback. It can be long, short, or anything in between. We just want to know your impressions and experience so far with our product. (Good feedback might include how our study material met your needs and ways we might be able to make it even better. You could highlight features that you found helpful or features that you think we should add.)

If you have any questions or concerns, please don't hesitate to contact me directly.

Thanks again!

Sincerely,

Jay Willis
Vice President
jay.willis@mometrix.com
1-800-673-8175

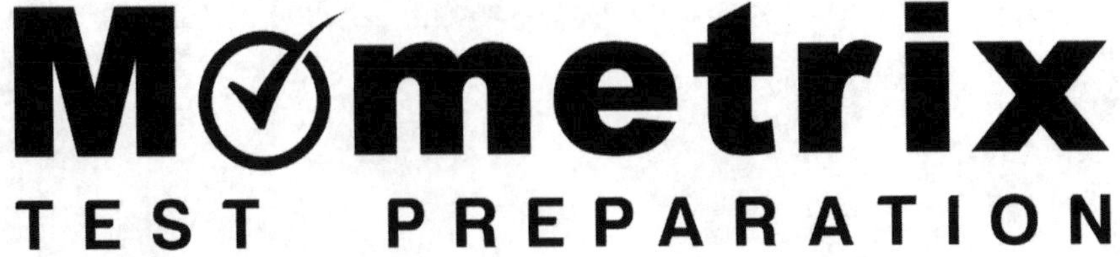

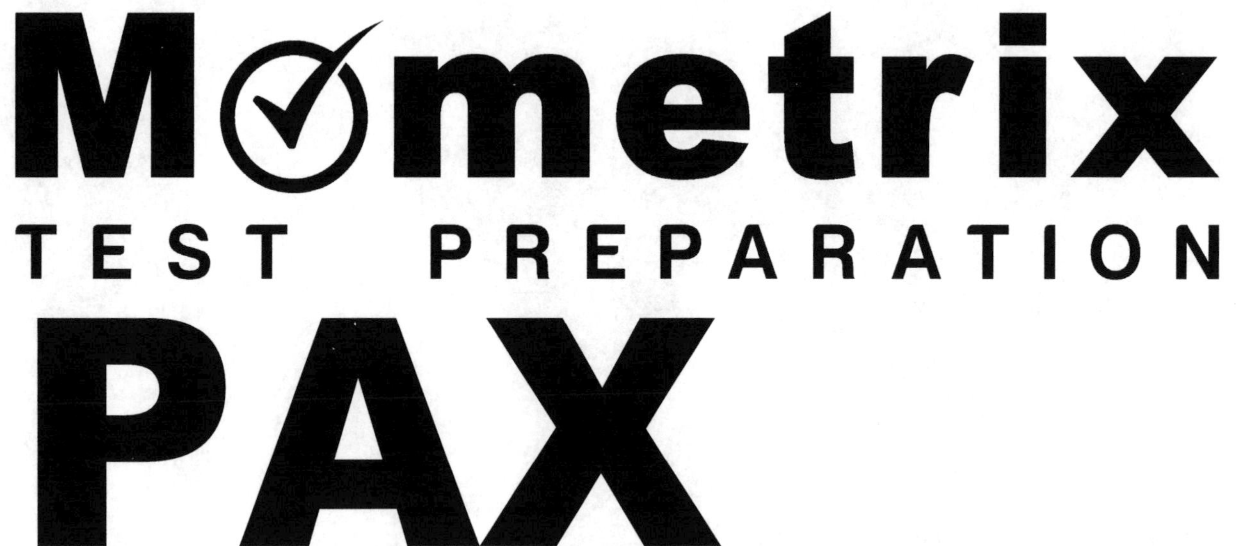

Study Guide Secrets 2022-2023

for the NLN Pre Entrance Exam

Full-Length Practice Test

**Step-by-Step
Video Tutorials**

5th Edition

Written and edited by the Mometrix Nursing School Admissions Test Team

Printed in the United States of America

This paper meets the requirements of ANSI/NISO Z39.48-1992 (Permanence of Paper).

Paperback
ISBN 13: 978-1-5167-1979-2
ISBN 10: 1-5167-1979-4

Dear Future Exam Success Story

First of all, **THANK YOU** for purchasing Mometrix study materials!

Second, congratulations! You are one of the few determined test-takers who are committed to doing whatever it takes to excel on your exam. **You have come to the right place.** We developed these study materials with one goal in mind: to deliver you the information you need in a format that's concise and easy to use.

In addition to optimizing your guide for the content of the test, we've outlined our recommended steps for breaking down the preparation process into small, attainable goals so you can make sure you stay on track.

We've also analyzed the entire test-taking process, identifying the most common pitfalls and showing how you can overcome them and be ready for any curveball the test throws you.

Standardized testing is one of the biggest obstacles on your road to success, which only increases the importance of doing well in the high-pressure, high-stakes environment of test day. Your results on this test could have a significant impact on your future, and this guide provides the information and practical advice to help you achieve your full potential on test day.

Your success is our success

We would love to hear from you! If you would like to share the story of your exam success or if you have any questions or comments in regard to our products, please contact us at **800-673-8175** or **support@mometrix.com**.

Thanks again for your business and we wish you continued success!

Sincerely,
The Mometrix Test Preparation Team

Need more help? Check out our flashcards at:
http://mometrixflashcards.com/nursing

TABLE OF CONTENTS

Introduction

Thank you for purchasing this resource! You have made the choice to prepare yourself for a test that could have a huge impact on your future, and this guide is designed to help you be fully ready for test day. Obviously, it's important to have a solid understanding of the test material, but you also need to be prepared for the unique environment and stressors of the test, so that you can perform to the best of your abilities.

For this purpose, the first section that appears in this guide is the **Secret Keys**. We've devoted countless hours to meticulously researching what works and what doesn't, and we've boiled down our findings to the five most impactful steps you can take to improve your performance on the test. We start at the beginning with study planning and move through the preparation process, all the way to the testing strategies that will help you get the most out of what you know when you're finally sitting in front of the test.

We recommend that you start preparing for your test as far in advance as possible. However, if you've bought this guide as a last-minute study resource and only have a few days before your test, we recommend that you skip over the first two Secret Keys since they address a long-term study plan.

If you struggle with **test anxiety**, we strongly encourage you to check out our recommendations for how you can overcome it. Test anxiety is a formidable foe, but it can be beaten, and we want to make sure you have the tools you need to defeat it.

Secret Key #1 – Plan Big, Study Small

There's a lot riding on your performance. If you want to ace this test, you're going to need to keep your skills sharp and the material fresh in your mind. You need a plan that lets you review everything you need to know while still fitting in your schedule. We'll break this strategy down into three categories.

Information Organization

Start with the information you already have: the official test outline. From this, you can make a complete list of all the concepts you need to cover before the test. Organize these concepts into groups that can be studied together, and create a list of any related vocabulary you need to learn so you can brush up on any difficult terms. You'll want to keep this vocabulary list handy once you actually start studying since you may need to add to it along the way.

Time Management

Once you have your set of study concepts, decide how to spread them out over the time you have left before the test. Break your study plan into small, clear goals so you have a manageable task for each day and know exactly what you're doing. Then just focus on one small step at a time. When you manage your time this way, you don't need to spend hours at a time studying. Studying a small block of content for a short period each day helps you retain information better and avoid stressing over how much you have left to do. You can relax knowing that you have a plan to cover everything in time. In order for this strategy to be effective though, you have to start studying early and stick to your schedule. Avoid the exhaustion and futility that comes from last-minute cramming!

Study Environment

The environment you study in has a big impact on your learning. Studying in a coffee shop, while probably more enjoyable, is not likely to be as fruitful as studying in a quiet room. It's important to keep distractions to a minimum. You're only planning to study for a short block of time, so make the most of it. Don't pause to check your phone or get up to find a snack. It's also important to **avoid multitasking**. Research has consistently shown that multitasking will make your studying dramatically less effective. Your study area should also be comfortable and well-lit so you don't have the distraction of straining your eyes or sitting on an uncomfortable chair.

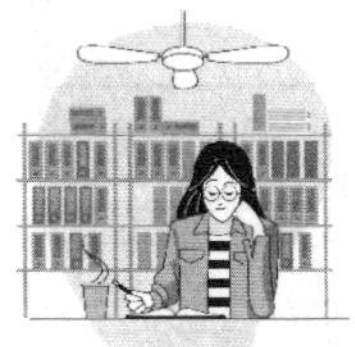

The time of day you study is also important. You want to be rested and alert. Don't wait until just before bedtime. Study when you'll be most likely to comprehend and remember. Even better, if you know what time of day your test will be, set that time aside for study. That way your brain will be used to working on that subject at that specific time and you'll have a better chance of recalling information.

Finally, it can be helpful to team up with others who are studying for the same test. Your actual studying should be done in as isolated an environment as possible, but the work of organizing the information and setting up the study plan can be divided up. In between study sessions, you can discuss with your teammates the concepts that you're all studying and quiz each other on the details. Just be sure that your teammates are as serious about the test as you are. If you find that your study time is being replaced with social time, you might need to find a new team.

Secret Key #2 – Make Your Studying Count

You're devoting a lot of time and effort to preparing for this test, so you want to be absolutely certain it will pay off. This means doing more than just reading the content and hoping you can remember it on test day. It's important to make every minute of study count. There are two main areas you can focus on to make your studying count.

Retention

It doesn't matter how much time you study if you can't remember the material. You need to make sure you are retaining the concepts. To check your retention of the information you're learning, try recalling it at later times with minimal prompting. Try carrying around flashcards and glance at one or two from time to time or ask a friend who's also studying for the test to quiz you.

To enhance your retention, look for ways to put the information into practice so that you can apply it rather than simply recalling it. If you're using the information in practical ways, it will be much easier to remember. Similarly, it helps to solidify a concept in your mind if you're not only reading it to yourself but also explaining it to someone else. Ask a friend to let you teach them about a concept you're a little shaky on (or speak aloud to an imaginary audience if necessary). As you try to summarize, define, give examples, and answer your friend's questions, you'll understand the concepts better and they will stay with you longer. Finally, step back for a big picture view and ask yourself how each piece of information fits with the whole subject. When you link the different concepts together and see them working together as a whole, it's easier to remember the individual components.

Finally, practice showing your work on any multi-step problems, even if you're just studying. Writing out each step you take to solve a problem will help solidify the process in your mind, and you'll be more likely to remember it during the test.

Modality

Modality simply refers to the means or method by which you study. Choosing a study modality that fits your own individual learning style is crucial. No two people learn best in exactly the same way, so it's important to know your strengths and use them to your advantage.

For example, if you learn best by visualization, focus on visualizing a concept in your mind and draw an image or a diagram. Try color-coding your notes, illustrating them, or creating symbols that will trigger your mind to recall a learned concept. If you learn best by hearing or discussing information, find a study partner who learns the same way or read aloud to yourself. Think about how to put the information in your own words. Imagine that you are giving a lecture on the topic and record yourself so you can listen to it later.

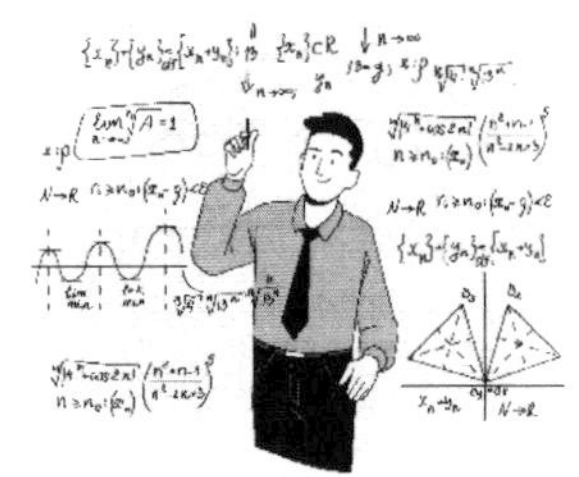

For any learning style, flashcards can be helpful. Organize the information so you can take advantage of spare moments to review. Underline key words or phrases. Use different colors for different categories. Mnemonic devices (such as creating a short list in which every item starts with the same letter) can also help with retention. Find what works best for you and use it to store the information in your mind most effectively and easily.

Secret Key #3 – Practice the Right Way

Your success on test day depends not only on how many hours you put into preparing, but also on whether you prepared the right way. It's good to check along the way to see if your studying is paying off. One of the most effective ways to do this is by taking practice tests to evaluate your progress. Practice tests are useful because they show exactly where you need to improve. Every time you take a practice test, pay special attention to these three groups of questions:

- The questions you got wrong
- The questions you had to guess on, even if you guessed right
- The questions you found difficult or slow to work through

This will show you exactly what your weak areas are, and where you need to devote more study time. Ask yourself why each of these questions gave you trouble. Was it because you didn't understand the material? Was it because you didn't remember the vocabulary? Do you need more repetitions on this type of question to build speed and confidence? Dig into those questions and figure out how you can strengthen your weak areas as you go back to review the material.

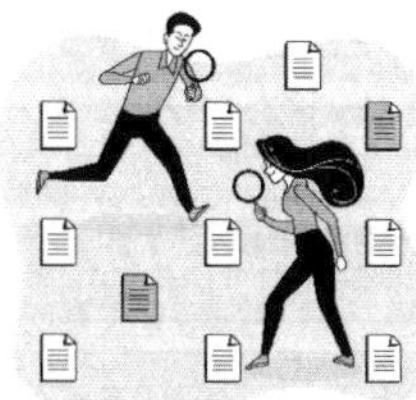

Additionally, many practice tests have a section explaining the answer choices. It can be tempting to read the explanation and think that you now have a good understanding of the concept. However, an explanation likely only covers part of the question's broader context. Even if the explanation makes perfect sense, **go back and investigate** every concept related to the question until you're positive you have a thorough understanding.

As you go along, keep in mind that the practice test is just that: practice. Memorizing these questions and answers will not be very helpful on the actual test because it is unlikely to have any of the same exact questions. If you only know the right answers to the sample questions, you won't be prepared for the real thing. **Study the concepts** until you understand them fully, and then you'll be able to answer any question that shows up on the test.

It's important to wait on the practice tests until you're ready. If you take a test on your first day of study, you may be overwhelmed by the amount of material covered and how much you need to learn. Work up to it gradually.

On test day, you'll need to be prepared for answering questions, managing your time, and using the test-taking strategies you've learned. It's a lot to balance, like a mental marathon that will have a big impact on your future. Like training for a marathon, you'll need to start slowly and work your way up. When test day arrives, you'll be ready.

Start with the strategies you've read in the first two Secret Keys—plan your course and study in the way that works best for you. If you have time, consider using multiple study resources to get different approaches to the same concepts. It can be helpful to see difficult concepts from more than one angle. Then find a good source for practice tests. Many times, the test website will suggest potential study resources or provide sample tests.

Practice Test Strategy

If you're able to find at least three practice tests, we recommend this strategy:

Untimed and Open-Book Practice

Take the first test with no time constraints and with your notes and study guide handy. Take your time and focus on applying the strategies you've learned.

Timed and Open-Book Practice

Take the second practice test open-book as well, but set a timer and practice pacing yourself to finish in time.

Timed and Closed-Book Practice

Take any other practice tests as if it were test day. Set a timer and put away your study materials. Sit at a table or desk in a quiet room, imagine yourself at the testing center, and answer questions as quickly and accurately as possible.

Keep repeating timed and closed-book tests on a regular basis until you run out of practice tests or it's time for the actual test. Your mind will be ready for the schedule and stress of test day, and you'll be able to focus on recalling the material you've learned.

Secret Key #4 – Pace Yourself

Once you're fully prepared for the material on the test, your biggest challenge on test day will be managing your time. Just knowing that the clock is ticking can make you panic even if you have plenty of time left. Work on pacing yourself so you can build confidence against the time constraints of the exam. Pacing is a difficult skill to master, especially in a high-pressure environment, so **practice is vital**.

Set time expectations for your pace based on how much time is available. For example, if a section has 60 questions and the time limit is 30 minutes, you know you have to average 30 seconds or less per question in order to answer them all. Although 30 seconds is the hard limit, set 25 seconds per question as your goal, so you reserve extra time to spend on harder questions. When you budget extra time for the harder questions, you no longer have any reason to stress when those questions take longer to answer.

Don't let this time expectation distract you from working through the test at a calm, steady pace, but keep it in mind so you don't spend too much time on any one question. Recognize that taking extra time on one question you don't understand may keep you from answering two that you do understand later in the test. If your time limit for a question is up and you're still not sure of the answer, mark it and move on, and come back to it later if the time and the test format allow. If the testing format doesn't allow you to return to earlier questions, just make an educated guess; then put it out of your mind and move on.

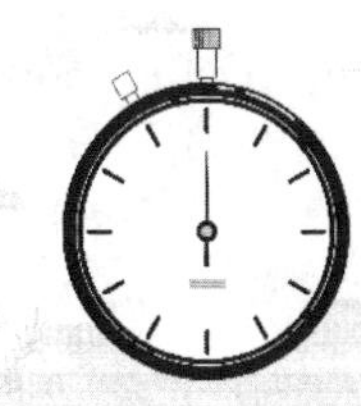

On the easier questions, be careful not to rush. It may seem wise to hurry through them so you have more time for the challenging ones, but it's not worth missing one if you know the concept and just didn't take the time to read the question fully. Work efficiently but make sure you understand the question and have looked at all of the answer choices, since more than one may seem right at first.

Even if you're paying attention to the time, you may find yourself a little behind at some point. You should speed up to get back on track, but do so wisely. Don't panic; just take a few seconds less on each question until you're caught up. Don't guess without thinking, but do look through the answer choices and eliminate any you know are wrong. If you can get down to two choices, it is often worthwhile to guess from those. Once you've chosen an answer, move on and don't dwell on any that you skipped or had to hurry through. If a question was taking too long, chances are it was one of the harder ones, so you weren't as likely to get it right anyway.

On the other hand, if you find yourself getting ahead of schedule, it may be beneficial to slow down a little. The more quickly you work, the more likely you are to make a careless mistake that will affect your score. You've budgeted time for each question, so don't be afraid to spend that time. Practice an efficient but careful pace to get the most out of the time you have.

Secret Key #5 – Have a Plan for Guessing

When you're taking the test, you may find yourself stuck on a question. Some of the answer choices seem better than others, but you don't see the one answer choice that is obviously correct. What do you do?

The scenario described above is very common, yet most test takers have not effectively prepared for it. Developing and practicing a plan for guessing may be one of the single most effective uses of your time as you get ready for the exam.

In developing your plan for guessing, there are three questions to address:

- When should you start the guessing process?
- How should you narrow down the choices?
- Which answer should you choose?

When to Start the Guessing Process

Unless your plan for guessing is to select C every time (which, despite its merits, is not what we recommend), you need to leave yourself enough time to apply your answer elimination strategies. Since you have a limited amount of time for each question, that means that if you're going to give yourself the best shot at guessing correctly, you have to decide quickly whether or not you will guess.

Of course, the best-case scenario is that you don't have to guess at all, so first, see if you can answer the question based on your knowledge of the subject and basic reasoning skills. Focus on the key words in the question and try to jog your memory of related topics. Give yourself a chance to bring the knowledge to mind, but once you realize that you don't have (or you can't access) the knowledge you need to answer the question, it's time to start the guessing process.

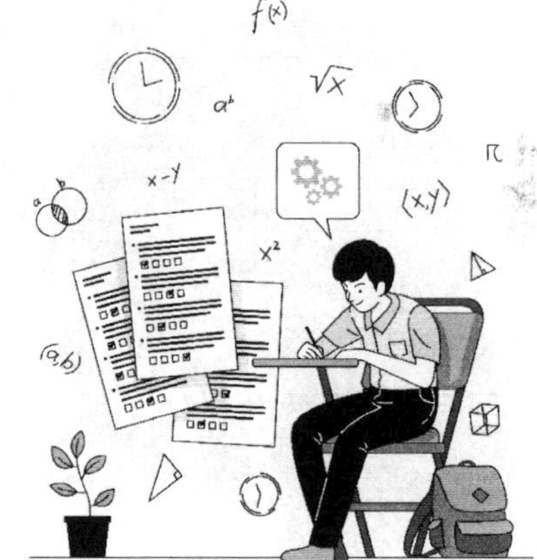

It's almost always better to start the guessing process too early than too late. It only takes a few seconds to remember something and answer the question from knowledge. Carefully eliminating wrong answer choices takes longer. Plus, going through the process of eliminating answer choices can actually help jog your memory.

Summary: Start the guessing process as soon as you decide that you can't answer the question based on your knowledge.

How to Narrow Down the Choices

The next chapter in this book (**Test-Taking Strategies**) includes a wide range of strategies for how to approach questions and how to look for answer choices to eliminate. You will definitely want to read those carefully, practice them, and figure out which ones work best for you. Here though, we're going to address a mindset rather than a particular strategy.

Your odds of guessing an answer correctly depend on how many options you are choosing from.

Number of options left	5	4	3	2	1
Odds of guessing correctly	20%	25%	33%	50%	100%

You can see from this chart just how valuable it is to be able to eliminate incorrect answers and make an educated guess, but there are two things that many test takers do that cause them to miss out on the benefits of guessing:

- Accidentally eliminating the correct answer
- Selecting an answer based on an impression

We'll look at the first one here, and the second one in the next section.

To avoid accidentally eliminating the correct answer, we recommend a thought exercise called **the $5 challenge**. In this challenge, you only eliminate an answer choice from contention if you are willing to bet $5 on it being wrong. Why $5? Five dollars is a small but not insignificant amount of money. It's an amount you could afford to lose but wouldn't want to throw away. And while losing $5 once might not hurt too much, doing it twenty times will set you back $100. In the same way, each small decision you make—eliminating a choice here, guessing on a question there—won't by itself impact your score very much, but when you put them all together, they can make a big difference. By holding each answer choice elimination decision to a higher standard, you can reduce the risk of accidentally eliminating the correct answer.

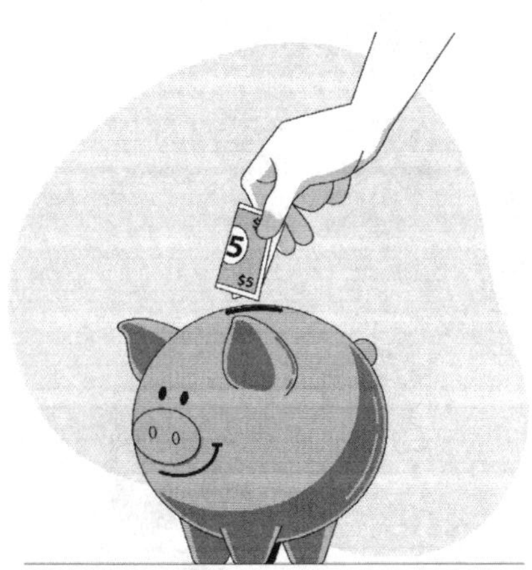

The $5 challenge can also be applied in a positive sense: If you are willing to bet $5 that an answer choice *is* correct, go ahead and mark it as correct.

Summary: Only eliminate an answer choice if you are willing to bet $5 that it is wrong.

Which Answer to Choose

You're taking the test. You've run into a hard question and decided you'll have to guess. You've eliminated all the answer choices you're willing to bet $5 on. Now you have to pick an answer. Why do we even need to talk about this? Why can't you just pick whichever one you feel like when the time comes?

The answer to these questions is that if you don't come into the test with a plan, you'll rely on your impression to select an answer choice, and if you do that, you risk falling into a trap. The test writers know that everyone who takes their test will be guessing on some of the questions, so they intentionally write wrong answer choices to seem plausible. You still have to pick an answer though, and if the wrong answer choices are designed to look right, how can you ever be sure that you're not falling for their trap? The best solution we've found to this dilemma is to take the decision out of your hands entirely. Here is the process we recommend:

Once you've eliminated any choices that you are confident (willing to bet $5) are wrong, select the first remaining choice as your answer.

Whether you choose to select the first remaining choice, the second, or the last, the important thing is that you use some preselected standard. Using this approach guarantees that you will not be enticed into selecting an answer choice that looks right, because you are not basing your decision on how the answer choices look.

A. This is wrong.
B. Also wrong.
C. Maybe?
D. Maybe?

This is not meant to make you question your knowledge. Instead, it is to help you recognize the difference between your knowledge and your impressions. There's a huge difference between thinking an answer is right because of what you know, and thinking an answer is right because it looks or sounds like it should be right.

Summary: To ensure that your selection is appropriately random, make a predetermined selection from among all answer choices you have not eliminated.

Test-Taking Strategies

This section contains a list of test-taking strategies that you may find helpful as you work through the test. By taking what you know and applying logical thought, you can maximize your chances of answering any question correctly!

It is very important to realize that every question is different and every person is different: no single strategy will work on every question, and no single strategy will work for every person. That's why we've included all of them here, so you can try them out and determine which ones work best for different types of questions and which ones work best for you.

Question Strategies

⊘ Read Carefully

Read the question and the answer choices carefully. Don't miss the question because you misread the terms. You have plenty of time to read each question thoroughly and make sure you understand what is being asked. Yet a happy medium must be attained, so don't waste too much time. You must read carefully and efficiently.

⊘ Contextual Clues

Look for contextual clues. If the question includes a word you are not familiar with, look at the immediate context for some indication of what the word might mean. Contextual clues can often give you all the information you need to decipher the meaning of an unfamiliar word. Even if you can't determine the meaning, you may be able to narrow down the possibilities enough to make a solid guess at the answer to the question.

⊘ Prefixes

If you're having trouble with a word in the question or answer choices, try dissecting it. Take advantage of every clue that the word might include. Prefixes can be a huge help. Usually, they allow you to determine a basic meaning. *Pre-* means before, *post-* means after, *pro-* is positive, *de-* is negative. From prefixes, you can get an idea of the general meaning of the word and try to put it into context.

⊘ Hedge Words

Watch out for critical hedge words, such as *likely, may, can, sometimes, often, almost, mostly, usually, generally, rarely*, and *sometimes*. Question writers insert these hedge phrases to cover every possibility. Often an answer choice will be wrong simply because it leaves no room for exception. Be on guard for answer choices that have definitive words such as *exactly* and *always*.

⊘ Switchback Words

Stay alert for *switchbacks*. These are the words and phrases frequently used to alert you to shifts in thought. The most common switchback words are *but, although*, and *however*. Others include *nevertheless, on the other hand, even though, while, in spite of, despite*, and *regardless of*. Switchback words are important to catch because they can change the direction of the question or an answer choice.

⊘ Face Value

When in doubt, use common sense. Accept the situation in the problem at face value. Don't read too much into it. These problems will not require you to make wild assumptions. If you have to go beyond creativity and warp time or space in order to have an answer choice fit the question, then you should move on and consider the other answer choices. These are normal problems rooted in reality. The applicable relationship or explanation may not be readily apparent, but it is there for you to figure out. Use your common sense to interpret anything that isn't clear.

Answer Choice Strategies

⊘ Answer Selection

The most thorough way to pick an answer choice is to identify and eliminate wrong answers until only one is left, then confirm it is the correct answer. Sometimes an answer choice may immediately seem right, but be careful. The test writers will usually put more than one reasonable answer choice on each question, so take a second to read all of them and make sure that the other choices are not equally obvious. As long as you have time left, it is better to read every answer choice than to pick the first one that looks right without checking the others.

⊘ Answer Choice Families

An answer choice family consists of two (in rare cases, three) answer choices that are very similar in construction and cannot all be true at the same time. If you see two answer choices that are direct opposites or parallels, one of them is usually the correct answer. For instance, if one answer choice says that quantity x increases and another either says that quantity x decreases (opposite) or says that quantity y increases (parallel), then those answer choices would fall into the same family. An answer choice that doesn't match the construction of the answer choice family is more likely to be incorrect. Most questions will not have answer choice families, but when they do appear, you should be prepared to recognize them.

⊘ Eliminate Answers

Eliminate answer choices as soon as you realize they are wrong, but make sure you consider all possibilities. If you are eliminating answer choices and realize that the last one you are left with is also wrong, don't panic. Start over and consider each choice again. There may be something you missed the first time that you will realize on the second pass.

⊘ Avoid Fact Traps

Don't be distracted by an answer choice that is factually true but doesn't answer the question. You are looking for the choice that answers the question. Stay focused on what the question is asking for so you don't accidentally pick an answer that is true but incorrect. Always go back to the question and make sure the answer choice you've selected actually answers the question and is not merely a true statement.

⊘ Extreme Statements

In general, you should avoid answers that put forth extreme actions as standard practice or proclaim controversial ideas as established fact. An answer choice that states the "process should be used in certain situations, if…" is much more likely to be correct than one that states the "process should be discontinued completely." The first is a calm rational statement and doesn't even make a definitive, uncompromising stance, using a hedge word *if* to provide wiggle room, whereas the second choice is far more extreme.

⊘ Benchmark

As you read through the answer choices and you come across one that seems to answer the question well, mentally select that answer choice. This is not your final answer, but it's the one that will help you evaluate the other answer choices. The one that you selected is your benchmark or standard for judging each of the other answer choices. Every other answer choice must be compared to your benchmark. That choice is correct until proven otherwise by another answer choice beating it. If you find a better answer, then that one becomes your new benchmark. Once you've decided that no other choice answers the question as well as your benchmark, you have your final answer.

☑ Predict the Answer

Before you even start looking at the answer choices, it is often best to try to predict the answer. When you come up with the answer on your own, it is easier to avoid distractions and traps because you will know exactly what to look for. The right answer choice is unlikely to be word-for-word what you came up with, but it should be a close match. Even if you are confident that you have the right answer, you should still take the time to read each option before moving on.

General Strategies

☑ Tough Questions

If you are stumped on a problem or it appears too hard or too difficult, don't waste time. Move on! Remember though, if you can quickly check for obviously incorrect answer choices, your chances of guessing correctly are greatly improved. Before you completely give up, at least try to knock out a couple of possible answers. Eliminate what you can and then guess at the remaining answer choices before moving on.

☑ Check Your Work

Since you will probably not know every term listed and the answer to every question, it is important that you get credit for the ones that you do know. Don't miss any questions through careless mistakes. If at all possible, try to take a second to look back over your answer selection and make sure you've selected the correct answer choice and haven't made a costly careless mistake (such as marking an answer choice that you didn't mean to mark). This quick double check should more than pay for itself in caught mistakes for the time it costs.

☑ Pace Yourself

It's easy to be overwhelmed when you're looking at a page full of questions; your mind is confused and full of random thoughts, and the clock is ticking down faster than you would like. Calm down and maintain the pace that you have set for yourself. Especially as you get down to the last few minutes of the test, don't let the small numbers on the clock make you panic. As long as you are on track by monitoring your pace, you are guaranteed to have time for each question.

☑ Don't Rush

It is very easy to make errors when you are in a hurry. Maintaining a fast pace in answering questions is pointless if it makes you miss questions that you would have gotten right otherwise. Test writers like to include distracting information and wrong answers that seem right. Taking a little extra time to avoid careless mistakes can make all the difference in your test score. Find a pace that allows you to be confident in the answers that you select.

☑ Keep Moving

Panicking will not help you pass the test, so do your best to stay calm and keep moving. Taking deep breaths and going through the answer elimination steps you practiced can help to break through a stress barrier and keep your pace.

Final Notes

The combination of a solid foundation of content knowledge and the confidence that comes from practicing your plan for applying that knowledge is the key to maximizing your performance on test day. As your foundation of content knowledge is built up and strengthened, you'll find that the strategies included in this chapter become more and more effective in helping you quickly sift through the distractions and traps of the test to isolate the correct answer.

Now that you're preparing to move forward into the test content chapters of this book, be sure to keep your goal in mind. As you read, think about how you will be able to apply this information on the test. If you've already seen sample questions for the test and you have an idea of the question format and style, try to come up with questions of your own that you can answer based on what you're reading. This will give you valuable practice applying your knowledge in the same ways you can expect to on test day.

Good luck and good studying!

Verbal

Transform passive reading into active learning! After immersing yourself in this chapter, put your comprehension to the test by taking a quiz. The insights you gained will stay with you longer this way. Scan the QR code to go directly to the chapter quiz interface for this study guide. If you're using a computer, simply visit the bonus page at **mometrix.com/bonus948/pax** and click the Chapter Quizzes link.

Reading in Context

COMMON ORGANIZATIONS OF TEXTS

ORGANIZATION OF THE TEXT

The way a text is organized can help readers understand the author's intent and his or her conclusions. There are various ways to organize a text, and each one has a purpose and use. Usually, authors will organize information logically in a passage so the reader can follow and locate the information within the text. However, since not all passages are written with the same logical structure, you need to be familiar with several different types of passage structure.

Review Video: Organizational Methods to Structure Text
Visit mometrix.com/academy and enter code: 606263

Review Video: Sequence of Events in a Story
Visit mometrix.com/academy and enter code: 807512

CHRONOLOGICAL

When using **chronological** order, the author presents information in the order that it happened. For example, biographies are typically written in chronological order. The subject's birth and childhood are presented first, followed by their adult life, and lastly the events leading up to the person's death.

CAUSE AND EFFECT

One of the most common text structures is **cause and effect**. A **cause** is an act or event that makes something happen, and an **effect** is the thing that happens as a result of the cause. A cause-and-effect relationship is not always explicit, but there are some terms in English that signal causes, such as *since*, *because*, and *due to*. Furthermore, terms that signal effects include *consequently, therefore, this leads to*. As an example, consider the sentence *Because the sky was clear, Ron did not bring an umbrella*. The cause is the clear sky, and the effect is that Ron did not bring an umbrella. However, readers may find that sometimes the cause-and-effect relationship will not be clearly noted. For instance, the sentence *He was late and missed the meeting* does not contain any signaling words, but the sentence still contains a cause (he was late) and an effect (he missed the meeting).

Review Video: Cause and Effect
Visit mometrix.com/academy and enter code: 868099

Review Video: Rhetorical Strategy of Cause and Effect Analysis
Visit mometrix.com/academy and enter code: 725944

MULTIPLE EFFECTS

Be aware of the possibility for a single cause to have **multiple effects.** (e.g., *Single cause*: Because you left your homework on the table, your dog engulfed the assignment. *Multiple effects*: As a result, you receive a failing grade, your parents do not allow you to go out with your friends, you miss out on the new movie, and one of your classmates spoils it for you before you have another chance to watch it).

Multiple Causes

Also, there is the possibility for a single effect to have **multiple causes.** (e.g., *Single effect*: Alan has a fever. *Multiple causes*: An unexpected cold front came through the area, and Alan forgot to take his multi-vitamin to avoid getting sick.) Additionally, an effect can in turn be the cause of another effect, in what is known as a cause-and-effect chain. (e.g., As a result of her disdain for procrastination, Lynn prepared for her exam. This led to her passing her test with high marks. Hence, her resume was accepted and her application was approved.)

Cause and Effect in Persuasive Essays

Persuasive essays, in which an author tries to make a convincing argument and change the minds of readers, usually include cause-and-effect relationships. However, these relationships should not always be taken at face value. Frequently, an author will assume a cause or take an effect for granted. To read a persuasive essay effectively, readers need to judge the cause-and-effect relationships that the author is presenting. For instance, imagine an author wrote the following: *The parking deck has been unprofitable because people would prefer to ride their bikes.* The relationship is clear: the cause is that people prefer to ride their bikes, and the effect is that the parking deck has been unprofitable. However, readers should consider whether this argument is conclusive. Perhaps there are other reasons for the failure of the parking deck: a down economy, excessive fees, etc. Too often, authors present causal relationships as if they are fact rather than opinion. Readers should be on the alert for these dubious claims.

Problem-Solution

Some nonfiction texts are organized to **present a problem** followed by a solution. For this type of text, the problem is often explained before the solution is offered. In some cases, as when the problem is well known, the solution may be introduced briefly at the beginning. Other passages may focus on the solution, and the problem will be referenced only occasionally. Some texts will outline multiple solutions to a problem, leaving readers to choose among them. If the author has an interest or an allegiance to one solution, he or she may fail to mention or describe accurately some of the other solutions. Readers should be careful of the author's agenda when reading a problem-solution text. Only by understanding the author's perspective and interests can one develop a proper judgment of the proposed solution.

Compare and Contrast

Many texts follow the **compare-and-contrast** model in which the similarities and differences between two ideas or things are explored. Analysis of the similarities between ideas is called **comparison**. In an ideal comparison, the author places ideas or things in an equivalent structure, i.e., the author presents the ideas in the same way. If an author wants to show the similarities between cricket and baseball, then he or she may do so by summarizing the equipment and rules for each game. Be mindful of the similarities as they appear in the passage and take note of any differences that are mentioned. Often, these small differences will only reinforce the more general similarity.

Review Video: Compare and Contrast
Visit mometrix.com/academy and enter code: 798319

Thinking critically about ideas and conclusions can seem like a daunting task. One way to ease this task is to understand the basic elements of ideas and writing techniques. Looking at the ways different ideas relate to each other can be a good way for readers to begin their analysis. For instance, sometimes authors will write about two ideas that are in opposition to each other. Or, one author will provide his or her ideas on a topic, and another author may respond in opposition. The analysis of these opposing ideas is known as **contrast**. Contrast is often marred by the author's obvious partiality to one of the ideas. A discerning reader will be put off by an author who does not engage in a fair fight. In an analysis of opposing ideas, both ideas should be presented in clear and reasonable terms. If the author does prefer a side, you need to read carefully to determine the areas where the author shows or avoids this preference. In an analysis of opposing ideas, you should proceed through the passage by marking the major differences point by point with an eye that is looking for an explanation of each side's view. For instance, in an analysis of capitalism and communism, there is an importance in outlining each side's view on labor, markets, prices, personal responsibility, etc. Additionally, as you read through the passages, you should note whether the opposing views present each side in a similar manner.

SEQUENCE

Readers must be able to identify a text's **sequence**, or the order in which things happen. Often, when the sequence is very important to the author, the text is indicated with signal words like *first, then, next,* and *last*. However, a sequence can be merely implied and must be noted by the reader. Consider the sentence *He walked through the garden and gave water and fertilizer to the plants.* Clearly, the man did not walk through the garden before he collected water and fertilizer for the plants. So, the implied sequence is that he first collected water, then he collected fertilizer, next he walked through the garden, and last he gave water or fertilizer as necessary to the plants. Texts do not always proceed in an orderly sequence from first to last. Sometimes they begin at the end and start over at the beginning. As a reader, you can enhance your understanding of the passage by taking brief notes to clarify the sequence.

Review Video: Sequence
Visit mometrix.com/academy and enter code: 489027

MAIN IDEAS AND SUPPORTING DETAILS

IDENTIFYING TOPICS AND MAIN IDEAS

One of the most important skills in reading comprehension is the identification of **topics** and **main ideas**. There is a subtle difference between these two features. The topic is the subject of a text (i.e., what the text is all about). The main idea, on the other hand, is the most important point being made by the author. The topic is usually expressed in a few words at the most while the main idea often needs a full sentence to be completely defined. As an example, a short passage might be written on the topic of penguins, and the main idea could be written as *Penguins are different from other birds in many ways.* In most nonfiction writing, the topic and the main idea will be **stated directly** and often appear in a sentence at the very beginning or end of the text. When being tested on an understanding of the author's topic, you may be able to skim the passage for the general idea by reading only the first sentence of each paragraph. A body paragraph's first sentence is often—but not always—the main **topic sentence** which gives you a summary of the content in the paragraph.

However, there are cases in which the reader must figure out an **unstated** topic or main idea. In these instances, you must read every sentence of the text and try to come up with an overarching idea that is supported by each of those sentences.

Note: The main idea should not be confused with the thesis statement. While the main idea gives a brief, general summary of a text, the thesis statement provides a **specific perspective** on an issue that the author supports with evidence.

Review Video: Topics and Main Ideas
Visit mometrix.com/academy and enter code: 407801

SUPPORTING DETAILS

Supporting details are smaller pieces of evidence that provide backing for the main point. In order to show that a main idea is correct or valid, an author must add details that prove their point. All texts contain details, but they are only classified as supporting details when they serve to reinforce some larger point. Supporting details are most commonly found in informative and persuasive texts. In some cases, they will be clearly indicated with terms like *for example* or *for instance*, or they will be enumerated with terms like *first, second,* and *last.* However, you need to be prepared for texts that do not contain those indicators. As a reader, you should consider whether the author's supporting details really back up his or her main point. Details can be factual and correct, yet they may not be **relevant** to the author's point. Conversely, details can be relevant, but be ineffective because they are based on opinion or assertions that cannot be proven.

Review Video: Supporting Details
Visit mometrix.com/academy and enter code: 396297

An example of a main idea is: *Giraffes live in the Serengeti of Africa.* A supporting detail about giraffes could be: *A giraffe in this region benefits from a long neck by reaching twigs and leaves on tall trees.* The main idea gives the general idea that the text is about giraffes. The supporting detail gives a specific fact about how the giraffes eat.

Recognizing an Author's Purpose

Author's Position and Purpose

In order to be an effective reader, one must pay attention to the author's **position** and **purpose**. Even those texts that seem objective and impartial, like textbooks, have a position and bias. Readers need to take these positions into account when considering the author's message. When an author uses emotional language or clearly favors one side of an argument, his or her position is clear. However, the author's position may be evident not only in what he or she writes, but also in what he or she doesn't write. In a normal setting, a reader would want to review some other texts on the same topic in order to develop a view of the author's position. If this was not possible, then you would want to at least acquire some background about the author. However, since you are in the middle of an exam and the only source of information is the text, you should look for language and argumentation that seems to indicate a particular stance on the subject.

Review Video: Author's Position
Visit mometrix.com/academy and enter code: 827954

Author's Purpose

Usually, identifying the author's **purpose** is easier than identifying his or her position. In most cases, the author has no interest in hiding his or her purpose. A text that is meant to entertain, for instance, should be written to please the reader. Most narratives, or stories, are written to entertain, though they may also inform or persuade. Informative texts are easy to identify, while the most difficult purpose of a text to identify is persuasion because the author has an interest in making this purpose hard to detect. When a reader discovers that the author is trying to persuade, he or she should be skeptical of the argument. For this reason, persuasive texts often try to establish an entertaining tone and hope to amuse the reader into agreement. On the other hand, an informative tone may be implemented to create an appearance of authority and objectivity.

An author's purpose is evident often in the organization of the text (e.g., section headings in bold font points to an informative text). However, you may not have such organization available to you in your exam. Instead, if the author makes his or her main idea clear from the beginning, then the likely purpose of the text is to inform. If the author begins by making a claim and provides various arguments to support that claim, then the purpose is probably to persuade. If the author tells a story or wants to gain the reader's attention more than to push a particular point or deliver information, then his or her purpose is most likely to entertain. As a reader, you must judge authors on how well they accomplish their purpose. In other words, you need to consider the type of passage (e.g., technical, persuasive, etc.) that the author has written and if the author has followed the requirements of the passage type.

Reading Comprehension and Connecting with Texts

Comparing Two Stories

When presented with two different stories, there will be **similarities** and **differences** between the two. A reader needs to make a list, or other graphic organizer, of the points presented in each story. Once the reader has written down the main point and supporting points for each story, the two sets of ideas can be compared. The reader can then present each idea and show how it is the same or different in the other story. This is called **comparing and contrasting ideas**.

The reader can compare ideas by stating, for example: "In Story 1, the author believes that humankind will one day land on Mars, whereas in Story 2, the author believes that Mars is too far away for humans to ever step foot on." Note that the two viewpoints are different in each story that the reader is comparing. A reader may state that: "Both stories discussed the likelihood of humankind landing on Mars." This statement shows how the viewpoint presented in both stories is based on the same topic, rather than how each viewpoint is different. The reader will complete a comparison of two stories with a conclusion.

> **Review Video: How to Compare and Contrast**
> Visit mometrix.com/academy and enter code: 833765

Outlining a Passage

As an aid to drawing conclusions, **outlining** the information contained in the passage should be a familiar skill to readers. An effective outline will reveal the structure of the passage and will lead to solid conclusions. An effective outline will have a title that refers to the basic subject of the text, though the title does not need to restate the main idea. In most outlines, the main idea will be the first major section. Each major idea in the passage will be established as the head of a category. For instance, the most common outline format calls for the main ideas of the passage to be indicated with Roman numerals. In an effective outline of this kind, each of the main ideas will be represented by a Roman numeral and none of the Roman numerals will designate minor details or secondary ideas. Moreover, all supporting ideas and details should be placed in the appropriate place on the outline. An outline does not need to include every detail listed in the text, but it should feature all of those that are central to the argument or message. Each of these details should be listed under the corresponding main idea.

> **Review Video: Outlining as an Aid to Drawing Conclusions**
> Visit mometrix.com/academy and enter code: 584445

Using Graphic Organizers

Ideas from a text can also be organized using **graphic organizers**. A graphic organizer is a way to simplify information and take key points from the text. A graphic organizer such as a timeline may have an event listed for a corresponding date on the timeline, while an outline may have an event listed under a key point that occurs in the text. Each reader needs to create the type of graphic organizer that works the best for him or her in terms of being able to recall information from a story. Examples include a spider-map, which takes a main idea from the story and places it in a bubble with supporting points branching off the main idea. An outline is useful for diagramming the main and supporting points of the entire story, and a Venn diagram compares and contrasts characteristics of two or more ideas.

> **Review Video: Graphic Organizers**
> Visit mometrix.com/academy and enter code: 665513

Making Logical Conclusions about a Passage

A reader should always be drawing conclusions from the text. Sometimes conclusions are **implied** from written information, and other times the information is **stated directly** within the passage. One should always aim to draw conclusions from information stated within a passage, rather than to draw them from mere implications. At times an author may provide some information and then describe a counterargument. Readers should be alert for direct statements that are subsequently rejected or weakened by the author. Furthermore, you should always read through the entire passage before drawing conclusions. Many readers are trained to expect the author's conclusions at either the beginning or the end of the passage, but many texts do not adhere to this format.

Drawing conclusions from information implied within a passage requires confidence on the part of the reader. **Implications** are things that the author does not state directly, but readers can assume based on what the author does say. Consider the following passage: *I stepped outside and opened my umbrella. By the time I got to work, the cuffs of my pants were soaked.* The author never states that it is raining, but this fact is clearly implied. Conclusions based on implication must be well supported by the text. In order to draw a solid conclusion, readers should have **multiple pieces of evidence**. If readers have only one piece, they must be assured that there is no other possible explanation than their conclusion. A good reader will be able to draw many conclusions from information implied by the text, which will be a great help on the exam.

Drawing Conclusions

A common type of inference that a reader has to make is **drawing a conclusion**. The reader makes this conclusion based on the information provided within a text. Certain facts are included to help a reader come to a specific conclusion. For example, a story may open with a man trudging through the snow on a cold winter day, dragging a sled behind him. The reader can logically **infer** from the setting of the story that the man is wearing heavy winter clothes in order to stay warm. Information is implied based on the setting of a story, which is why **setting** is an important element of the text. If the same man in the example was trudging down a beach on a hot summer day, dragging a surf board behind him, the reader would assume that the man is not wearing heavy clothes. The reader makes inferences based on their own experiences and the information presented to them in the story.

Test-taking tip: When asked to identify a conclusion that may be drawn, look for critical "hedge" phrases, such as *likely*, *may*, *can*, and *will often*, among many others. When you are being tested on this knowledge, remember the question that writers insert into these hedge phrases to cover every possibility. Often an answer will be wrong simply because there is no room for exception. Extreme positive or negative answers (such as always or never) are usually not correct. When answering these questions, the reader **should not** use any outside knowledge that is not gathered directly or reasonably inferred from the passage. Correct answers can be derived straight from the passage.

Example

Read the following sentence from *Little Women* by Louisa May Alcott and draw a conclusion based upon the information presented:

> *You know the reason Mother proposed not having any presents this Christmas was because it is going to be a hard winter for everyone; and she thinks we ought not to spend money for pleasure, when our men are suffering so in the army.*

Based on the information in the sentence, the reader can conclude, or **infer**, that the men are away at war while the women are still at home. The pronoun *our* gives a clue to the reader that the character is speaking about men she knows. In addition, the reader can assume that the character is speaking to a brother or sister, since the term "Mother" is used by the character while speaking to another person. The reader can also come to the conclusion that the characters celebrate Christmas, since it is mentioned in the **context** of the sentence. In the sentence, the mother is presented as an unselfish character who is opinionated and thinks about the wellbeing of other people.

Summarizing

A helpful tool is the ability to **summarize** the information that you have read in a paragraph or passage format. This process is similar to creating an effective outline. First, a summary should accurately define the main idea of the passage, though the summary does not need to explain this main idea in exhaustive detail. The summary should continue by laying out the most important supporting details or arguments from the passage. All of the significant supporting details should be included, and none of the details included should be irrelevant or insignificant. Also, the summary should accurately report all of these details. Too often, the desire for brevity in a summary leads to the sacrifice of clarity or accuracy. Summaries are often difficult to read because they omit all of the graceful language, digressions, and asides that distinguish great writing. However, an effective summary should communicate the same overall message as the original text.

Review Video: Summarizing Text
Visit mometrix.com/academy and enter code: 172903

Paraphrasing

Paraphrasing is another method that the reader can use to aid in comprehension. When paraphrasing, one puts what they have read into their own words by rephrasing what the author has written, or one "translates" all of what the author shared into their own words by including as many details as they can.

Evaluating a Passage

It is important to understand the logical conclusion of the ideas presented in an informational text. **Identifying a logical conclusion** can help you determine whether you agree with the writer or not. Coming to this conclusion is much like making an inference: the approach requires you to combine the information given by the text with what you already know and make a logical conclusion. If the author intended for the reader to draw a certain conclusion, then you can expect the author's argumentation and detail to be leading in that direction.

One way to approach the task of drawing conclusions is to make brief **notes** of all the points made by the author. When the notes are arranged on paper, they may clarify the logical conclusion. Another way to approach conclusions is to consider whether the reasoning of the author raises any pertinent questions. Sometimes you will be able to draw several conclusions from a passage. On occasion these will be conclusions that were never imagined by the author. Therefore, be aware that these conclusions must be **supported directly by the text**.

Evaluation of Summaries

A summary of a literary passage is a condensation in the reader's own words of the passage's main points. Several guidelines can be used in evaluating a summary. The summary should be complete yet concise. It should be accurate, balanced, fair, neutral, and objective, excluding the reader's own opinions or reactions. It should reflect in similar proportion how much each point summarized was covered in the original passage. Summary writers should include tags of attribution, like "Macaulay argues that" to reference the original author whose ideas are represented in the summary. Summary writers should not overuse quotations; they should only quote central concepts or phrases they cannot precisely convey in words other than those of the original author. Another aspect of evaluating a summary is considering whether it can stand alone as a coherent, unified composition. In addition, evaluation of a summary should include whether its writer has cited the original source of the passage they have summarized so that readers can find it.

Making Connections to Enhance Comprehension

Reading involves thinking. For good comprehension, readers make **text-to-self**, **text-to-text**, and **text-to-world connections**. Making connections helps readers understand text better and predict what might occur next based on what they already know, such as how characters in the story feel or what happened in another text. Text-to-self connections with the reader's life and experiences make literature more personally relevant and meaningful to readers. Readers can make connections before, during, and after reading—including whenever the text reminds them of something similar they have encountered in life or other texts. The genre, setting, characters, plot elements, literary structure and devices, and themes an author uses allow a reader to make connections to other works of literature or to people and events in their own lives. Venn diagrams and other graphic organizers help visualize connections. Readers can also make double-entry notes: key content, ideas, events, words, and quotations on one side, and the connections with these on the other.

Finding the Meaning and Assessing the Text

Persuasion and Rhetoric

Persuasive Techniques

To **appeal using reason**, writers present logical arguments, such as using "If... then... because" statements. To **appeal to emotions**, authors may ask readers how they would feel about something or to put themselves in another's place, present their argument as one that will make the audience feel good, or tell readers how they should feel. To **appeal to character**, **morality**, or **ethics**, authors present their points to readers as the right or most moral choices. Authors cite expert opinions to show readers that someone very knowledgeable about the subject or viewpoint agrees with the author's claims. **Testimonials**, usually via anecdotes or quotations regarding the author's subject, help build the audience's trust in an author's message through positive support from ordinary people. **Bandwagon appeals** claim that everybody else agrees with the author's argument and persuade readers to conform and agree, also. Authors **appeal to greed** by presenting their choice as cheaper, free, or more valuable for less cost. They **appeal to laziness** by presenting their views as more convenient, easy, or relaxing. Authors also anticipate potential objections and argue against them before audiences think of them, thereby depicting those objections as weak.

Authors can use **comparisons** like analogies, similes, and metaphors to persuade audiences. For example, a writer might represent excessive expenses as "hemorrhaging" money, which the author's recommended solution will stop. Authors can use negative word connotations to make some choices unappealing to readers, and positive word connotations to make others more appealing. Using **humor** can relax readers and garner their agreement. However, writers must take care: ridiculing opponents can be a successful strategy for appealing to readers who already agree with the author, but can backfire by angering other readers. **Rhetorical questions** need no answer, but create effect that can force agreement, such as asking the question, "Wouldn't you rather be paid more than less?" **Generalizations** persuade readers by being impossible to disagree with. Writers can easily make generalizations that appear to support their viewpoints, like saying, "We all want peace, not war" regarding more specific political arguments. **Transfer** and **association** persuade by example: if advertisements show attractive actors enjoying their products, audiences imagine they will experience the same. **Repetition** can also sometimes effectively persuade audiences.

Review Video: Using Rhetorical Strategies for Persuasion
Visit mometrix.com/academy and enter code: 302658

Classical Author Appeals

In his *On Rhetoric,* ancient Greek philosopher Aristotle defined three basic types of appeal used in writing, which he called *pathos*, *ethos*, and *logos*. ***Pathos*** means suffering or experience and refers to appeals to the emotions (the English word *pathetic* comes from this root). Writing that is meant to entertain audiences, by making them either happy, as with comedy, or sad, as with tragedy, uses *pathos*. Aristotle's *Poetics* states that evoking the emotions of terror and pity is one of the criteria for writing tragedy. ***Ethos*** means character and connotes ideology (the English word *ethics* comes from this root). Writing that appeals to credibility, based on academic, professional, or personal merit, uses *ethos*. ***Logos*** means "I say" and refers to a plea, opinion, expectation, word or speech, account, opinion, or reason (the English word *logic* comes from this root.) Aristotle used it to mean persuasion that appeals to the audience through reasoning and logic to influence their opinions.

Critical Evaluation of Effectiveness of Persuasive Methods

First, readers should identify the author's **thesis**—what he or she argues for or against. They should consider the argument's content and the author's reason for presenting it. Does the author offer **solutions** to problems raised? If so, are they realistic? Note all central ideas and evidence supporting the author's thesis. Research any unfamiliar subjects or vocabulary. Readers should then outline or summarize the work in their own words. Identify which types of appeals the author uses. Readers should evaluate how well the author communicated meaning from the reader's perspective: Did they respond to emotional appeals with anger, concern, happiness, etc.? If so, why? Decide if the author's reasoning sufficed for changing the reader's mind. Determine whether the content and presentation were accurate, cohesive, and clear. Readers should also ask themselves whether they found the author believable or not, and why or why not.

Evaluating an Argument

Argumentative and persuasive passages take a stand on a debatable issue, seek to explore all sides of the issue, and find the best possible solution. Argumentative and persuasive passages should not be combative or abusive. The word *argument* may remind you of two or more people shouting at each other and walking away in anger. However, an argumentative or persuasive passage should be a calm and reasonable presentation of an author's ideas for others to consider. When an author writes reasonable arguments, his or her goal is not to win or have the last word. Instead, authors want to reveal current understanding of the question at hand and suggest a solution to a problem. The purpose of argument and persuasion in a free society is to reach the best solution.

Evidence

The term **text evidence** refers to information that supports a main point or minor points and can help lead the reader to a conclusion about the text's credibility. Information used as text evidence is precise, descriptive, and factual. A main point is often followed by supporting details that provide evidence to back up a claim. For example, a passage may include the claim that winter occurs during opposite months in the Northern and Southern hemispheres. Text evidence for this claim may include examples of countries where winter occurs in opposite months. Stating that the tilt of the Earth as it rotates around the sun causes winter to occur at different times in separate hemispheres is another example of text evidence. Text evidence can come from common knowledge, but it is also valuable to include text evidence from credible, relevant outside sources.

Review Video: Textual Evidence
Visit mometrix.com/academy and enter code: 486236

Evidence that supports the thesis and additional arguments needs to be provided. Most arguments must be supported by facts or statistics. A fact is something that is known with certainty, has been verified by several independent individuals, and can be proven to be true. In addition to facts, examples and illustrations can support an argument by adding an emotional component. With this component, you persuade readers in ways that facts and statistics cannot. The emotional component is effective when used alongside objective information that can be confirmed.

Credibility

The text used to support an argument can be the argument's downfall if the text is not credible. A text is **credible**, or believable, when its author is knowledgeable and objective, or unbiased. The author's motivations for writing the text play a critical role in determining the credibility of the text and must be evaluated when assessing that credibility. Reports written about the ozone layer by an environmental scientist and a hairdresser will have a different level of credibility.

Review Video: Author Credibility
Visit mometrix.com/academy and enter code: 827257

Appeal to Emotion

Sometimes, authors will appeal to the reader's emotion in an attempt to persuade or to distract the reader from the weakness of the argument. For instance, the author may try to inspire the pity of the reader by delivering a heart-rending story. An author also might use the bandwagon approach, in which he suggests that his opinion is correct because it is held by the majority. Some authors resort to name-calling, in which insults and harsh words are delivered to the opponent in an attempt to distract. In advertising, a common appeal is the celebrity testimonial, in which a famous person endorses a product. Of course, the fact that a famous person likes something should not really mean anything to the reader. These and other emotional appeals are usually evidence of poor reasoning and a weak argument.

Review Video: Emotional Language in Literature
Visit mometrix.com/academy and enter code: 759390

Counter Arguments

When authors give both sides to the argument, they build trust with their readers. As a reader, you should start with an undecided or neutral position. If an author presents only his or her side to the argument, then they are not exhibiting credibility and are weakening their argument.

Building common ground with readers can be effective for persuading neutral, skeptical, or opposed readers. Sharing values with undecided readers can allow people to switch positions without giving up what they feel is important. People who may oppose a position need to feel that they can change their minds without betraying who they are as a person. This appeal to having an open mind can be a powerful tool in arguing a position without antagonizing other views. Objections can be countered on a point-by-point basis or in a summary paragraph. Be mindful of how an author points out flaws in counter arguments. If they are unfair to the other side of the argument, then you should lose trust with the author.

Rhetorical Devices

- An **anecdote** is a brief story authors may relate to their argument, which can illustrate their points in a more real and relatable way.
- **Aphorisms** concisely state common beliefs and may rhyme. For example, Benjamin Franklin's "Early to bed and early to rise / Makes a man healthy, wealthy, and wise" is an aphorism.
- **Allusions** refer to literary or historical figures to impart symbolism to a thing or person and to create reader resonance. In John Steinbeck's *Of Mice and Men,* protagonist George's last name is Milton. This alludes to John Milton, who wrote *Paradise Lost,* and symbolizes George's eventual loss of his dream.
- **Satire** exaggerates, ridicules, or pokes fun at human flaws or ideas, as in the works of Jonathan Swift and Mark Twain.
- A **parody** is a form of satire that imitates another work to ridicule its topic or style.
- A **paradox** is a statement that is true despite appearing contradictory.
- **Hyperbole** is overstatement using exaggerated language.
- An **oxymoron** combines seeming contradictions, such as "deafening silence."
- **Analogies** compare two things that share common elements.
- **Similes** (stated comparisons using the words *like* or *as*) and **metaphors** (stated comparisons that do not use *like* or *as*) are considered forms of analogy.
- When using logic to reason with audiences, **syllogism** refers either to deductive reasoning or a deceptive, very sophisticated, or subtle argument.
- **Deductive reasoning** moves from general to specific, **inductive reasoning** from specific to general.
- **Diction** is author word choice that establishes tone and effect.
- **Understatement** achieves effects like contrast or irony by downplaying or describing something more subtly than warranted.
- **Chiasmus** uses parallel clauses, the second reversing the order of the first. Examples include T. S. Eliot's "Has the Church failed mankind, or has mankind failed the Church?" and John F. Kennedy's "Ask not what your country can do for you; ask what you can do for your country."
- **Anaphora** regularly repeats a word or phrase at the beginnings of consecutive clauses or phrases to add emphasis to an idea. A classic example of anaphora was Winston Churchill's emphasis of determination: "[W]e shall fight on the beaches, we shall fight on the landing grounds, we shall fight in the fields and in the streets, we shall fight in the hills; we shall never surrender..."

Reading Argumentative Writing

Author's Argument in Argumentative Writing

In argumentative writing, the argument is a belief, position, or opinion that the author wants to convince readers to believe as well. For the first step, readers should identify the **issue**. Some issues are controversial, meaning people disagree about them. Gun control, foreign policy, and the death penalty are all controversial issues. The next step is to determine the **author's position** on the issue. That position or viewpoint constitutes the author's argument. Readers should then identify the **author's assumptions**: things he or she accepts, believes, or takes for granted without needing proof. Inaccurate or illogical assumptions produce flawed arguments and can mislead readers. Readers should identify what kinds of **supporting evidence** the author offers, such as research results, personal observations or experiences, case studies, facts, examples, expert testimony and opinions, and comparisons. Readers should decide how relevant this support is to the argument.

Review Video: Argumentative Writing
Visit mometrix.com/academy and enter code: 561544

Evaluating an Author's Argument

The first three reader steps to **evaluate an author's argument** are to identify the **author's assumptions**, identify the **supporting evidence**, and decide **whether the evidence is relevant**. For example, if an author is not an expert on a particular topic, then that author's personal experience or opinion might not be relevant. The fourth step is to assess the **author's objectivity**. For example, consider whether the author introduces clear, understandable supporting evidence and facts to support the argument. The fifth step is evaluating whether the author's **argument is complete**. When authors give sufficient support for their arguments and also anticipate and respond effectively to opposing arguments or objections to their points, their arguments are complete. However, some authors omit information that could detract from their arguments. If instead they stated this information and refuted it, it would strengthen their arguments. The sixth step in evaluating an author's argumentative writing is to assess whether the **argument is valid**. Providing clear, logical reasoning makes an author's argument valid. Readers should ask themselves whether the author's points follow a sequence that makes sense, and whether each point leads to the next. The seventh step is to determine whether the author's **argument is credible**, meaning that it is convincing and believable. Arguments that are not valid are not credible, so step seven depends on step six. Readers should be mindful of their own biases as they evaluate and should not expect authors to conclusively prove their arguments, but rather to provide effective support and reason.

Evaluating an Author's Method of Appeal

To evaluate the effectiveness of an appeal, it is important to consider the author's purpose for writing. Any appeals an author uses in their argument must be relevant to the argument's goal. For example, a writer that argues for the reclassification of Pluto, but primarily uses appeals to emotion, will not have an effective argument. This writer should focus on using appeals to logic and support their argument with provable facts. While most arguments should include appeals to logic, emotion, and credibility, some arguments only call for one or two of these types of appeal. Evidence can support an appeal, but the evidence must be relevant to truly strengthen the appeal's effectiveness. If the writer arguing for Pluto's reclassification uses the reasons for Jupiter's classification as evidence, their argument would be weak. This information may seem relevant because it is related to the classification of planets. However, this classification is highly dependent on the size of the celestial object, and Jupiter is significantly bigger than Pluto. This use of evidence is illogical and does not support the appeal. Even when appropriate evidence and appeals are used, appeals and arguments lose their effectiveness when they create logical fallacies.

Opinions, Facts, and Fallacies

Critical thinking skills are mastered through understanding various types of writing and the different purposes of authors can have for writing different passages. Every author writes for a purpose. When you understand their purpose and how they accomplish their goal, you will be able to analyze their writing and determine whether or not you agree with their conclusions.

Readers must always be aware of the difference between fact and opinion. A **fact** can be subjected to analysis and proven to be true. An **opinion**, on the other hand, is the author's personal thoughts or feelings and may not be altered by research or evidence. If the author writes that the distance from New York City to Boston is about two hundred miles, then he or she is stating a fact. If the author writes that New York City is too crowded, then he or she is giving an opinion because there is no objective standard for overpopulation. Opinions are often supported by facts. For instance, an author might use a comparison between the population density of New York City and that of other major American cities as evidence of an overcrowded population. An opinion supported by facts tends to be more convincing. On the other hand, when authors support their opinions with other opinions, readers should employ critical thinking and approach the argument with skepticism.

Review Video: Distinguishing Fact and Opinion
Visit mometrix.com/academy and enter code: 870899

Reliable Sources

When you have an argumentative passage, you need to be sure that facts are presented to the reader from **reliable sources**. An opinion is what the author thinks about a given topic. An opinion is not common knowledge or proven by expert sources, instead the information is the personal beliefs and thoughts of the author. To distinguish between fact and opinion, a reader needs to consider the type of source that is presenting information, the information that backs-up a claim, and the author's motivation to have a certain point-of-view on a given topic. For example, if a panel of scientists has conducted multiple studies on the effectiveness of taking a certain vitamin, then the results are more likely to be factual than those of a company that is selling a vitamin and simply claims that taking the vitamin can produce positive effects. The company is motivated to sell their product, and the scientists are using the scientific method to prove a theory. Remember, if you find sentences that contain phrases such as "I think...", then the statement is an opinion.

Biases

In their attempts to persuade, writers often make mistakes in their thought processes and writing choices. These processes and choices are important to understand so you can make an informed decision about the author's credibility. Every author has a point of view, but authors demonstrate a **bias** when they ignore reasonable counterarguments or distort opposing viewpoints. A bias is evident whenever the author's claims are presented in a way that is unfair or inaccurate. Bias can be intentional or unintentional, but readers should be skeptical of the author's argument in either case. Remember that a biased author may still be correct. However, the author will be correct in spite of, not because of, his or her bias.

A **stereotype** is a bias applied specifically to a group of people or a place. Stereotyping is considered to be particularly abhorrent because it promotes negative, misleading generalizations about people. Readers should be very cautious of authors who use stereotypes in their writing. These faulty assumptions typically reveal the author's ignorance and lack of curiosity.

Review Video: Bias and Stereotype
Visit mometrix.com/academy and enter code: 644829

Making Predictions and Inferences

Making Predictions

When we read literature, **making predictions** about what will happen in the writing reinforces our purpose for reading and prepares us mentally. A **prediction** is a guess about what will happen next. Readers constantly make predictions based on what they have read and what they already know. We can make predictions before we begin reading and during our reading. Consider the following sentence: *Staring at the computer screen in shock, Kim blindly reached over for the brimming glass of water on the shelf to her side.* The sentence suggests that Kim is distracted, and that she is not looking at the glass that she is going to pick up. So, a reader might predict that Kim is going to knock over the glass. Of course, not every prediction will be accurate: perhaps Kim will pick the glass up cleanly. Nevertheless, the author has certainly created the expectation that the water might be spilled.

As we read on, we can test the accuracy of our predictions, revise them in light of additional reading, and confirm or refute our predictions. Predictions are always subject to revision as the reader acquires more information. A reader can make predictions by observing the title and illustrations; noting the structure, characters, and subject; drawing on existing knowledge relative to the subject; and asking "why" and "who" questions. Connecting reading to what we already know enables us to learn new information and construct meaning. For example, before third-graders read a book about Johnny Appleseed, they may start a KWL chart—a list of what they *Know*, what they *Want* to know or learn, and what they have *Learned* after reading. Activating existing background knowledge and thinking about the text before reading improves comprehension.

Review Video: Predictive Reading
Visit mometrix.com/academy and enter code: 437248

Test-taking tip: To respond to questions requiring future predictions, your answers should be based on evidence of past or present behavior and events.

Evaluating Predictions

When making predictions, readers should be able to explain how they developed their prediction. One way readers can defend their thought process is by citing textual evidence. Textual evidence to evaluate reader predictions about literature includes specific synopses of the work, paraphrases of the work or parts of it, and direct quotations from the work. These references to the text must support the prediction by indicating, clearly or unclearly, what will happen later in the story. A text may provide these indications through literary devices such as foreshadowing. Foreshadowing is anything in a text that gives the reader a hint about what is to come by emphasizing the likelihood of an event or development. Foreshadowing can occur through descriptions, exposition, and dialogue. Foreshadowing in dialogue usually occurs when a character gives a warning or expresses a strong feeling that a certain event will occur. Foreshadowing can also occur through irony. However, unlike other forms of foreshadowing, the events that seem the most likely are the opposite of what actually happens. Instances of foreshadowing and irony can be summarized, paraphrased, or quoted to defend a reader's prediction.

Review Video: Textual Evidence for Predictions
Visit mometrix.com/academy and enter code: 261070

Drawing Conclusions from Inferences

Inferences about literary text are logical conclusions that readers make based on their observations and previous knowledge. An inference is based on both what is found in a passage or a story and what is known from personal experience. For instance, a story may say that a character is frightened and can hear howling in the distance. Based on both what is in the text and personal knowledge, it is a logical conclusion that the character is frightened because he hears the sound of wolves. A good inference is supported by the information in a passage.

Implicit and Explicit Information

By inferring, readers construct meanings from text that are personally relevant. By combining their own schemas or concepts and their background information pertinent to the text with what they read, readers interpret it according to both what the author has conveyed and their own unique perspectives. Inferences are different from **explicit information**, which is clearly stated in a passage. Authors do not always explicitly spell out every meaning in what they write; many meanings are implicit. Through inference, readers can comprehend implied meanings in the text, and also derive personal significance from it, making the text meaningful and memorable to them. Inference is a natural process in everyday life. When readers infer, they can draw conclusions about what the author is saying, predict what may reasonably follow, amend these predictions as they continue to read, interpret the import of themes, and analyze the characters' feelings and motivations through their actions.

EXAMPLE OF DRAWING CONCLUSIONS FROM INFERENCES

Read the excerpt and decide why Jana finally relaxed.

> Jana loved her job, but the work was very demanding. She had trouble relaxing. She called a friend, but she still thought about work. She ordered a pizza, but eating it did not help. Then, her kitten jumped on her lap and began to purr. Jana leaned back and began to hum a little tune. She felt better.

You can draw the conclusion that Jana relaxed because her kitten jumped on her lap. The kitten purred, and Jana leaned back and hummed a tune. Then she felt better. The excerpt does not explicitly say that this is the reason why she was able to relax. The text leaves the matter unclear, but the reader can infer or make a "best guess" that this is the reason she is relaxing. This is a logical conclusion based on the information in the passage. It is the best conclusion a reader can make based on the information he or she has read. Inferences are based on the information in a passage, but they are not directly stated in the passage.

Test-taking tip: While being tested on your ability to make correct inferences, you must look for **contextual clues.** An answer can be true, but not the best or most correct answer. The contextual clues will help you find the answer that is the **best answer** out of the given choices. Be careful in your reading to understand the context in which a phrase is stated. When asked for the implied meaning of a statement made in the passage, you should immediately locate the statement and read the **context** in which the statement was made. Also, look for an answer choice that has a similar phrase to the statement in question.

Review Video: Inference
Visit mometrix.com/academy and enter code: 379203

Review Video: How to Support a Conclusion
Visit mometrix.com/academy and enter code: 281653

Additional Reading Concepts

SOURCES OF INFORMATION

PRIMARY SOURCES

In literature review, one may examine both primary and secondary sources. Primary sources contain original information that was witnessed, gathered, or otherwise produced by the source's author. **Primary sources** can include firsthand accounts, found in sources such as books, autobiographies, transcripts, speeches, videos, photos, and personal journals or diaries. Primary sources may also include records of information, such as government documents, or personally-conducted research in sources like reports and essays. They may be found in academic books, journals and other periodicals, and authoritative databases. Using primary sources allows researchers to develop their own conclusions about the subject. Primary sources are also reliable for finding information about a person or their personal accounts and experiences. Primary sources such as photos, videos, audio recordings, transcripts, and government documents are often reliable, as they are usually objective and can be used to confirm information from other sources.

SECONDARY SOURCES

Secondary sources are sources that reference information originally provided by another source. The original source may be cited, quoted, paraphrased, or described in a secondary source. **Secondary sources** may be articles, essays, videos, or books found in periodicals, magazines, newspapers, films, databases, or websites. A secondary source can be used to reference another researcher's analysis or conclusion from a primary source.

This information can inform the researcher of the existing discussions regarding their subject. These types of sources may also support the researcher's claims by providing a credible argument that contributes to the researcher's argument. Secondary sources may also highlight connections between primary sources or criticize both primary and other secondary sources. These types of secondary sources are valuable because they provide information and conclusions the researcher may not have considered or found, otherwise.

Review Video: Primary and Secondary Sources
Visit mometrix.com/academy and enter code: 383328

Types of Sources

- **Textbooks** are specialized materials that are designed to thoroughly instruct readers on a particular topic. Textbooks often include features such as a table of contents, visuals, an index, a glossary, headings, and practice questions and exercises.
- **Newspapers** are collections of several written pieces and are primarily used to distribute news stories to their audience. In addition to news articles, newspapers may also include advertisements or pieces meant to entertain their audience, such as comic strips, columns, and letters from readers. Newspapers are written for a variety of audiences, as they are published on both the local and national levels.
- **Manuals** are instructional documents that accompany a product or explain an important procedure. Manuals include a table of contents, guidelines, and instructional content. Instructional manuals often include information about safe practices, risks, and product warranty. The instructions in manuals are often presented as step-by-step instructions, as they are meant to help users properly use a product or complete a task.
- **Electronic texts** are written documents that are read digitally and are primarily accessed online or through a network. Many electronic texts have characteristics similar to printed texts, such as a table of contents, publication information, a main text, and supplemental materials. However, electronic texts are more interactive and can be navigated more quickly. Electronic texts can also provide more accessibility, as they can be easily resized or narrated by text-to-speech software.

Finding Sources

Finding sources for a research project may be intimidating or difficult. There are numerous sources available, and several research tools to help researchers find them. Starting with one of these tools can help narrow down the number of sources a researcher is working with at one time.

- **Libraries** house independent, printed publications that are organized by subject. This makes finding sources easy, since researchers can visit sections with sources relevant to their topic and immediately see what sources are available. Many libraries also offer printed journals and collections that include sources related to a common subject or written by the same author.
- **Databases** offer digital access to sources from a wide variety of libraries and online containers. To use a database, users search for keywords related to their topic or the type of source they want to use. The database then lists results related to or featuring those key words. Users can narrow their results using filters that will limit their results based on factors such as publication year, source type, or whether the sources are peer-reviewed. Database search results also list individual articles and methods of accessing the article directly. While databases help users find sources, they do not guarantee users access to each source.
- **Academic Journals** are collections of articles that cover a particular topic or fit within a certain category. These journals are often offered both online and in print. Academic journals typically contain peer-reviewed works or works that have undergone another type of reviewing process.

Credibility

There are innumerable primary and secondary sources available in print and online. However, not every published or posted source is appropriate for a research project. When finding sources, the researcher must know how to evaluate each source for credibility and relevance. Not only must the sources be reliable and relevant to the research subject, but they must also be appropriate and help form an answer to the research question. As researchers progress in their research and composition, the relevance of each source will become clear. Appropriate sources will contribute valuable information and arguments to the researcher's own thoughts and conclusions, providing useful evidence to bolster the researcher's claims. The researcher has the freedom to choose which sources they reference or even change their research topic and question in response to the sources they find. However, the researcher should not use unreliable sources, and determining a source's credibility is not always easy.

Considerations for Evaluating the Credibility of a Source

- The author and their purpose for writing the source
- The author's qualifications to write on the topic
- Whether the source is peer-reviewed or included in a scholarly publication
- The publisher
- The target audience
- The jargon or dialect the source is written in (e.g., academic, technical)
- The presence of bias or manipulation of information
- The date of publication
- The author's use of other sources to support their claims
- Whether any outside sources are cited appropriately in the source
- The accuracy of information presented

Author's Purpose and Credibility

Knowing who wrote a source and why they wrote it is important to determine whether a source is appropriate for a research project. The author should be qualified to write on the subject of the material. Their purpose may be to inform their audience of information, to present and defend an analysis, or even to criticize a work or other argument. The researcher must decide whether the author's purpose makes the source appropriate to use. The source's container and publisher are important to note because they indicate the source's reputability and whether other qualified individuals have reviewed the information in the source. Credible secondary sources should also reference other sources, primary or secondary, that support or inform the source's content. Evaluating the accuracy of the information or the presence of bias in a source will require careful reading and critical thinking on the part of the researcher. However, a source with excellent credentials may still contain pieces of inaccurate information or bias, so it is the researcher's responsibility to be careful in their use of each source.

Citing Sources

Integrating References and Quotations

In research papers, one can include studies whose conclusions agree with one's position (Reed 284; Becker and Fagen 93), as well as studies that disagree (Limbaugh 442, Beck 69) by including parenthetical citations as demonstrated in this sentence. Quotations should be selective: writers should compose an original sentence and incorporate only a few words from a research source. If students cannot use more original words than quotation, they are likely padding their compositions. However, including quotations appropriately increases the credibility of the writer and their argument.

Properly Integrating Quotations

When using sources in a research paper, it is important to integrate information so that the flow of the composition is not interrupted as the two compositions are combined. When quoting outside sources, it is necessary to lead into the quote and ensure that the whole sentence is logical, is grammatically correct, and flows well. Below is an example of an incorrectly integrated quote.

> During the Industrial Revolution, many unions organized labor strikes "child labor, unregulated working conditions, and excessive working hours" in America.

Below is the same sentence with a properly integrated quote.

> During the Industrial Revolution, many unions organized labor strikes to protest the presence of "child labor, unregulated working conditions, and excessive working hours" in America.

In the first example, the connection between "strikes" and the quoted list is unclear. In the second example, the phrase "to protest the presence of" link the ideas together and successfully creates a suitable place for the quotation.

When quoting sources, writers should work quotations and references seamlessly into their sentences instead of interrupting the flow of their own argument to summarize a source. Summarizing others' content is often a ploy to bolster word counts. Writing that analyzes the content, evaluates it, and synthesizes material from various sources demonstrates critical thinking skills and is thus more valuable.

Properly Incorporating Outside Sources

Writers do better to include short quotations rather than long. For example, quoting six to eight long passages in a 10-page paper is excessive. It is also better to avoid wording like "This quotation shows," "As you can see from this quotation," or "It talks about." These are amateur, feeble efforts to interact with other authors' ideas. Also, writing about sources and quotations wastes words that should be used to develop one's own ideas. Quotations should be used to stimulate discussion rather than taking its place. Ending a paragraph, section, or paper with a quotation is not incorrect per se, but using it to prove a point, without including anything more in one's own words regarding the point or subject, suggests a lack of critical thinking about the topic and consideration of multiple alternatives. It can also be a tactic to dissuade readers from challenging one's propositions. Writers should include references and quotations that challenge as well as support their thesis statements. Presenting evidence on both sides of an issue makes it easier for reasonably skeptical readers to agree with a writer's viewpoint.

Textual Evidence

No analysis is complete without textual evidence. Summaries, paraphrases, and quotes are all forms of textual evidence, but direct quotes from the text are the most effective form of evidence. The best textual evidence is relevant, accurate, and clearly supports the writer's claim. This can include pieces of descriptions, dialogue, or exposition that shows the applicability of the analysis to the text. Analysis that is average, or sufficient, shows an understanding of the text; contains supporting textual evidence that is relevant and accurate, if not strong; and shows a specific and clear response. Analysis that partially meets criteria also shows understanding, but the textual evidence is generalized, incomplete, only partly relevant or accurate, or connected only weakly. Inadequate analysis is vague, too general, or incorrect. It may give irrelevant or incomplete textual evidence, or may simply summarize the plot rather than analyzing the work. It is important to incorporate textual evidence from the work being analyzed and any supplemental materials and to provide appropriate attribution for these sources.

Citing Sources

Formal research writers must **cite all sources used**—books, articles, interviews, conversations, and anything else that contributed to the research. One reason is to **avoid plagiarism** and give others credit for their ideas. Another reason is to help readers find the sources consulted in the research and access more information about the subject for further reading and research. Additionally, citing sources helps to make a paper academically authoritative. To prepare, research writers should keep a running list of sources consulted, in an electronic file or on file cards. For every source used, the writer needs specific information. For books, a writer needs to record the author's and editor's names, book title, publication date, city, and publisher name. For articles, one needs the author's name, article title, journal (or magazine or newspaper) name, volume and issue number, publication date, and page numbers. For electronic resources, a writer will need the author's name, article information plus the URL, database name, name of the database's publisher, and the date of access.

Common Reference Styles

Three common reference styles are **MLA** (Modern Language Association), **APA** (American Psychological Association), and **Turabian** (created by author Kate Turabian, also known as the Chicago Manual of Style). Each style formats citation information differently. Professors and instructors often specify that students use one of these. Generally, APA style is used in psychology and sociology papers, and MLA style is used in English literature papers and similar scholarly projects. To understand how these styles differ, consider an imaginary article cited in each of these styles. This article is titled "Ten Things You Won't Believe Dragons Do," written by author Andra Gaines, included in the journal *Studies in Fantasy Fiction*, and published by Quest for Knowledge Publishing.

MLA:

Gaines, Andra. "Ten Things You Won't Believe Dragons Do." Studies in Fantasy Fiction, vol. 3, no. 8, Quest for Knowledge Publishing, 21 Aug. 2019.

APA:

Gaines, A. (2019). Ten Things You Won't Believe Dragons Do. *Studies in Fantasy Fiction, 3(8)*, 42-65.

Chicago:

Gaines, Andra. "Ten Things You Won't Believe Dragons Do," *Studies in Fantasy Fiction* 3, no. 8 (2019): 42-65.

Within each of these styles, citations, though they vary according to the type of source and how its used, generally follow a structure and format similar to those above. For example, citations for whole books will probably not include a container title or a volume number, but will otherwise look very similar.

Review Video: Citing Sources
Visit mometrix.com/academy and enter code: 993637

Setting, Mood, Tone, and Perspective in Literary Texts

Setting and Time Frame

A literary text has both a setting and time frame. A **setting** is the place in which the story as a whole is set. The **time frame** is the period in which the story is set. This may refer to the historical period the story takes place in or if the story takes place over a single day. Both setting and time frame are relevant to a text's meaning because they help the reader place the story in time and space. An author uses setting and time frame to anchor a text, create a mood, and enhance its meaning. This helps a reader understand why a character acts the way he does, or why certain events in the story are important. The setting impacts the **plot** and character **motivations**, while the time frame helps place the story in **chronological context**.

Example

Read the following excerpt from The Adventures of Huckleberry Finn by Mark Twain and analyze the relevance of setting to the text's meaning:

> We said there warn't no home like a raft, after all. Other places do seem so cramped up and smothery, but a raft don't. You feel mighty free and easy and comfortable on a raft.

This excerpt from *The Adventures of Huckleberry Finn* by Mark Twain reveals information about the **setting** of the book. By understanding that the main character, Huckleberry Finn, lives on a raft, the reader can place the story on a river, in this case, the Mississippi River in the South before the Civil War. The information about the setting also gives the reader clues about the **character** of Huck Finn: he clearly values independence and freedom, and he likes the outdoors. The information about the setting in the quote helps the reader to better understand the rest of the text.

SYNTAX AND WORD CHOICE

Authors use words and **syntax**, or sentence structure, to make their texts unique, convey their own writing style, and sometimes to make a point or emphasis. They know that word choice and syntax contribute to the reader's understanding of the text as well as to the tone and mood of a text.

Review Video: What is Syntax?
Visit mometrix.com/academy and enter code: 242280

MOOD AND TONE

Mood is a story's atmosphere, or the feelings the reader gets from reading it. The way authors set the mood in writing is comparable to the way filmmakers use music to set the mood in movies. Instead of music, though, writers judiciously select descriptive words to evoke certain **moods**. The mood of a work may convey joy, anger, bitterness, hope, gloom, fear, apprehension, or any other emotion the author wants the reader to feel. In addition to vocabulary choices, authors also use figurative expressions, particular sentence structures, and choices of diction that project and reinforce the moods they want to create. Whereas mood is the reader's emotions evoked by reading what is written, **tone** is the emotions and attitudes of the writer that she or he expresses in the writing. Authors use the same literary techniques to establish tone as they do to establish mood. An author may use a humorous tone, an angry or sad tone, a sentimental or unsentimental tone, or something else entirely.

MOOD AND TONE IN THE GREAT GATSBY

To understand the difference between mood and tone, look at this excerpt from F. Scott Fitzgerald's *The Great Gatsby*. In this passage, Nick Caraway, the novel's narrator, is describing his affordable house, which sits in a neighborhood full of expensive mansions.

> "I lived at West Egg, the—well the less fashionable of the two, though this is a most superficial tag to express the bizarre and not a little sinister contrast between them. My house was at the very tip of the egg, only fifty yard from the Sound, and squeezed between two huge places that rented for twelve or fifteen thousand a season ... My own house was an eyesore, but it was a small eyesore, and it had been overlooked, so I had a view of the water, a partial view of my neighbor's lawn, and the consoling proximity of millionaires—all for eighty dollars a month."

In this description, the mood created for the reader does not match the tone created through the narrator. The mood in this passage is one of dissatisfaction and inferiority. Nick compares his home to his neighbors', saying he lives in the "less fashionable" neighborhood and that his house is "overlooked," an "eyesore," and "squeezed between two huge" mansions. He also adds that his placement allows him the "consoling proximity of millionaires." A literal reading of these details leads the reader to have negative feelings toward Nick's house and his economic inferiority to his neighbors, creating the mood.

However, Fitzgerald also conveys an opposing attitude, or tone, through Nick's description. Nick calls the distinction between the neighborhoods "superficial," showing a suspicion of the value suggested by the neighborhoods' titles, properties, and residents. Nick also undermines his critique of his own home by calling it "a small eyesore" and claiming it has "been overlooked." However, he follows these statements with a description of his surroundings, claiming that he has "a view of the water" and can see some of his wealthy neighbor's property from his home, and a comparison between the properties' rent. While the mental image created for the reader depicts a small house shoved between looming mansions, the tone suggests that Nick enjoys these qualities about his home, or at least finds it charming. He acknowledges its shortcomings, but includes the benefits of his home's unassuming appearance.

Review Video: Style, Tone, and Mood
Visit mometrix.com/academy and enter code: 416961

POINT OF VIEW

Another element that impacts a text is the author's point of view. The **point of view** of a text is the perspective from which a passage is told. An author will always have a point of view about a story before he or she draws up a plot line. The author will know what events they want to take place, how they want the characters to interact, and how they want the story to resolve. An author will also have an opinion on the topic or series of events which is presented in the story that is based on their prior experience and beliefs.

The two main points of view that authors use, especially in a work of fiction, are first person and third person. If the narrator of the story is also the main character, or *protagonist*, the text is written in first-person point of view. In first person, the author writes from the perspective of *I*. Third-person point of view is probably the most common that authors use in their passages. Using third person, authors refer to each character by using *he* or *she*. In third-person omniscient, the narrator is not a character in the story and tells the story of all of the characters at the same time.

Review Video: Point of View
Visit mometrix.com/academy and enter code: 383336

FIRST-PERSON NARRATION

First-person narratives let narrators express inner feelings and thoughts, especially when the narrator is the protagonist as Lemuel Gulliver is in Jonathan Swift's *Gulliver's Travels.* The narrator may be a close friend of the protagonist, like Dr. Watson in Sir Arthur Conan Doyle's *Sherlock Holmes.* Or, the narrator can be less involved with the main characters and plot, like Nick Carraway in F. Scott Fitzgerald's *The Great Gatsby.* When a narrator reports others' narratives, she or he is a "**frame narrator**," like the nameless narrator of Joseph Conrad's *Heart of Darkness* or Mr. Lockwood in Emily Brontë's *Wuthering Heights.* **First-person plural** is unusual but can be effective. Isaac Asimov's *I, Robot*, William Faulkner's *A Rose for Emily*, Maxim Gorky's *Twenty-Six Men and a Girl*, and Jeffrey Eugenides' *The Virgin Suicides* all use first-person plural narration. Author Kurt Vonnegut is the first-person narrator in his semi-autobiographical novel *Timequake.* Also unusual, but effective, is a **first-person omniscient** (rather than the more common third-person omniscient) narrator, like Death in Markus Zusak's *The Book Thief* and the ghost in Alice Sebold's *The Lovely Bones.*

SECOND-PERSON NARRATION

While **second-person** address is very commonplace in popular song lyrics, it is the least used form of narrative voice in literary works. Popular serial books of the 1980s like *Fighting Fantasy* or *Choose Your Own Adventure* employed second-person narratives. In some cases, a narrative combines both second-person and first-person voices, using the pronouns *you* and *I*. This can draw readers into the story, and it can also enable the authors to compare directly "your" and "my" feelings, thoughts, and actions. When the narrator is also a character in the story, as in Edgar Allan Poe's short story "The Tell-Tale Heart" or Jay McInerney's novel *Bright Lights, Big City,* the narrative is better defined as first-person despite it also addressing "you."

THIRD-PERSON NARRATION

Narration in the third person is the most prevalent type, as it allows authors the most flexibility. It is so common that readers simply assume without needing to be informed that the narrator is not a character in the story, or involved in its events. **Third-person singular** is used more frequently than **third-person plural**, though some authors have also effectively used plural. However, both singular and plural are most often included in stories according to which characters are being described. The third-person narrator may be either objective or subjective, and either omniscient or limited. **Objective third-person** narration does not include what the characters described are thinking or feeling, while **subjective third-person** narration does. The **third-person omniscient** narrator knows everything about all characters, including their thoughts and emotions, and all related places, times, and events. However, the **third-person limited** narrator may know everything about a particular character, but is limited to that character. In other words, the narrator cannot speak about anything that character does not know.

Alternating-Person Narration

Although authors more commonly write stories from one point of view, there are also instances wherein they alternate the narrative voice within the same book. For example, they may sometimes use an omniscient third-person narrator and a more intimate first-person narrator at other times. In J. K. Rowling's series of *Harry Potter* novels, she often writes in a third-person limited narrative, but sometimes changes to narration by characters other than the protagonist. George R. R. Martin's series *A Song of Ice and Fire* changes the point of view to coincide with divisions between chapters. The same technique is used by Erin Hunter (a pseudonym for several authors of the *Warriors, Seekers,* and *Survivors* book series). Authors using first-person narrative sometimes switch to third-person to describe significant action scenes, especially those where the narrator was absent or uninvolved, as Barbara Kingsolver does in her novel *The Poisonwood Bible.*

Historical and Social Context

Fiction that is heavily influenced by a historical or social context cannot be comprehended as the author intended if the reader does not keep this context in mind. Many important elements of the text will be influenced by any context, including symbols, allusions, settings, and plot events. These contexts, as well as the identity of the work's author, can help to inform the reader about the author's concerns and intended meanings. For example, George Orwell published his novel *1984* in the year 1949, soon after the end of World War II. At that time, following the defeat of the Nazis, the Cold War began between the Western Allied nations and the Eastern Soviet Communists. People were therefore concerned about the conflict between the freedoms afforded by Western democracies versus the oppression represented by Communism. Orwell had also previously fought in the Spanish Civil War against a Spanish regime that he and his fellows viewed as oppressive. From this information, readers can infer that Orwell was concerned about oppression by totalitarian governments. This informs *1984*'s story of Winston Smith's rebellion against the oppressive "Big Brother" government, of the fictional dictatorial state of Oceania, and his capture, torture, and ultimate conversion by that government. Some literary theories also seek to use historical and social contexts to reveal deeper meanings and implications in a text.

Plot and Story Structure

Theme

The **theme** of a passage is what the reader learns from the text or the passage. It is the lesson or **moral** contained in the passage. It also is a unifying idea that is used throughout the text; it can take the form of a common setting, idea, symbol, design, or recurring event. A passage can have two or more themes that convey its overall idea. The theme or themes of a passage are often based on **universal themes**. They can frequently be expressed using well-known sayings about life, society, or human nature, such as "Hard work pays off" or "Good triumphs over evil." Themes are not usually stated **explicitly**. The reader must figure them out by carefully reading the passage. Themes are often the reason why passages are written; they give a passage unity and meaning. Themes are created through **plot development**. The events of a story help shape the themes of a passage.

Example

Explain why "Take care of what you care about" accurately describes the theme of the following excerpt.

> Luca collected baseball cards, but he wasn't very careful with them. He left them around the house. His dog liked to chew. One day, Luca and his friend Bart were looking at his collection. Then they went outside. When Luca got home, he saw his dog chewing on his cards. They were ruined.

This excerpt tells the story of a boy who is careless with his baseball cards and leaves them lying around. His dog ends up chewing them and ruining them. The lesson is that if you care about something, you need to take care of it. This is the theme, or point, of the story. Some stories have more than one theme, but this is not really true of this excerpt. The reader needs to figure out the theme based on what happens in the story. Sometimes, as in the case of fables, the theme is stated directly in the text. However, this is not usually the case.

Review Video: Themes in Literature
Visit mometrix.com/academy and enter code: 732074

PLOT AND STORY STRUCTURE

The **plot** includes the events that happen in a story and the order in which they are told to the reader. There are several types of plot structures, as stories can be told in many ways. The most common plot structure is the chronological plot, which presents the events to the reader in the same order they occur for the characters in the story. Chronological plots usually have five main parts, the **exposition**, **rising action**, the **climax**, **falling action**, and the **resolution**. This type of plot structure guides the reader through the story's events as the characters experience them and is the easiest structure to understand and identify. While this is the most common plot structure, many stories are nonlinear, which means the plot does not sequence events in the same order the characters experience them. Such stories might include elements like flashbacks that cause the story to be nonlinear.

Review Video: How to Make a Story Map
Visit mometrix.com/academy and enter code: 261719

EXPOSITION

The **exposition** is at the beginning of the story and generally takes place before the rising action begins. The purpose of the exposition is to give the reader context for the story, which the author may do by introducing one or more characters, describing the setting or world, or explaining the events leading up to the point where the story begins. The exposition may still include events that contribute to the plot, but the **rising action** and main conflict of the story are not part of the exposition. Some narratives skip the exposition and begin the story with the beginning of the rising action, which causes the reader to learn the context as the story intensifies.

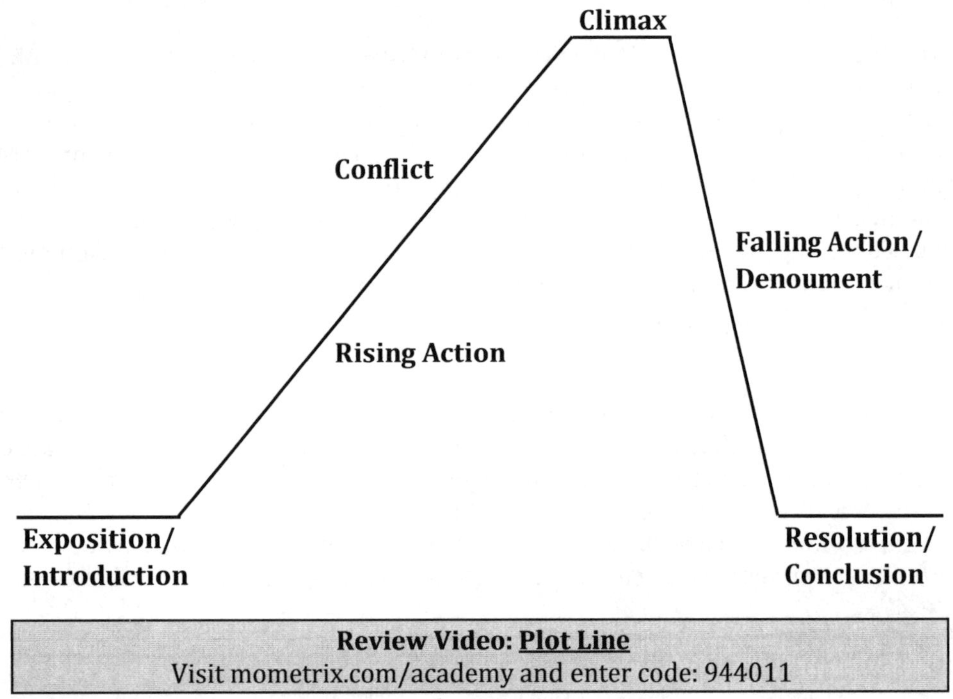

Review Video: Plot Line
Visit mometrix.com/academy and enter code: 944011

CONFLICT

A **conflict** is a problem to be solved. Literary plots typically include one conflict or more. Characters' attempts to resolve conflicts drive the narrative's forward movement. **Conflict resolution** is often the protagonist's primary occupation. Physical conflicts like exploring, wars, and escapes tend to make plots most suspenseful and exciting. Emotional, mental, or moral conflicts tend to make stories more personally gratifying or rewarding for many audiences. Conflicts can be external or internal. A major type of internal conflict is some inner personal battle, or **man versus self**. Major types of external conflicts include **man versus nature**, **man versus man**, and **man versus society**. Readers can identify conflicts in literary plots by identifying the protagonist and antagonist and asking why they conflict, what events develop the conflict, where the climax occurs, and how they identify with the characters.

Read the following paragraph and discuss the type of conflict present:

> Timothy was shocked out of sleep by the appearance of a bear just outside his tent. After panicking for a moment, he remembered some advice he had read in preparation for this trip: he should make noise so the bear would not be startled. As Timothy started to hum and sing, the bear wandered away.

There are three main types of conflict in literature: **man versus man**, **man versus nature**, and **man versus self**. This paragraph is an example of man versus nature. Timothy is in conflict with the bear. Even though no physical conflict like an attack exists, Timothy is pitted against the bear. Timothy uses his knowledge to "defeat" the bear and keep himself safe. The solution to the conflict is that Timothy makes noise, the bear wanders away, and Timothy is safe.

Review Video: Conflict
Visit mometrix.com/academy and enter code: 559550

Review Video: Determining Relationships in a Story
Visit mometrix.com/academy and enter code: 929925

Rising Action

The **rising action** is the part of the story where conflict **intensifies**. The rising action begins with an event that prompts the main conflict of the story. This may also be called the **inciting incident**. The main conflict generally occurs between the protagonist and an antagonist, but this is not the only type of conflict that may occur in a narrative. After this event, the protagonist works to resolve the main conflict by preparing for an altercation, pursuing a goal, fleeing an antagonist, or doing some other action that will end the conflict. The rising action is composed of several additional events that increase the story's tension. Most often, other developments will occur alongside the growth of the main conflict, such as character development or the development of minor conflicts. The rising action ends with the **climax**, which is the point of highest tension in the story.

Climax

The **climax** is the event in the narrative that marks the height of the story's conflict or tension. The event that takes place at the story's climax will end the rising action and bring about the results of the main conflict. If the conflict was between a good protagonist and an evil antagonist, the climax may be a final battle between the two characters. If the conflict is an adventurer looking for heavily guarded treasure, the climax may be the adventurer's encounter with the final obstacle that protects the treasure. The climax may be made of multiple scenes, but can usually be summarized as one event. Once the conflict and climax are complete, the **falling action** begins.

Falling Action

The **falling action** shows what happens in the story between the climax and the resolution. The falling action often composes a much smaller portion of the story than the rising action does. While the climax includes the end of the main conflict, the falling action may show the results of any minor conflicts in the story. For example, if the protagonist encountered a troll on the way to find some treasure, and the troll demanded the protagonist share the treasure after retrieving it, the falling action would include the protagonist returning to share the treasure with the troll. Similarly, any unexplained major events are usually made clear during the falling action. Once all significant elements of the story are resolved or addressed, the story's resolution will occur. The **resolution** is the end of the story, which shows the final result of the plot's events and shows what life is like for the main characters once they are no longer experiencing the story's conflicts.

Resolution

The way the conflict is **resolved** depends on the type of conflict. The plot of any book starts with the lead up to the conflict, then the conflict itself, and finally the solution, or **resolution**, to the conflict. In **man versus man** conflicts, the conflict is often resolved by two parties coming to some sort of agreement or by one party triumphing over the other party. In **man versus nature** conflicts, the conflict is often resolved by man coming to some realization about some aspect of nature. In **man versus self** conflicts, the conflict is often resolved by the character growing or coming to an understanding about part of himself.

Character Development

When depicting characters or figures in a written text, authors generally use actions, dialogue, and descriptions as characterization techniques. Characterization can occur in both fiction and nonfiction and is used to show a character or figure's personality, demeanor, and thoughts. This helps create a more engaging experience for the reader by providing a more concrete picture of a character or figure's tendencies and features. Characterizations also gives authors the opportunity to integrate elements such as dialects, activities, attire, and attitudes into their writing.

To understand the meaning of a story, it is vital to understand the characters as the author describes them. We can look for contradictions in what a character thinks, says, and does. We can notice whether the author's observations about a character differ from what other characters in the story say about that character. A character may be dynamic, meaning they change significantly during the story, or static, meaning they remain the same from beginning to end. Characters may be two-dimensional, not fully developed, or may be well developed with characteristics that stand out vividly. Characters may also symbolize universal properties. Additionally, readers can compare and contrast characters to analyze how each one developed.

A well-known example of character development can be found in Charles Dickens's *Great Expectations*. The novel's main character, Pip, is introduced as a young boy, and he is depicted as innocent, kind, and humble. However, as Pip grows up and is confronted with the social hierarchy of Victorian England, he becomes arrogant and rejects his loved ones in pursuit of his own social advancement. Once he achieves his social goals, he realizes the merits of his former lifestyle, and lives with the wisdom he gained in both environments and life stages. Dickens shows Pip's ever-changing character through his interactions with others and his inner thoughts, which evolve as his personal values and personality shift.

Review Video: Character Changes
Visit mometrix.com/academy and enter code: 408719

Dialogue

Effectively written dialogue serves at least one, but usually several, purposes. It advances the story and moves the plot, develops the characters, sheds light on the work's theme or meaning, and can, often subtly, account for the passage of time not otherwise indicated. It can alter the direction that the plot is taking, typically by introducing some new conflict or changing existing ones. **Dialogue** can establish a work's narrative voice and the characters' voices and set the tone of the story or of particular characters. When fictional characters display enlightenment or realization, dialogue can give readers an understanding of what those characters have discovered and how. Dialogue can illuminate the motivations and wishes of the story's characters. By using consistent thoughts and syntax, dialogue can support character development. Skillfully created, it can also represent real-life speech rhythms in written form. Via conflicts and ensuing action, dialogue also provides drama.

Dialogue in Fiction

In fictional works, effectively written dialogue does more than just break up or interrupt sections of narrative. While **dialogue** may supply exposition for readers, it must nonetheless be believable. Dialogue should be dynamic, not static, and it should not resemble regular prose. Authors should not use dialogue to write clever similes or metaphors, or to inject their own opinions. Nor should they use dialogue at all when narrative would be better. Most importantly, dialogue should not slow the plot movement. Dialogue must seem natural, which means careful construction of phrases rather than actually duplicating natural speech, which does not necessarily translate well to the written word. Finally, all dialogue must be pertinent to the story, rather than just added conversation.

Figurative Language and Literary Devices

Literary Analysis

The best literary analysis shows special insight into at least one important aspect of a text. When analyzing literary texts, it can be difficult to find a starting place. Many texts can be analyzed several different ways, often leaving an overwhelming number of options for writers to consider. However, narrowing the focus to a particular element of literature can be helpful when preparing to analyze a text. Symbolism, themes, and motifs are common starting points for literary analysis. These three methods of analysis can lead to a holistic analysis of a text, since they involve elements that are often distributed throughout the text. However, not all texts feature these elements in a way that facilitates a strong analysis, if they are present at all. It is also common to focus on character or plot development for analysis. These elements are compatible with theme, symbolism, and allusion. Setting and imagery, figurative language, and any external contexts can also contribute to analysis or complement one of these other elements. The application of a critical, or literary, theory to a text can also provide a thorough and strong analysis.

LITERAL AND FIGURATIVE MEANING

When language is used **literally**, the words mean exactly what they say and nothing more. When language is used **figuratively**, the words mean something beyond their literal meaning. For example, "The weeping willow tree has long, trailing branches and leaves" is a literal description. But "The weeping willow tree looks as if it is bending over and crying" is a figurative description—specifically, a **simile** or stated comparison. Another figurative language form is **metaphor**, or an implied comparison. A good example is the metaphor of a city, state, or city-state as a ship, and its governance as sailing that ship. Ancient Greek lyrical poet Alcaeus is credited with first using this metaphor, and ancient Greek tragedian Aeschylus then used it in *Seven Against Thebes,* and then Plato used it in the *Republic.*

FIGURES OF SPEECH

A **figure of speech** is a verbal expression whose meaning is figurative rather than literal. For example, the phrase "butterflies in the stomach" does not refer to actual butterflies in a person's stomach. It is a metaphor representing the fluttery feelings experienced when a person is nervous or excited—or when one "falls in love," which does not mean physically falling. "Hitting a sales target" does not mean physically hitting a target with arrows as in archery; it is a metaphor for meeting a sales quota. "Climbing the ladder of success" metaphorically likens advancing in one's career to ascending ladder rungs. Similes, such as "light as a feather" (meaning very light, not a feather's actual weight), and hyperbole, like "I'm starving/freezing/roasting," are also figures of speech. Figures of speech are often used and crafted for emphasis, freshness of expression, or clarity.

Review Video: Figures of Speech
Visit mometrix.com/academy and enter code: 111295

FIGURATIVE LANGUAGE

Figurative language extends past the literal meanings of words. It offers readers new insight into the people, things, events, and subjects covered in a work of literature. Figurative language also enables readers to feel they are sharing the authors' experiences. It can stimulate the reader's senses, make comparisons that readers find intriguing or even startling, and enable readers to view the world in different ways. When looking for figurative language, it is important to consider the context of the sentence or situation. Phrases that appear out of place or make little sense when read literally are likely instances of figurative language. Once figurative language has been recognized, context is also important to determining the type of figurative language being used and its function. For example, when a comparison is being made, a metaphor or simile is likely being used. This means the comparison may emphasize or create irony through the things being compared. Seven specific types of figurative language include: alliteration, onomatopoeia, personification, imagery, similes, metaphors, and hyperbole.

Review Video: Figurative Language
Visit mometrix.com/academy and enter code: 584902

ALLITERATION AND ONOMATOPOEIA

Alliteration describes a series of words beginning with the same sounds. **Onomatopoeia** uses words imitating the sounds of things they name or describe. For example, in his poem "Come Down, O Maid," Alfred Tennyson writes of "The moan of doves in immemorial elms, / And murmuring of innumerable bees." The word "moan" sounds like some sounds doves make, "murmuring" represents the sounds of bees buzzing. Onomatopoeia also includes words that are simply meant to represent sounds, such as "meow," "kaboom," and "whoosh."

Review Video: Alliteration in Everyday Expressions
Visit mometrix.com/academy and enter code: 462837

PERSONIFICATION

Another type of figurative language is **personification**. This is describing a non-human thing, like an animal or an object, as if it were human. The general intent of personification is to describe things in a manner that will be comprehensible to readers. When an author states that a tree *groans* in the wind, he or she does not mean that the tree is emitting a low, pained sound from a mouth. Instead, the author means that the tree is making a noise similar to a human groan. Of course, this personification establishes a tone of sadness or suffering. A different tone would be established if the author said that the tree was *swaying* or *dancing*. Alfred Tennyson's poem "The Eagle" uses all of these types of figurative language: "He clasps the crag with crooked hands." Tennyson used alliteration, repeating /k/ and /kr/ sounds. These hard-sounding consonants reinforce the imagery, giving visual and tactile impressions of the eagle.

> **Review Video: Personification**
> Visit mometrix.com/academy and enter code: 260066

SIMILES AND METAPHORS

Similes are stated comparisons using "like" or "as." Similes can be used to stimulate readers' imaginations and appeal to their senses. Because a simile includes *like* or *as,* the device creates more space between the description and the thing being described than a metaphor does. If an author says that *a house was like a shoebox*, then the tone is different than the author saying that the house *was* a shoebox. Authors will choose between a metaphor and a simile depending on their intended tone.

Similes also help compare fictional characters to well-known objects or experiences, so the reader can better relate to them. William Wordsworth's poem about "Daffodils" begins, "I wandered lonely as a cloud." This simile compares his loneliness to that of a cloud. It is also personification, giving a cloud the human quality loneliness. In his novel *Lord Jim* (1900), Joseph Conrad writes in Chapter 33, "I would have given anything for the power to soothe her frail soul, tormenting itself in its invincible ignorance like a small bird beating about the cruel wires of a cage." Conrad uses the word "like" to compare the girl's soul to a small bird. His description of the bird beating at the cage shows the similar helplessness of the girl's soul to gain freedom.

> **Review Video: Similes**
> Visit mometrix.com/academy and enter code: 642949

A **metaphor** is a type of figurative language in which the writer equates something with another thing that is not particularly similar, instead of using *like* or *as*. For instance, *the bird was an arrow arcing through the sky*. In this sentence, the arrow is serving as a metaphor for the bird. The point of a metaphor is to encourage the reader to consider the item being described in a *different way*. Let's continue with this metaphor for a flying bird. You are asked to envision the bird's flight as being similar to the arc of an arrow. So, you imagine the flight to be swift and bending. Metaphors are a way for the author to describe an item *without being direct and obvious*. This literary device is a lyrical and suggestive way of providing information. Note that the reference for a metaphor will not always be mentioned explicitly by the author. Consider the following description of a forest in winter: *Swaying skeletons reached for the sky and groaned as the wind blew through them*. In this example, the author is using *skeletons* as a metaphor for leafless trees. This metaphor creates a spooky tone while inspiring the reader's imagination.

LITERARY EXAMPLES OF METAPHOR

A **metaphor** is an implied comparison, i.e., it compares something to something else without using "like", "as", or other comparative words. For example, in "The Tyger" (1794), William Blake writes, "Tyger Tyger, burning bright, / In the forests of the night." Blake compares the tiger to a flame not by saying it is like a fire, but by simply describing it as "burning." Henry Wadsworth Longfellow's poem "O Ship of State" (1850) uses an extended metaphor by referring consistently throughout the entire poem to the state, union, or republic as a seagoing vessel, referring to its keel, mast, sail, rope, anchors, and to its braving waves, rocks, gale, tempest, and "false lights on the shore." Within the extended metaphor, Wordsworth uses a specific metaphor: "the anchors of thy hope!"

Ted Hughes' Animal Metaphors

Ted Hughes frequently used animal metaphors in his poetry. In "The Thought Fox," a model of concise, structured beauty, Hughes characterizes the poet's creative process with succinct, striking imagery of an idea entering his head like a wild fox. Repeating "loneliness" in the first two stanzas emphasizes the poet's lonely work: "Something else is alive / Beside the clock's loneliness." He treats an idea's arrival as separate from himself. Three stanzas detail in vivid images a fox's approach from the outside winter forest at starless midnight—its nose, "Cold, delicately" touching twigs and leaves; "neat" paw prints in snow; "bold" body; brilliant green eyes; and self-contained, focused progress—"Till, with a sudden sharp hot stink of fox," he metaphorically depicts poetic inspiration as the fox's physical entry into "the dark hole of the head." Hughes ends by summarizing his vision of a poet as an interior, passive idea recipient, with the outside world unchanged: "The window is starless still; the clock ticks, / The page is printed."

> **Review Video: Metaphors in Writing**
> Visit mometrix.com/academy and enter code: 133295

Metonymy

Metonymy is naming one thing with words or phrases of a closely related thing. This is similar to metaphor. However, the comparison has a close connection, unlike metaphor. An example of metonymy is to call the news media *the press*. Of course, *the press* is the machine that prints newspapers. Metonymy is a way of naming something without using the same name constantly.

Synecdoche

Synecdoche points to the whole by naming one of the parts. An example of synecdoche would be calling a construction worker a *hard hat*. Like metonymy, synecdoche is an easy way of naming something without having to overuse a name. The device allows writers to highlight pieces of the thing being described. For example, referring to businessmen as *suits* suggests professionalism and unity.

Hyperbole

Hyperbole is excessive exaggeration used for humor or emphasis rather than for literal meaning. For example, in *To Kill a Mockingbird*, Harper Lee wrote, "People moved slowly then. There was no hurry, for there was nowhere to go, nothing to buy and no money to buy it with, nothing to see outside the boundaries of Maycomb County." This was not literally true; Lee exaggerates the scarcity of these things for emphasis. In "Old Times on the Mississippi," Mark Twain wrote, "I... could have hung my hat on my eyes, they stuck out so far." This is not literal, but makes his description vivid and funny. In his poem "As I Walked Out One Evening", W. H. Auden wrote, "I'll love you, dear, I'll love you / Till China and Africa meet, / And the river jumps over the mountain / And the salmon sing in the street." He used things not literally possible to emphasize the duration of his love.

Understatement

Understatement is the opposite of hyperbole. This device discounts or downplays something. Think about someone who climbs Mount Everest. Then, they say that the journey was *a little stroll*. As with other types of figurative language, understatement has a range of uses. The device may show self-defeat or modesty as in the Mount Everest example. However, some may think of understatement as false modesty (i.e., an attempt to bring attention to you or a situation). For example, a woman is praised on her diamond engagement ring. The woman says, *Oh, this little thing?* Her understatement might be heard as stuck-up or unfeeling.

> **Review Video: Hyperbole and Understatement**
> Visit mometrix.com/academy and enter code: 308470

LITERARY IRONY

In literature, irony demonstrates the opposite of what is said or done. The three types of irony are **verbal irony**, **situational irony**, and **dramatic irony**. Verbal irony uses words opposite to the meaning. Sarcasm may use verbal irony. One common example is describing something that is confusing as "clear as mud." For example, in his 1986 movie *Hannah and Her Sisters,* author, director, and actor Woody Allen says to his character's date, "I had a great evening; it was like the Nuremburg Trials." Notice these employ similes. In situational irony, what happens contrasts with what was expected. O. Henry's short story *The Gift of the Magi* uses situational irony: a husband and wife each sacrifice their most prized possession to buy each other a Christmas present. The irony is that she sells her long hair to buy him a watch fob, while he sells his heirloom pocket-watch to buy her the jeweled combs for her hair she had long wanted; in the end, neither of them can use their gifts. In dramatic irony, narrative informs audiences of more than its characters know. For example, in *Romeo and Juliet,* the audience is made aware that Juliet is only asleep, while Romeo believes her to be dead, which then leads to Romeo's death.

Review Video: What is Irony?
Visit mometrix.com/academy and enter code: 374204

IDIOMS

Idioms create comparisons, and often take the form of similes or metaphors. Idioms are always phrases and are understood to have a meaning that is different from its individual words' literal meaning. For example, "break a leg" is a common idiom that is used to wish someone luck or tell them to perform well. Literally, the phrase "break a leg" means to injure a person's leg, but the phrase takes on a different meaning when used as an idiom. Another example is "call it a day," which means to temporarily stop working on a task, or find a stopping point, rather than literally referring to something as "a day." Many idioms are associated with a region or group. For example, an idiom commonly used in the American South is "'til the cows come home." This phrase is often used to indicate that something will take or may last for a very long time, but not that it will literally last until the cows return to where they reside.

ALLUSION

An allusion is an uncited but recognizable reference to something else. Authors use language to make allusions to places, events, artwork, and other books in order to make their own text richer. For example, an author may allude to a very important text in order to make his own text seem more important. Martin Luther King, Jr. started his "I Have a Dream" speech by saying "Five score years ago…" This is a clear allusion to President Abraham Lincoln's "Gettysburg Address" and served to remind people of the significance of the event. An author may allude to a place to ground his text or make a cultural reference to make readers feel included. There are many reasons that authors make allusions.

Review Video: Allusions
Visit mometrix.com/academy and enter code: 294065

COMIC RELIEF

Comic relief is the use of comedy by an author to break up a dramatic or tragic scene and infuse it with a bit of **lightheartedness**. In William Shakespeare's *Hamlet,* two gravediggers digging the grave for Ophelia share a joke while they work. The death and burial of Ophelia are tragic moments that directly follow each other. Shakespeare uses an instance of comedy to break up the tragedy and give his audience a bit of a break from the tragic drama. Authors sometimes use comic relief so that their work will be less depressing; other times they use it to create irony or contrast between the darkness of the situation and the lightness of the joke. Often, authors will use comedy to parallel what is happening in the tragic scenes.

Review Video: Comic Relief
Visit mometrix.com/academy and enter code: 779604

Foreshadowing

Foreshadowing is a device authors use to give readers **hints** about events that will take place later in a story. Foreshadowing most often takes place through a character's dialogue or actions. Sometimes the character will know what is going to happen and will purposefully allude to future events. For example, consider a protagonist who is about to embark on a journey through the woods. Just before the protagonist begins the trip, another character says, "Be careful, you never know what could be out in those woods!" This alerts the reader that the woods may be dangerous and prompts the reader to expect something to attack the protagonist in the woods. This is an example of foreshadowing through warning. Alternatively, a character may unknowingly foreshadow later events. For example, consider a story where a brother and sister run through their house and knock over a vase and break it. The brother says, "Don't worry, we'll clean it up! Mom will never know!" However, the reader knows that their mother will most likely find out what they have done, so the reader expects the siblings to later get in trouble for running, breaking the vase, and hiding it from their mother.

Symbolism

Symbolism describes an author's use of a **symbol**, an element of the story that **represents** something else. Symbols can impact stories in many ways, including deepening the meaning of a story or its elements, comparing a story to another work, or foreshadowing later events in a story. Symbols can be objects, characters, colors, numbers, or anything else the author establishes as a symbol. Symbols can be clearly established through direct comparison or repetition, but they can also be established subtly or gradually over a large portion of the story. Another form of symbolism is **allusion**, which is when something in a story is used to prompt the reader to think about another work. Many well-known works use **Biblical allusions**, which are allusions to events or details in the Bible that inform a work or an element within it.

Word Knowledge

Word Roots and Prefixes and Suffixes

Affixes

Affixes in the English language are morphemes that are added to words to create related but different words. Derivational affixes form new words based on and related to the original words. For example, the affix *-ness* added to the end of the adjective *happy* forms the noun *happiness.* Inflectional affixes form different grammatical versions of words. For example, the plural affix *-s* changes the singular noun *book* to the plural noun *books*, and the past tense affix *-ed* changes the present tense verb *look* to the past tense *looked.* Prefixes are affixes placed in front of words. For example, *heat* means to make hot; *preheat* means to heat in advance. Suffixes are affixes placed at the ends of words. The *happiness* example above contains the suffix *-ness.* Circumfixes add parts both before and after words, such as how *light* becomes *enlighten* with the prefix *en-* and the suffix *-en.* Interfixes create compound words via central affixes: *speed* and *meter* become *speedometer* via the interfix *-o-*.

Review Video: Affixes
Visit mometrix.com/academy and enter code: 782422

Word Roots, Prefixes, and Suffixes to Help Determine Meanings of Words

Many English words were formed from combining multiple sources. For example, the Latin *habēre* means "to have," and the prefixes *in-* and *im-* mean a lack or prevention of something, as in *insufficient* and *imperfect.* Latin combined *in-* with *habēre* to form *inhibēre,* whose past participle was *inhibitus*. This is the origin of the English word *inhibit,* meaning to prevent from having. Hence by knowing the meanings of both the prefix and the root, one can decipher the word meaning. In Greek, the root *enkephalo-* refers to the brain. Many medical terms are based on this root, such as encephalitis and hydrocephalus. Understanding the prefix and suffix meanings (*-itis* means inflammation; *hydro-* means water) allows a person to deduce that encephalitis refers to brain inflammation and hydrocephalus refers to water (or other fluid) in the brain.

Review Video: Determining Word Meanings
Visit mometrix.com/academy and enter code: 894894

PREFIXES

While knowing prefix meanings helps ESL and beginning readers learn new words, other readers take for granted the meanings of known words. However, prefix knowledge will also benefit them for determining meanings or definitions of unfamiliar words. For example, native English speakers and readers familiar with recipes know what *preheat* means. Knowing that *pre-* means in advance can also inform them that *presume* means to assume in advance, that *prejudice* means advance judgment, and that this understanding can be applied to many other words beginning with *pre-*. Knowing that the prefix *dis-* indicates opposition informs the meanings of words like *disbar, disagree, disestablish,* and many more. Knowing *dys-* means bad, impaired, abnormal, or difficult informs *dyslogistic, dysfunctional, dysphagia,* and *dysplasia.*

SUFFIXES

In English, certain suffixes generally indicate both that a word is a noun, and that the noun represents a state of being or quality. For example, *-ness* is commonly used to change an adjective into its noun form, as with *happy* and *happiness, nice* and *niceness,* and so on. The suffix *–tion* is commonly used to transform a verb into its noun form, as with *converse* and *conversation or move* and *motion*. Thus, if readers are unfamiliar with the second form of a word, knowing the meaning of the transforming suffix can help them determine meaning.

PREFIXES FOR NUMBERS

Prefix	Definition	Examples
bi-	two	bisect, biennial
mono-	one, single	monogamy, monologue
poly-	many	polymorphous, polygamous
semi-	half, partly	semicircle, semicolon
uni-	one	uniform, unity

Prefixes for Time, Direction, and Space

Prefix	Definition	Examples
a-	in, on, of, up, to	abed, afoot
ab-	from, away, off	abdicate, abjure
ad-	to, toward	advance, adventure
ante-	before, previous	antecedent, antedate
anti-	against, opposing	antipathy, antidote
cata-	down, away, thoroughly	catastrophe, cataclysm
circum-	around	circumspect, circumference
com-	with, together, very	commotion, complicate
contra-	against, opposing	contradict, contravene
de-	from	depart
dia-	through, across, apart	diameter, diagnose
dis-	away, off, down, not	dissent, disappear
epi-	upon	epilogue
ex-	out	extract, excerpt
hypo-	under, beneath	hypodermic, hypothesis
inter-	among, between	intercede, interrupt
intra-	within	intramural, intrastate
ob-	against, opposing	objection
per-	through	perceive, permit
peri-	around	periscope, perimeter
post-	after, following	postpone, postscript
pre-	before, previous	prevent, preclude
pro-	forward, in place of	propel, pronoun
retro-	back, backward	retrospect, retrograde
sub-	under, beneath	subjugate, substitute
super-	above, extra	supersede, supernumerary
trans-	across, beyond, over	transact, transport
ultra-	beyond, excessively	ultramodern, ultrasonic

Negative Prefixes

Prefix	Definition	Examples
a-	without, lacking	atheist, agnostic
in-	not, opposing	incapable, ineligible
non-	not	nonentity, nonsense
un-	not, reverse of	unhappy, unlock

EXTRA PREFIXES

Prefix	Definition	Examples
for-	away, off, from	forget, forswear
fore-	previous	foretell, forefathers
homo-	same, equal	homogenized, homonym
hyper-	excessive, over	hypercritical, hypertension
in-	in, into	intrude, invade
mal-	bad, poorly, not	malfunction, malpractice
mis-	bad, poorly, not	misspell, misfire
neo-	new	Neolithic, neoconservative
omni-	all, everywhere	omniscient, omnivore
ortho-	right, straight	orthogonal, orthodox
over-	above	overbearing, oversight
pan-	all, entire	panorama, pandemonium
para-	beside, beyond	parallel, paradox
re-	backward, again	revoke, recur
sym-	with, together	sympathy, symphony

Below is a list of common suffixes and their meanings:

ADJECTIVE SUFFIXES

Suffix	Definition	Examples
-able (-ible)	capable of being	toler*able*, ed*ible*
-esque	in the style of, like	picturesque, grotesque
-ful	filled with, marked by	thankful, zestful
-ific	make, cause	terrific, beatific
-ish	suggesting, like	churlish, childish
-less	lacking, without	hopeless, countless
-ous	marked by, given to	religious, riotous

NOUN SUFFIXES

Suffix	Definition	Examples
-acy	state, condition	accuracy, privacy
-ance	act, condition, fact	acceptance, vigilance
-ard	one that does excessively	drunkard, sluggard
-ation	action, state, result	occupation, starvation
-dom	state, rank, condition	serfdom, wisdom
-er (-or)	office, action	teach*er*, elevat*or*, hon*or*
-ess	feminine	waitress, duchess
-hood	state, condition	manhood, statehood
-ion	action, result, state	union, fusion
-ism	act, manner, doctrine	barbarism, socialism
-ist	worker, follower	monopolist, socialist
-ity (-ty)	state, quality, condition	acid*ity*, civil*ity*, twen*ty*
-ment	result, action	Refreshment
-ness	quality, state	greatness, tallness
-ship	position	internship, statesmanship
-sion (-tion)	state, result	revi*sion*, expedi*tion*
-th	act, state, quality	warmth, width
-tude	quality, state, result	magnitude, fortitude

VERB SUFFIXES

Suffix	Definition	Examples
-ate	having, showing	separate, desolate
-en	cause to be, become	deepen, strengthen
-fy	make, cause to have	glorify, fortify
-ize	cause to be, treat with	sterilize, mechanize

DETERMINING WORD MEANINGS

SYNONYMS AND ANTONYMS

When you understand how words relate to each other, you will discover more in a passage. This is explained by understanding **synonyms** (e.g., words that mean the same thing) and **antonyms** (e.g., words that mean the opposite of one another). As an example, *dry* and *arid* are synonyms, and *dry* and *wet* are antonyms.

There are many pairs of words in English that can be considered synonyms, despite having slightly different definitions. For instance, the words *friendly* and *collegial* can both be used to describe a warm interpersonal relationship, and one would be correct to call them synonyms. However, *collegial* (kin to *colleague*) is often used in reference to professional or academic relationships, and *friendly* has no such connotation.

If the difference between the two words is too great, then they should not be called synonyms. *Hot* and *warm* are not synonyms because their meanings are too distinct. A good way to determine whether two words are synonyms is to substitute one word for the other word and verify that the meaning of the sentence has not changed. Substituting *warm* for *hot* in a sentence would convey a different meaning. Although warm and hot may seem close in meaning, warm generally means that the temperature is moderate, and hot generally means that the temperature is excessively high.

Antonyms are words with opposite meanings. *Light* and *dark*, *up* and *down*, *right* and *left*, *good* and *bad*: these are all sets of antonyms. Be careful to distinguish between antonyms and pairs of words that are simply different. *Black* and *gray*, for instance, are not antonyms because gray is not the opposite of black. *Black* and *white*, on the other hand, are antonyms.

Not every word has an antonym. For instance, many nouns do not. What would be the antonym of *chair*? During your exam, the questions related to antonyms are more likely to concern adjectives. You will recall that adjectives are words that describe a noun. Some common adjectives include *purple*, *fast*, *skinny*, and *sweet*. From those four adjectives, *purple* is the item that lacks a group of obvious antonyms.

Review Video: What Are Synonyms and Antonyms?
Visit mometrix.com/academy and enter code: 105612

DENOTATIVE VS. CONNOTATIVE MEANING

The **denotative** meaning of a word is the literal meaning. The **connotative** meaning goes beyond the denotative meaning to include the emotional reaction that a word may invoke. The connotative meaning often takes the denotative meaning a step further due to associations the reader makes with the denotative meaning. Readers can differentiate between the denotative and connotative meanings by first recognizing how authors use each meaning. Most non-fiction, for example, is fact-based and authors do not use flowery, figurative language. The reader can assume that the writer is using the denotative meaning of words. In fiction, the author may use the connotative meaning. Readers can determine whether the author is using the denotative or connotative meaning of a word by implementing context clues.

Review Video: Connotation and Denotation
Visit mometrix.com/academy and enter code: 310092

Nuances of Word Meaning Relative to Connotation, Denotation, Diction, and Usage

A word's denotation is simply its objective dictionary definition. However, its connotation refers to the subjective associations, often emotional, that specific words evoke in listeners and readers. Two or more words can have the same dictionary meaning, but very different connotations. Writers use diction (word choice) to convey various nuances of thought and emotion by selecting synonyms for other words that best communicate the associations they want to trigger for readers. For example, a car engine is naturally greasy; in this sense, "greasy" is a neutral term. But when a person's smile, appearance, or clothing is described as "greasy," it has a negative connotation. Some words have even gained additional or different meanings over time. For example, *awful* used to be used to describe things that evoked a sense of awe. When *awful* is separated into its root word, awe, and suffix, -ful, it can be understood to mean "full of awe." However, the word is now commonly used to describe things that evoke repulsion, terror, or another intense, negative reaction.

> **Review Video: Word Usage in Sentences**
> Visit mometrix.com/academy and enter code: 197863

Context Clues

Readers of all levels will encounter words that they have either never seen or have encountered only on a limited basis. The best way to define a word in **context** is to look for nearby words that can assist in revealing the meaning of the word. For instance, unfamiliar nouns are often accompanied by examples that provide a definition. Consider the following sentence: *Dave arrived at the party in hilarious garb: a leopard-print shirt, buckskin trousers, and bright green sneakers.* If a reader was unfamiliar with the meaning of garb, he or she could read the examples (i.e., a leopard-print shirt, buckskin trousers, and high heels) and quickly determine that the word means *clothing*. Examples will not always be this obvious. Consider this sentence: *Parsley, lemon, and flowers were just a few of the items he used as garnishes.* Here, the word *garnishes* is exemplified by parsley, lemon, and flowers. Readers who have eaten in a variety of restaurants will probably be able to identify a garnish as something used to decorate a plate.

> **Review Video: Reading Comprehension: Using Context Clues**
> Visit mometrix.com/academy and enter code: 613660

Using Contrast in Context Clues

In addition to looking at the context of a passage, readers can use contrast to define an unfamiliar word in context. In many sentences, the author will not describe the unfamiliar word directly; instead, he or she will describe the opposite of the unfamiliar word. Thus, you are provided with some information that will bring you closer to defining the word. Consider the following example: *Despite his intelligence, Hector's low brow and bad posture made him look obtuse.* The author writes that Hector's appearance does not convey intelligence. Therefore, *obtuse* must mean unintelligent. Here is another example: *Despite the horrible weather, we were beatific about our trip to Alaska*. The word *despite* indicates that the speaker's feelings were at odds with the weather. Since the weather is described as *horrible*, then *beatific* must mean something positive.

Substitution to Find Meaning

In some cases, there will be very few contextual clues to help a reader define the meaning of an unfamiliar word. When this happens, one strategy that readers may employ is **substitution**. A good reader will brainstorm some possible synonyms for the given word, and he or she will substitute these words into the sentence. If the sentence and the surrounding passage continue to make sense, then the substitution has revealed at least some information about the unfamiliar word. Consider the sentence: *Frank's admonition rang in her ears as she climbed the mountain.* A reader unfamiliar with *admonition* might come up with some substitutions like *vow, promise, advice, complaint,* or *compliment.* All of these words make general sense of the sentence, though their meanings are diverse. However, this process has suggested that an admonition is some sort of message. The substitution strategy is rarely able to pinpoint a precise definition, but this process can be effective as a last resort.

Occasionally, you will be able to define an unfamiliar word by looking at the descriptive words in the context. Consider the following sentence: *Fred dragged the recalcitrant boy kicking and screaming up the stairs.* The words *dragged*, *kicking*, and *screaming* all suggest that the boy does not want to go up the stairs. The reader may assume that *recalcitrant* means something like unwilling or protesting. In this example, an unfamiliar adjective was identified.

Additionally, using description to define an unfamiliar noun is a common practice compared to unfamiliar adjectives, as in this sentence: *Don's wrinkled frown and constantly shaking fist identified him as a curmudgeon of the first order.* Don is described as having a *wrinkled frown and constantly shaking fist*, suggesting that a *curmudgeon* must be a grumpy person. Contrasts do not always provide detailed information about the unfamiliar word, but they at least give the reader some clues.

Words with Multiple Meanings

When a word has more than one meaning, readers can have difficulty determining how the word is being used in a given sentence. For instance, the verb *cleave*, can mean either *join* or *separate*. When readers come upon this word, they will have to select the definition that makes the most sense. Consider the following sentence: *Hermione's knife cleaved the bread cleanly.* Since a knife cannot join bread together, the word must indicate separation. A slightly more difficult example would be the sentence: *The birds cleaved to one another as they flew from the oak tree.* Immediately, the presence of the words *to one another* should suggest that in this sentence *cleave* is being used to mean *join*. Discovering the intent of a word with multiple meanings requires the same tricks as defining an unknown word: look for contextual clues and evaluate the substituted words.

Context Clues to Help Determine Meanings of Words

If readers simply bypass unknown words, they can reach unclear conclusions about what they read. However, looking for the definition of every unfamiliar word in the dictionary can slow their reading progress. Moreover, the dictionary may list multiple definitions for a word, so readers must search the word's context for meaning. Hence context is important to new vocabulary regardless of reader methods. Four types of context clues are examples, definitions, descriptive words, and opposites. Authors may use a certain word, and then follow it with several different examples of what it describes. Sometimes authors actually supply a definition of a word they use, which is especially true in informational and technical texts. Authors may use descriptive words that elaborate upon a vocabulary word they just used. Authors may also use opposites with negation that help define meaning.

Examples and Definitions

An author may use a word and then give examples that illustrate its meaning. Consider this text: "Teachers who do not know how to use sign language can help students who are deaf or hard of hearing understand certain instructions by using gestures instead, like pointing their fingers to indicate which direction to look or go; holding up a hand, palm outward, to indicate stopping; holding the hands flat, palms up, curling a finger toward oneself in a beckoning motion to indicate 'come here'; or curling all fingers toward oneself repeatedly to indicate 'come on', 'more', or 'continue.'" The author of this text has used the word "gestures" and then followed it with examples, so a reader unfamiliar with the word could deduce from the examples that "gestures" means "hand motions." Readers can find examples by looking for signal words "for example," "for instance," "like," "such as," and "e.g."

While readers sometimes have to look for definitions of unfamiliar words in a dictionary or do some work to determine a word's meaning from its surrounding context, at other times an author may make it easier for readers by defining certain words. For example, an author may write, "The company did not have sufficient capital, that is, available money, to continue operations." The author defined "capital" as "available money," and heralded the definition with the phrase "that is." Another way that authors supply word definitions is with appositives. Rather than being introduced by a signal phrase like "that is," "namely," or "meaning," an appositive comes after the vocabulary word it defines and is enclosed within two commas. For example, an author may write, "The Indians introduced the Pilgrims to pemmican, cakes they made of lean meat dried and mixed with fat, which proved greatly beneficial to keep settlers from starving while trapping." In this example, the appositive phrase following "pemmican" and preceding "which" defines the word "pemmican."

Descriptions

When readers encounter a word they do not recognize in a text, the author may expand on that word to illustrate it better. While the author may do this to make the prose more picturesque and vivid, the reader can also take advantage of this description to provide context clues to the meaning of the unfamiliar word. For example, an author may write, "The man sitting next to me on the airplane was obese. His shirt stretched across his vast expanse of flesh, strained almost to bursting." The descriptive second sentence elaborates on and helps to define the previous sentence's word "obese" to mean extremely fat. A reader unfamiliar with the word "repugnant" can decipher its meaning through an author's accompanying description: "The way the child grimaced and shuddered as he swallowed the medicine showed that its taste was particularly repugnant."

Opposites

Text authors sometimes introduce a contrasting or opposing idea before or after a concept they present. They may do this to emphasize or heighten the idea they present by contrasting it with something that is the reverse. However, readers can also use these context clues to understand familiar words. For example, an author may write, "Our conversation was not cheery. We sat and talked very solemnly about his experience and a number of similar events." The reader who is not familiar with the word "solemnly" can deduce by the author's preceding use of "not cheery" that "solemn" means the opposite of cheery or happy, so it must mean serious or sad. Or if someone writes, "Don't condemn his entire project because you couldn't find anything good to say about it," readers unfamiliar with "condemn" can understand from the sentence structure that it means the opposite of saying anything good, so it must mean reject, dismiss, or disapprove. "Entire" adds another context clue, meaning total or complete rejection.

Syntax to Determine Part of Speech and Meanings of Words

Syntax refers to sentence structure and word order. Suppose that a reader encounters an unfamiliar word when reading a text. To illustrate, consider an invented word like "splunch." If this word is used in a sentence like "Please splunch that ball to me," the reader can assume from syntactic context that "splunch" is a verb. We would not use a noun, adjective, adverb, or preposition with the object "that ball," and the prepositional phrase "to me" further indicates "splunch" represents an action. However, in the sentence, "Please hand that splunch to me," the reader can assume that "splunch" is a noun. Demonstrative adjectives like "that" modify nouns. Also, we hand someone some*thing*—a thing being a noun; we do not hand someone a verb, adjective, or adverb. Some sentences contain further clues. For example, from the sentence, "The princess wore the glittering splunch on her head," the reader can deduce that it is a crown, tiara, or something similar from the syntactic context, without knowing the word.

Syntax to Indicate Different Meanings of Similar Sentences

The syntax, or structure, of a sentence affords grammatical cues that aid readers in comprehending the meanings of words, phrases, and sentences in the texts that they read. Seemingly minor differences in how the words or phrases in a sentence are ordered can make major differences in meaning. For example, two sentences can use exactly the same words but have different meanings based on the word order:

- "The man with a broken arm sat in a chair."
- "The man sat in a chair with a broken arm."

While both sentences indicate that a man sat in a chair, differing syntax indicates whether the man's or chair's arm was broken.

Determining Meaning of Phrases and Paragraphs

Like unknown words, the meanings of phrases, paragraphs, and entire works can also be difficult to discern. Each of these can be better understood with added context. However, for larger groups of words, more context is needed. Unclear phrases are similar to unclear words, and the same methods can be used to understand their meaning. However, it is also important to consider how the individual words in the phrase work together. Paragraphs are a bit more complicated. Just as words must be compared to other words in a sentence, paragraphs must be compared to other paragraphs in a composition or a section.

Determining Meaning in Various Types of Compositions

To understand the meaning of an entire composition, the type of composition must be considered. **Expository writing** is generally organized so that each paragraph focuses on explaining one idea, or part of an idea, and its relevance. **Persuasive writing** uses paragraphs for different purposes to organize the parts of the argument. **Unclear paragraphs** must be read in the context of the paragraphs around them for their meaning to be fully understood. The meaning of full texts can also be unclear at times. The purpose of composition is also important for understanding the meaning of a text. To quickly understand the broad meaning of a text, look to the introductory and concluding paragraphs. Fictional texts are different. Some fictional works have implicit meanings, but some do not. The target audience must be considered for understanding texts that do have an implicit meaning, as most children's fiction will clearly state any lessons or morals. For other fiction, the application of literary theories and criticism may be helpful for understanding the text.

Additional Resources for Determining Word Meaning and Usage

While these strategies are useful for determining the meaning of unknown words and phrases, sometimes additional resources are needed to properly use the terms in different contexts. Some words have multiple definitions, and some words are inappropriate in particular contexts or modes of writing. The following tools are helpful for understanding all meanings and proper uses for words and phrases.

- **Dictionaries** provide the meaning of a multitude of words in a language. Many dictionaries include additional information about each word, such as its etymology, its synonyms, or variations of the word.
- **Glossaries** are similar to dictionaries, as they provide the meanings of a variety of terms. However, while dictionaries typically feature an extensive list of words and comprise an entire publication, glossaries are often included at the end of a text and only include terms and definitions that are relevant to the text they follow.
- **Spell Checkers** are used to detect spelling errors in typed text. Some spell checkers may also detect the misuse of plural or singular nouns, verb tenses, or capitalization. While spell checkers are a helpful tool, they are not always reliable or attuned to the author's intent, so it is important to review the spell checker's suggestions before accepting them.
- **Style Manuals** are guidelines on the preferred punctuation, format, and grammar usage according to different fields or organizations. For example, the Associated Press Stylebook is a style guide often used for media writing. The guidelines within a style guide are not always applicable across different contexts and usages, as the guidelines often cover grammatical or formatting situations that are not objectively correct or incorrect.

Chapter Quiz

Ready to see how well you retained what you just read? Scan the QR code to go directly to the chapter quiz interface for this study guide. If you're using a computer, simply visit the bonus page at **mometrix.com/bonus948/pax** and click the Chapter Quizzes link.

Mathematics

Integers

Subtraction with Regrouping

A great way to make use of some of the features built into the decimal system would be regrouping when attempting longform subtraction operations. When subtracting within a place value, sometimes the minuend is smaller than the subtrahend, **regrouping** enables you to 'borrow' a unit from a place value to the left in order to get a positive difference. For example, consider subtracting 189 from 525 with regrouping.

First, set up the subtraction problem in vertical form:

	525
-	189

Notice that the numbers in the ones and tens columns of 525 are smaller than the numbers in the ones and tens columns of 189. This means you will need to use regrouping to perform subtraction:

	5	2	5
-	1	8	9

To subtract 9 from 5 in the ones column you will need to borrow from the 2 in the tens columns:

	5	1	15
-	1	8	9
			6

Next, to subtract 8 from 1 in the tens column you will need to borrow from the 5 in the hundreds column:

	4	11	15
-	1	8	9
		3	6

Last, subtract the 1 from the 4 in the hundreds column:

	4	11	15
-	1	8	9
	3	3	6

Review Video: Subtracting Large Numbers
Visit mometrix.com/academy and enter code: 603350

Order of Operations

The **order of operations** is a set of rules that dictates the order in which we must perform each operation in an expression so that we will evaluate it accurately. If we have an expression that includes multiple different operations, the order of operations tells us which operations to do first. The most common mnemonic for the order of operations is **PEMDAS**, or "Please Excuse My Dear Aunt Sally." PEMDAS stands for parentheses, exponents, multiplication, division, addition, and subtraction. It is important to understand that multiplication and division have equal precedence, as do addition and subtraction, so those pairs of operations are simply worked from left to right in order.

For example, evaluating the expression $5 + 20 \div 4 \times (2 + 3)^2 - 6$ using the correct order of operations would be done like this:

- **P:** Perform the operations inside the parentheses: $(2 + 3) = 5$
- **E:** Simplify the exponents: $(5)^2 = 5 \times 5 = 25$
    - The expression now looks like this: $5 + 20 \div 4 \times 25 - 6$
- **MD:** Perform multiplication and division from left to right: $20 \div 4 = 5$; then $5 \times 25 = 125$
    - The expression now looks like this: $5 + 125 - 6$
- **AS:** Perform addition and subtraction from left to right: $5 + 125 = 130$; then $130 - 6 = 124$

Review Video: Order of Operations
Visit mometrix.com/academy and enter code: 259675

Decimals, Fractions, and Percentages

Fractions, Decimals, and Percentages

Fractions

A **fraction** is a number that is expressed as one integer written above another integer, with a dividing line between them $\left(\frac{x}{y}\right)$. It represents the **quotient** of the two numbers "x divided by y." It can also be thought of as x out of y equal parts.

The top number of a fraction is called the **numerator**, and it represents the number of parts under consideration. The 1 in $\frac{1}{4}$ means that 1 part out of the whole is being considered in the calculation. The bottom number of a fraction is called the **denominator**, and it represents the total number of equal parts. The 4 in $\frac{1}{4}$ means that the whole consists of 4 equal parts. A fraction cannot have a denominator of zero; this is referred to as "*undefined.*"

Fractions can be manipulated, without changing the value of the fraction, by multiplying or dividing (but not adding or subtracting) both the numerator and denominator by the same number. If you divide both numbers by a common factor, you are **reducing** or simplifying the fraction. Two fractions that have the same value but are expressed differently are known as **equivalent fractions**. For example, $\frac{2}{10}, \frac{3}{15}, \frac{4}{20}$, and $\frac{5}{25}$ are all equivalent fractions. They can also all be reduced or simplified to $\frac{1}{5}$.

When two fractions are manipulated so that they have the same denominator, this is known as finding a **common denominator**. The number chosen to be that common denominator should be the least common multiple of the two original denominators. Example: $\frac{3}{4}$ and $\frac{5}{6}$; the least common multiple of 4 and 6 is 12. Manipulating to achieve the common denominator: $\frac{3}{4} = \frac{9}{12}; \frac{5}{6} = \frac{10}{12}$.

Review Video: Overview of Fractions
Visit mometrix.com/academy and enter code: 262335

Proper Fractions and Mixed Numbers

A fraction whose denominator is greater than its numerator is known as a **proper fraction**, while a fraction whose numerator is greater than its denominator is known as an **improper fraction**. Proper fractions have values *less than one* and improper fractions have values *greater than one.*

A **mixed number** is a number that contains both an integer and a fraction. Any improper fraction can be rewritten as a mixed number. Example: $\frac{8}{3} = \frac{6}{3} + \frac{2}{3} = 2 + \frac{2}{3} = 2\frac{2}{3}$. Similarly, any mixed number can be rewritten as an improper fraction. Example: $1\frac{3}{5} = 1 + \frac{3}{5} = \frac{5}{5} + \frac{3}{5} = \frac{8}{5}$.

Review Video: Proper and Improper Fractions and Mixed Numbers
Visit mometrix.com/academy and enter code: 211077

Adding and Subtracting Fractions

If two fractions have a common denominator, they can be added or subtracted simply by adding or subtracting the two numerators and retaining the same denominator. If the two fractions do not already have the same denominator, one or both of them must be manipulated to achieve a common denominator before they can be added or subtracted. Example: $\frac{1}{2} + \frac{1}{4} = \frac{2}{4} + \frac{1}{4} = \frac{3}{4}$.

Review Video: Adding and Subtracting Fractions
Visit mometrix.com/academy and enter code: 378080

Multiplying Fractions

Two fractions can be multiplied by multiplying the two numerators to find the new numerator and the two denominators to find the new denominator. Example: $\frac{1}{3} \times \frac{2}{3} = \frac{1\times2}{3\times3} = \frac{2}{9}$.

Dividing Fractions

Two fractions can be divided by flipping the numerator and denominator of the second fraction and then proceeding as though it were a multiplication problem. Example: $\frac{2}{3} \div \frac{3}{4} = \frac{2}{3} \times \frac{4}{3} = \frac{8}{9}$.

Review Video: Multiplying and Dividing Fractions
Visit mometrix.com/academy and enter code: 473632

Multiplying a Mixed Number by a Whole Number or a Decimal

When multiplying a mixed number by something, it is usually best to convert it to an improper fraction first. Additionally, if the multiplicand is a decimal, it is most often simplest to convert it to a fraction. For instance, to multiply $4\frac{3}{8}$ by 3.5, begin by rewriting each quantity as a whole number plus a proper fraction. Remember, a mixed number is a fraction added to a whole number and a decimal is a representation of the sum of fractions, specifically tenths, hundredths, thousandths, and so on:

$$4\frac{3}{8} \times 3.5 = \left(4 + \frac{3}{8}\right) \times \left(3 + \frac{1}{2}\right)$$

Next, the quantities being added need to be expressed with the same denominator. This is achieved by multiplying and dividing the whole number by the denominator of the fraction. Recall that a whole number is equivalent to that number divided by 1:

$$= \left(\frac{4}{1} \times \frac{8}{8} + \frac{3}{8}\right) \times \left(\frac{3}{1} \times \frac{2}{2} + \frac{1}{2}\right)$$

When multiplying fractions, remember to multiply the numerators and denominators separately:

$$= \left(\frac{4 \times 8}{1 \times 8} + \frac{3}{8}\right) \times \left(\frac{3 \times 2}{1 \times 2} + \frac{1}{2}\right)$$
$$= \left(\frac{32}{8} + \frac{3}{8}\right) \times \left(\frac{6}{2} + \frac{1}{2}\right)$$

Now that the fractions have the same denominators, they can be added:

$$= \frac{35}{8} \times \frac{7}{2}$$

Finally, perform the last multiplication and then simplify:

$$= \frac{35 \times 7}{8 \times 2} = \frac{245}{16} = \frac{240}{16} + \frac{5}{16} = 15\frac{5}{16}$$

Comparing Fractions

It is important to master the ability to compare and order fractions. This skill is relevant to many real-world scenarios. For example, carpenters often compare fractional construction nail lengths when preparing for a project, and bakers often compare fractional measurements to have the correct ratio of ingredients. There are three commonly used strategies when comparing fractions. These strategies are referred to as the common denominator approach, the decimal approach, and the cross-multiplication approach.

Using a Common Denominator to Compare Fractions

The fractions $\frac{2}{3}$ and $\frac{4}{7}$ have different denominators. $\frac{2}{3}$ has a denominator of 3, and $\frac{4}{7}$ has a denominator of 7. In order to precisely compare these two fractions, it is necessary to use a common denominator. A common denominator is a common multiple that is shared by both denominators. In this case, the denominators 3 and 7 share a multiple of 21. In general, it is most efficient to select the least common multiple for the two denominators.

Rewrite each fraction with the common denominator of 21. Then, calculate the new numerators as illustrated below.

$$\frac{2}{3} \xrightarrow{\times 7} \frac{\mathbf{14}}{21} \qquad \frac{4}{7} \xrightarrow{\times 3} \frac{\mathbf{12}}{21}$$

×7 ×3

$$\frac{2}{3} = \frac{\mathbf{14}}{21} \qquad \frac{4}{7} = \frac{\mathbf{12}}{21}$$

×7 ×3

For $\frac{2}{3}$, multiply the numerator and denominator by 7. The result is $\frac{14}{21}$.

For $\frac{4}{7}$, multiply the numerator and denominator by 3. The result is $\frac{12}{21}$.

Now that both fractions have a denominator of 21, the fractions can accurately be compared by comparing the numerators. Since 14 is greater than 12, the fraction $\frac{14}{21}$ is greater than $\frac{12}{21}$. This means that $\frac{2}{3}$ is greater than $\frac{4}{7}$.

Using Decimals to Compare Fractions

Sometimes decimal values are easier to compare than fraction values. For example, $\frac{5}{8}$ is equivalent to 0.625 and $\frac{3}{5}$ is equivalent to 0.6. This means that the comparison of $\frac{5}{8}$ and $\frac{3}{5}$ can be determined by comparing the decimals 0.625 and 0.6. When both decimal values are extended to the thousandths place, they become 0.625 and 0.600, respectively. It becomes clear that 0.625 is greater than 0.600 because 625 thousandths is greater than 600 thousandths. In other words, $\frac{5}{8}$ is greater than $\frac{3}{5}$ because 0.625 is greater than 0.6.

Using Cross-Multiplication to Compare Fractions

Cross-multiplication is an efficient strategy for comparing fractions. This is a shortcut for the common denominator strategy. Start by writing each fraction next to one another. Multiply the numerator of the fraction on the left by the denominator of the fraction on the right. Write down the result next to the fraction on the left. Now multiply the numerator of the fraction on the right by the denominator of the fraction on the left. Write down the result next to the fraction on the right. Compare both products. The fraction with the larger result is the larger fraction.

Consider the fractions $\frac{4}{7}$ and $\frac{5}{9}$.

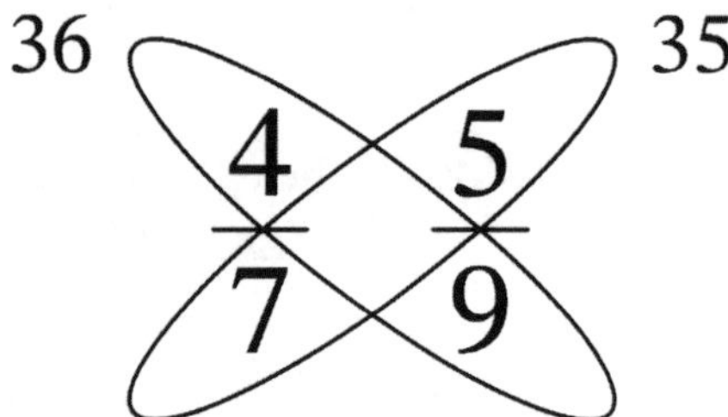

36 is greater than 35. Therefore, $\frac{4}{7}$ is greater than $\frac{5}{9}$.

Decimals

Decimals are one way to represent parts of a whole. Using the place value system, each digit to the right of a decimal point denotes the number of units of a corresponding *negative* power of ten. For example, consider the decimal 0.24. We can use a model to represent the decimal. Since a dime is worth one-tenth of a dollar and a penny is worth one-hundredth of a dollar, one possible model to represent this fraction is to have 2 dimes representing the 2 in the tenths place and 4 pennies representing the 4 in the hundredths place:

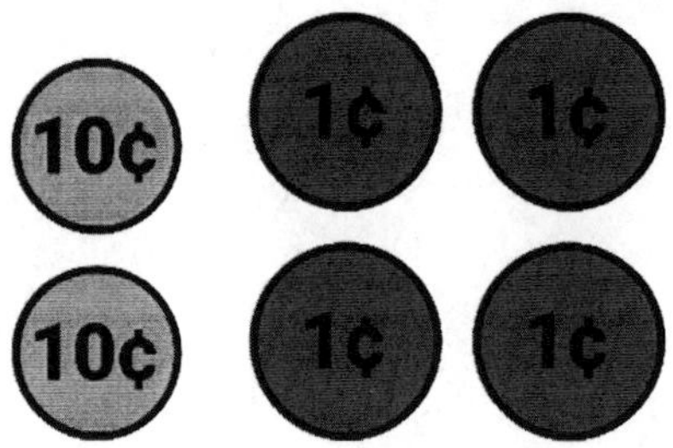

To write the decimal as a fraction, put the decimal in the numerator with 1 in the denominator. Multiply the numerator and denominator by tens until there are no more decimal places. Then simplify the fraction to lowest terms. For example, converting 0.24 to a fraction:

$$0.24 = \frac{0.24}{1} = \frac{0.24 \times 100}{1 \times 100} = \frac{24}{100} = \frac{6}{25}$$

Review Video: Decimals
Visit mometrix.com/academy and enter code: 837268

Operations with Decimals

Adding and Subtracting Decimals

When adding and subtracting decimals, the decimal points must always be aligned. Adding decimals is just like adding regular whole numbers. Example: $4.5 + 2.0 = 6.5$.

If the problem-solver does not properly align the decimal points, an incorrect answer of 4.7 may result. An easy way to add decimals is to align all of the decimal points in a vertical column visually. This will allow you to see exactly where the decimal should be placed in the final answer. Begin adding from right to left. Add each column in turn, making sure to carry the number to the left if a column adds up to more than 9. The same rules apply to the subtraction of decimals.

Review Video: Adding and Subtracting Decimals
Visit mometrix.com/academy and enter code: 381101

Multiplying Decimals

A simple multiplication problem has two components: a **multiplicand** and a **multiplier**. When multiplying decimals, work as though the numbers were whole rather than decimals. Once the final product is calculated, count the number of places to the right of the decimal in both the multiplicand and the multiplier. Then, count that number of places from the right of the product and place the decimal in that position.

For example, 12.3×2.56 has a total of three places to the right of the respective decimals. Multiply 123×256 to get 31,488. Now, beginning on the right, count three places to the left and insert the decimal. The final product will be 31.488.

Review Video: How to Multiply Decimals
Visit mometrix.com/academy and enter code: 731574

Dividing Decimals

Every division problem has a **divisor** and a **dividend**. The dividend is the number that is being divided. In the problem $14 \div 7$, 14 is the dividend and 7 is the divisor. In a division problem with decimals, the divisor must be converted into a whole number. Begin by moving the decimal in the divisor to the right until a whole number is created. Next, move the decimal in the dividend the same number of spaces to the right. For example, 4.9 into 24.5 would become 49 into 245. The decimal was moved one space to the right to create a whole number in the divisor, and then the same was done for the dividend. Once the whole numbers are created, the problem is carried out normally: $245 \div 49 = 5$.

Review Video: Dividing Decimals
Visit mometrix.com/academy and enter code: 560690

Review Video: Dividing Decimals by Whole Numbers
Visit mometrix.com/academy and enter code: 535669

Percentages

Percentages can be thought of as fractions that are based on a whole of 100; that is, one whole is equal to 100%. The word **percent** means "per hundred." Percentage problems are often presented in three main ways:

- Find what percentage of some number another number is.
    - Example: What percentage of 40 is 8?
- Find what number is some percentage of a given number.
    - Example: What number is 20% of 40?
- Find what number another number is a given percentage of.
    - Example: What number is 8 20% of?

There are three components in each of these cases: a **whole** (W), a **part** (P), and a **percentage** (%). These are related by the equation: $P = W \times \%$. This can easily be rearranged into other forms that may suit different questions better: $\% = \frac{P}{W}$ and $W = \frac{P}{\%}$. Percentage problems are often also word problems. As such, a large part of solving them is figuring out which quantities are what. For example, consider the following word problem:

In a school cafeteria, 7 students choose pizza, 9 choose hamburgers, and 4 choose tacos. What percentage of student choose tacos?

To find the whole, you must first add all of the parts: $7 + 9 + 4 = 20$. The percentage can then be found by dividing the part by the whole $\left(\% = \frac{P}{W}\right)$: $\frac{4}{20} = \frac{20}{100} = 20\%$.

Review Video: Computation with Percentages Visit mometrix.com/academy and enter code: 693099

Converting Between Percentages, Fractions, and Decimals

Converting decimals to percentages and percentages to decimals is as simple as moving the decimal point. To *convert from a decimal to a percentage*, move the decimal point **two places to the right**. To *convert from a percentage to a decimal*, move it **two places to the left**. It may be helpful to remember that the percentage number will always be larger than the equivalent decimal number. Example:

$$0.23 = 23\% \qquad 5.34 = 534\% \qquad 0.007 = 0.7\%$$
$$700\% = 7.00 \qquad 86\% = 0.86 \qquad 0.15\% = 0.0015$$

To convert a fraction to a decimal, simply divide the numerator by the denominator in the fraction. To convert a decimal to a fraction, put the decimal in the numerator with 1 in the denominator. Multiply the numerator and denominator by tens until there are no more decimal places. Then simplify the fraction to lowest terms. For example, converting 0.24 to a fraction:

$$0.24 = \frac{0.24}{1} = \frac{0.24 \times 100}{1 \times 100} = \frac{24}{100} = \frac{6}{25}$$

Fractions can be converted to a percentage by finding equivalent fractions with a denominator of 100. Example:

$$\frac{7}{10} = \frac{70}{100} = 70\% \quad \frac{1}{4} = \frac{25}{100} = 25\%$$

To convert a percentage to a fraction, divide the percentage number by 100 and reduce the fraction to its simplest possible terms. Example:

$$60\% = \frac{60}{100} = \frac{3}{5} \quad 96\% = \frac{96}{100} = \frac{24}{25}$$

Review Video: Converting Fractions to Percentages and Decimals
Visit mometrix.com/academy and enter code: 306233

Review Video: Converting Percentages to Decimals and Fractions
Visit mometrix.com/academy and enter code: 287297

Review Video: Converting Decimals to Fractions and Percentages
Visit mometrix.com/academy and enter code: 986765

Review Video: Converting Decimals, Improper Fractions, and Mixed Numbers
Visit mometrix.com/academy and enter code: 696924

Ratio Conversion

Proportions and Ratios

Proportions

A proportion is a relationship between two quantities that dictates how one changes when the other changes. A **direct proportion** describes a relationship in which a quantity increases by a set amount for every increase in the other quantity, or decreases by that same amount for every decrease in the other quantity. Example: Assuming a constant driving speed, the time required for a car trip increases as the distance of the trip increases. The distance to be traveled and the time required to travel are directly proportional.

An **inverse proportion** is a relationship in which an increase in one quantity is accompanied by a decrease in the other, or vice versa. Example: the time required for a car trip decreases as the speed increases and increases as the speed decreases, so the time required is inversely proportional to the speed of the car.

Review Video: Proportions
Visit mometrix.com/academy and enter code: 505355

Ratios

A **ratio** is a comparison of two quantities in a particular order. Example: If there are 14 computers in a lab, and the class has 20 students, there is a student to computer ratio of 20 to 14, commonly written as $20{:}\ 14$. Ratios are normally reduced to their smallest whole number representation, so $20{:}\ 14$ would be reduced to $10{:}\ 7$ by dividing both sides by 2.

Review Video: Ratios
Visit mometrix.com/academy and enter code: 996914

CONSTANT OF PROPORTIONALITY

When two quantities have a proportional relationship, there exists a **constant of proportionality** between the quantities. The product of this constant and one of the quantities is equal to the other quantity. For example, if one lemon costs $0.25, two lemons cost $0.50, and three lemons cost $0.75, there is a proportional relationship between the total cost of lemons and the number of lemons purchased. The constant of proportionality is the **unit price**, namely $0.25/lemon. Notice that the total price of lemons, t, can be found by multiplying the unit price of lemons, p, and the number of lemons, n: $t = pn$.

WORK/UNIT RATE

Unit rate expresses a quantity of one thing in terms of one unit of another. For example, if you travel 30 miles every two hours, a unit rate expresses this comparison in terms of one hour: in one hour you travel 15 miles, so your unit rate is 15 miles per hour. Other examples are how much one ounce of food costs (price per ounce) or figuring out how much one egg costs out of the dozen (price per 1 egg, instead of price per 12 eggs). The denominator of a unit rate is always 1. Unit rates are used to compare different situations to solve problems. For example, to make sure you get the best deal when deciding which kind of soda to buy, you can find the unit rate of each. If soda #1 costs $1.50 for a 1-liter bottle, and soda #2 costs $2.75 for a 2-liter bottle, it would be a better deal to buy soda #2, because its unit rate is only $1.375 per 1-liter, which is cheaper than soda #1. Unit rates can also help determine the length of time a given event will take. For example, if you can paint 2 rooms in 4.5 hours, you can determine how long it will take you to paint 5 rooms by solving for the unit rate per room and then multiplying that by 5.

Review Video: Rates and Unit Rates
Visit mometrix.com/academy and enter code: 185363

Measurement Conversion

METRIC AND CUSTOMARY MEASUREMENTS

METRIC MEASUREMENT PREFIXES

Giga-	One billion	1 *giga*watt is one billion watts
Mega-	One million	1 *mega*hertz is one million hertz
Kilo-	One thousand	1 *kilo*gram is one thousand grams
Deci-	One-tenth	1 *deci*meter is one-tenth of a meter
Centi-	One-hundredth	1 *centi*meter is one-hundredth of a meter
Milli-	One-thousandth	1 *milli*liter is one-thousandth of a liter
Micro-	One-millionth	1 *micro*gram is one-millionth of a gram

Review Video: Metric System Conversion - How the Metric System Works
Visit mometrix.com/academy and enter code: 163709

MEASUREMENT CONVERSION

When converting between units, the goal is to maintain the same meaning but change the way it is displayed. In order to go from a larger unit to a smaller unit, multiply the number of the known amount by the equivalent amount. When going from a smaller unit to a larger unit, divide the number of the known amount by the equivalent amount.

For complicated conversions, it may be helpful to set up conversion fractions. In these fractions, one fraction is the **conversion factor**. The other fraction has the unknown amount in the numerator. So, the known value is placed in the denominator. Sometimes, the second fraction has the known value from the problem in the numerator and the unknown in the denominator. Multiply the two fractions to get the converted measurement. Note that since the numerator and the denominator of the factor are equivalent, the value of the fraction is 1. That is why we can say that the result in the new units is equal to the result in the old units even though they have different numbers.

It can often be necessary to chain known conversion factors together. As an example, consider converting 512 square inches to square meters. We know that there are 2.54 centimeters in an inch and 100 centimeters in a meter, and we know we will need to square each of these factors to achieve the conversion we are looking for.

$$\frac{512\text{ in}^2}{1} \times \left(\frac{2.54\text{ cm}}{1\text{ in}}\right)^2 \times \left(\frac{1\text{ m}}{100\text{ cm}}\right)^2 = \frac{512\,\cancel{\text{in}^2}}{1} \times \left(\frac{6.4516\,\cancel{\text{cm}^2}}{1\,\cancel{\text{in}^2}}\right) \times \left(\frac{1\text{ m}^2}{10{,}000\,\cancel{\text{cm}^2}}\right) = 0.330\text{ m}^2$$

Review Video: Measurement Conversions
Visit mometrix.com/academy and enter code: 316703

Common Units and Equivalents

Metric Equivalents

1000 μg (microgram)	1 mg
1000 mg (milligram)	1 g
1000 g (gram)	1 kg
1000 kg (kilogram)	1 metric ton
1000 mL (milliliter)	1 L
1000 μm (micrometer)	1 mm
1000 mm (millimeter)	1 m
100 cm (centimeter)	1 m
1000 m (meter)	1 km

Distance and Area Measurement

Unit	Abbreviation	US equivalent	Metric equivalent
Inch	in	1 inch	2.54 centimeters
Foot	ft	12 inches	0.305 meters
Yard	yd	3 feet	0.914 meters
Mile	mi	5280 feet	1.609 kilometers
Acre	ac	4840 square yards	0.405 hectares
Square Mile	sq. mi. or mi.^{2}	640 acres	2.590 square kilometers

Capacity Measurements

Unit	Abbreviation	US equivalent	Metric equivalent
Fluid Ounce	fl oz	8 fluid drams	29.573 milliliters
Cup	c	8 fluid ounces	0.237 liter
Pint	pt.	16 fluid ounces	0.473 liter
Quart	qt.	2 pints	0.946 liter
Gallon	gal.	4 quarts	3.785 liters
Teaspoon	t or tsp.	1 fluid dram	5 milliliters
Tablespoon	T or tbsp.	4 fluid drams	15 or 16 milliliters
Cubic Centimeter	cc or cm^3	0.271 drams	1 milliliter

Weight Measurements

Unit	Abbreviation	US equivalent	Metric equivalent
Ounce	oz	16 drams	28.35 grams
Pound	lb	16 ounces	453.6 grams
Ton	tn.	2,000 pounds	907.2 kilograms

Volume and Weight Measurement Clarifications

Always be careful when using ounces and fluid ounces. They are not equivalent.

1 pint = 16 fluid ounces	1 fluid ounce ≠ 1 ounce
1 pound = 16 ounces	1 pint ≠ 1 pound

Having one pint of something does not mean you have one pound of it. In the same way, just because something weighs one pound does not mean that its volume is one pint.

In the United States, the word "ton" by itself refers to a short ton or a net ton. Do not confuse this with a long ton (also called a gross ton) or a metric ton (also spelled *tonne*), which have different measurement equivalents.

$$1 \text{ US ton} = 2000 \text{ pounds} \quad \neq \quad 1 \text{ metric ton} = 1000 \text{ kilograms}$$

Algebra

Linear Expressions

Terms and Coefficients

Mathematical expressions consist of a combination of one or more values arranged in terms that are added together. As such, an expression could be just a single number, including zero. A **variable term** is the product of a real number, also called a **coefficient**, and one or more variables, each of which may be raised to an exponent. Expressions may also include numbers without a variable, called **constants** or **constant terms**. The expression $6s^2$, for example, is a single term where the coefficient is the real number 6 and the variable term is s^2. Note that if a term is written as simply a variable to some exponent, like t^2, then the coefficient is 1, because $t^2 = 1t^2$.

Linear Expressions

A **single variable linear expression** is the sum of a single variable term, where the variable has no exponent, and a constant, which may be zero. For instance, the expression $2w + 7$ has $2w$ as the variable term and 7 as the constant term. It is important to realize that terms are separated by addition or subtraction. Since an expression is a sum of terms, expressions such as $5x - 3$ can be written as $5x + (-3)$ to emphasize that the constant term is negative. A real-world example of a single variable linear expression is the perimeter of a square, four times the side length, often expressed: $4s$.

In general, a **linear expression** is the sum of any number of variable terms so long as none of the variables have an exponent. For example, $3m + 8n - \frac{1}{4}p + 5.5q - 1$ is a linear expression, but $3y^3$ is not. In the same way, the expression for the perimeter of a general triangle, the sum of the side lengths $(a + b + c)$ is considered to be linear, but the expression for the area of a square, the side length squared $(s^2)$is not.

Slope

On a graph with two points, (x_1, y_1) and (x_2, y_2), the **slope** is found with the formula $m = \frac{y_2 - y_1}{x_2 - x_1}$; where $x_1 \neq x_2$ and m stands for slope. If the value of the slope is **positive**, the line has an *upward direction* from left to right. If the value of the slope is **negative**, the line has a *downward direction* from left to right. Consider the following example:

A new book goes on sale in bookstores and online stores. In the first month, 5,000 copies of the book are sold. Over time, the book continues to grow in popularity. The data for the number of copies sold is in the table below.

# of Months on Sale	1	2	3	4	5
# of Copies Sold (In Thousands)	5	10	15	20	25

So, the number of copies that are sold and the time that the book is on sale is a proportional relationship. In this example, an equation can be used to show the data: $y = 5x$, where x is the number of months that the book is on sale. Also, y is the number of copies sold. So, the slope of the corresponding line is $\frac{\text{rise}}{\text{run}} = \frac{5}{1} = 5$.

Review Video: Finding the Slope of a Line
Visit mometrix.com/academy and enter code: 766664

Linear Equations

Equations that can be written as $ax + b = 0$, where $a \neq 0$, are referred to as **one variable linear equations**. A solution to such an equation is called a **root**. In the case where we have the equation $5x + 10 = 0$, if we solve for x we get a solution of $x = -2$. In other words, the root of the equation is -2. This is found by first subtracting 10 from both sides, which gives $5x = -10$. Next, simply divide both sides by the coefficient of the variable, in this case 5, to get $x = -2$. This can be checked by plugging -2 back into the original equation $(5)(-2) + 10 = -10 + 10 = 0$.

The **solution set** is the set of all solutions of an equation. In our example, the solution set would simply be -2. If there were more solutions (there usually are in multivariable equations) then they would also be included in the solution set. When an equation has no true solutions, it is referred to as an **empty set**. Equations with identical solution sets are **equivalent equations**. An **identity** is a term whose value or determinant is equal to 1.

Linear equations can be written many ways. Below is a list of some forms linear equations can take:

- **Standard Form**: $Ax + By = C$; the slope is $\frac{-A}{B}$ and the y-intercept is $\frac{C}{B}$
- **Slope Intercept Form**: $y = mx + b$, where m is the slope and b is the y-intercept
- **Point-Slope Form**: $y - y_1 = m(x - x_1)$, where m is the slope and (x_1, y_1) is a point on the line
- **Two-Point Form**: $\frac{y-y_1}{x-x_1} = \frac{y_2-y_1}{x_2-x_1}$, where (x_1, y_1) and (x_2, y_2) are two points on the given line
- **Intercept Form**: $\frac{x}{x_1} + \frac{y}{y_1} = 1$, where $(x_1, 0)$ is the point at which a line intersects the x-axis, and $(0, y_1)$ is the point at which the same line intersects the y-axis

Review Video: Slope-Intercept and Point-Slope Forms
Visit mometrix.com/academy and enter code: 113216

Review Video: Linear Equations Basics
Visit mometrix.com/academy and enter code: 793005

Solving Equations

Solving One-Variable Linear Equations

Multiply all terms by the lowest common denominator to eliminate any fractions. Look for addition or subtraction to undo so you can isolate the variable on one side of the equal sign. Divide both sides by the coefficient of the variable. When you have a value for the variable, substitute this value into the original equation to make sure you have a true equation. Consider the following example:

Kim's savings are represented by the table below. Represent her savings, using an equation.

X (Months)	Y (Total Savings)
2	$1,300
5	$2,050
9	$3,050
11	$3,550
16	$4,800

The table shows a function with a constant rate of change, or slope, of 250. Given the points on the table, the slopes can be calculated as $\frac{(2{,}050-1300)}{(5-2)}$, $\frac{(3{,}050-2{,}050)}{(9-5)}$, $\frac{(3{,}550-3{,}050)}{(11-9)}$, and $\frac{(4{,}800-3{,}550)}{(16-11)}$, each of which equals 250. Thus, the table shows a constant rate of change, indicating a linear function. The slope-intercept form of a linear equation is written as $y = mx + b$, where m represents the slope and b represents the y-intercept. Substituting the slope into this form gives $y = 250x + b$. Substituting corresponding x- and y-values from any point into this equation will give the y-intercept, or b. Using the point, (2, 1,300), gives $1{,}300 = 250(2) + b$, which simplifies as $b = 800$. Thus, her savings may be represented by the equation, $y = 250x + 800$.

Rules for Manipulating Equations

Like Terms

Like terms are terms in an equation that have the same variable, regardless of whether or not they also have the same coefficient. This includes terms that *lack* a variable; all constants (i.e., numbers without variables) are considered like terms. If the equation involves terms with a variable raised to different powers, the like terms are those that have the variable raised to the same power.

For example, consider the equation $x^2 + 3x + 2 = 2x^2 + x - 7 + 2x$. In this equation, 2 and -7 are like terms; they are both constants. $3x$, x, and $2x$ are like terms, they all include the variable x raised to the first power. x^2 and $2x^2$ are like terms, they both include the variable x, raised to the second power. $2x$ and $2x^2$ are not like terms; although they both involve the variable x, the variable is not raised to the same power in both terms. The fact that they have the same coefficient, 2, is not relevant.

Review Video: Rules for Manipulating Equations
Visit mometrix.com/academy and enter code: 838871

Carrying Out the Same Operation on Both Sides of an Equation

When solving an equation, the general procedure is to carry out a series of operations on both sides of an equation, choosing operations that will tend to simplify the equation when doing so. The reason why the same operation must be carried out on both sides of the equation is because that leaves the meaning of the equation unchanged, and yields a result that is equivalent to the original equation. This would not be the case if we carried out an operation on one side of an equation and not the other. Consider what an equation means: it is a statement that two values or expressions are equal. If we carry out the same operation on both sides of the equation—add 3 to both sides, for example—then the two sides of the equation are changed in the same way, and so remain equal. If we do that to only one side of the equation—add 3 to one side but not the other—then that wouldn't be true; if we change one side of the equation but not the other then the two sides are no longer equal.

Advantage of Combining Like Terms

Combining like terms refers to adding or subtracting like terms—terms with the same variable—and therefore reducing sets of like terms to a single term. The main advantage of doing this is that it simplifies the equation. Often, combining like terms can be done as the first step in solving an equation, though it can also be done later, such as after distributing terms in a product.

For example, consider the equation $2(x+3)+3(2+x+3)=-4$. The 2 and the 3 in the second set of parentheses are like terms, and we can combine them, yielding $2(x+3)+3(x+5)=-4$. Now we can carry out the multiplications implied by the parentheses, distributing the outer 2 and 3 accordingly: $2x+6+3x+15=-4$. The $2x$ and the $3x$ are like terms, and we can add them together: $5x+6+15=-4$. Now, the constants 6, 15, and -4 are also like terms, and we can combine them as well: subtracting 6 and 15 from both sides of the equation, we get $5x=-4-6-15$, or $5x=-25$, which simplifies further to $x=-5$.

Review Video: Solving Equations by Combining Like Terms
Visit mometrix.com/academy and enter code: 668506

Canceling Terms on Opposite Sides of an Equation

Two terms on opposite sides of an equation can be canceled if and only if they *exactly* match each other. They must have the same variable raised to the same power and the same coefficient. For example, in the equation $3x+2x^2+6=2x^2-6$, $2x^2$ appears on both sides of the equation and can be canceled, leaving $3x+6=-6$. The 6 on each side of the equation *cannot* be canceled, because it is added on one side of the equation and subtracted on the other. While they cannot be canceled, however, the 6 and -6 are like terms and can be combined, yielding $3x=-12$, which simplifies further to $x=-4$.

It's also important to note that the terms to be canceled must be independent terms and cannot be part of a larger term. For example, consider the equation $2(x+6)=3(x+4)+1$. We cannot cancel the x's, because even though they match each other they are part of the larger terms $2(x+6)$ and $3(x+4)$. We must first distribute the 2 and 3, yielding $2x+12=3x+12+1$. Now we see that the terms with the x's do not match, but the 12s do, and can be canceled, leaving $2x=3x+1$, which simplifies to $x=-1$.

Process for Manipulating Equations

Isolating Variables

To **isolate a variable** means to manipulate the equation so that the variable appears by itself on one side of the equation, and does not appear at all on the other side. Generally, an equation or inequality is considered to be solved once the variable is isolated and the other side of the equation or inequality is simplified as much as possible. In the case of a two-variable equation or inequality, only one variable needs to be isolated; it will not usually be possible to simultaneously isolate both variables.

For a linear equation—an equation in which the variable only appears raised to the first power—isolating a variable can be done by first moving all the terms with the variable to one side of the equation and all other terms to the other side. (*Moving* a term really means adding the inverse of the term to both sides; when a term is *moved* to the other side of the equation its sign is flipped.) Then combine like terms on each side. Finally, divide both sides by the coefficient of the variable, if applicable. The steps need not necessarily be done in this order, but this order will always work.

Review Video: Solving One-Step Equations
Visit mometrix.com/academy and enter code: 777004

Equations with More Than One Solution

Some types of non-linear equations, such as equations involving squares of variables, may have more than one solution. For example, the equation $x^2=4$ has two solutions: 2 and -2. Equations with absolute values can also have multiple solutions: $|x|=1$ has the solutions $x=1$ and $x=-1$.

It is also possible for a linear equation to have more than one solution, but only if the equation is true regardless of the value of the variable. In this case, the equation is considered to have infinitely many solutions, because any possible value of the variable is a solution. We know a linear equation has infinitely many solutions if when we combine like terms the variables cancel, leaving a true statement. For example, consider the equation $2(3x + 5) = x + 5(x + 2)$. Distributing, we get $6x + 10 = x + 5x + 10$; combining like terms gives $6x + 10 = 6x + 10$, and the $6x$-terms cancel to leave $10 = 10$. This is clearly true, so the original equation is true for any value of x. We could also have canceled the 10s leaving $0 = 0$, but again this is clearly true—in general if both sides of the equation match exactly, it has infinitely many solutions.

Equations with No Solution

Some types of non-linear equations, such as equations involving squares of variables, may have no solution. For example, the equation $x^2 = -2$ has no solutions in the real numbers, because the square of any real number must be positive. Similarly, $|x| = -1$ has no solution, because the absolute value of a number is always positive.

It is also possible for an equation to have no solution even if does not involve any powers greater than one, absolute values, or other special functions. For example, the equation $2(x + 3) + x = 3x$ has no solution. We can see that if we try to solve it: first we distribute, leaving $2x + 6 + x = 3x$. But now if we try to combine all the terms with the variable, we find that they cancel: we have $3x$ on the left and $3x$ on the right, canceling to leave us with $6 = 0$. This is clearly false. In general, whenever the variable terms in an equation cancel leaving different constants on both sides, it means that the equation has no solution. (If we are left with the *same* constant on both sides, the equation has infinitely many solutions instead.)

Features of Equations That Require Special Treatment

Linear Equations

A linear equation is an equation in which variables only appear by themselves: not multiplied together, not with exponents other than one, and not inside absolute value signs or any other functions. For example, the equation $x + 1 - 3x = 5 - x$ is a linear equation; while x appears multiple times, it never appears with an exponent other than one, or inside any function. The two-variable equation $2x - 3y = 5 + 2x$ is also a linear equation. In contrast, the equation $x^2 - 5 = 3x$ is *not* a linear equation, because it involves the term x^2. $\sqrt{x} = 5$ is not a linear equation, because it involves a square root. $(x - 1)^2 = 4$ is not a linear equation because even though there's no exponent on the x directly, it appears as part of an expression that is squared. The two-variable equation $x + xy - y = 5$ is not a linear equation because it includes the term xy, where two variables are multiplied together.

Linear equations can always be solved (or shown to have no solution) by combining like terms and performing simple operations on both sides of the equation. Some non-linear equations can be solved by similar methods, but others may require more advanced methods of solution, if they can be solved analytically at all.

Solving Equations Involving Roots

In an equation involving roots, the first step is to isolate the term with the root, if possible, and then raise both sides of the equation to the appropriate power to eliminate it. Consider an example equation, $2\sqrt{x + 1} - 1 = 3$. In this case, begin by adding 1 to both sides, yielding $2\sqrt{x + 1} = 4$, and then dividing both sides by 2, yielding $\sqrt{x + 1} = 2$. Now square both sides, yielding $x + 1 = 4$. Finally, subtracting 1 from both sides yields $x = 3$.

Squaring both sides of an equation may, however, yield a spurious solution—a solution to the squared equation that is *not* a solution of the original equation. It's therefore necessary to plug the solution back into the original equation to make sure it works. In this case, it does: $2\sqrt{3 + 1} - 1 = 2\sqrt{4} - 1 = 2(2) - 1 = 4 - 1 = 3$.

The same procedure applies for other roots as well. For example, given the equation $3 + \sqrt[3]{2x} = 5$, we can first subtract 3 from both sides, yielding $\sqrt[3]{2x} = 2$ and isolating the root. Raising both sides to the third power yields $2x = 2^3$; i.e., $2x = 8$. We can now divide both sides by 2 to get $x = 4$.

> **Review Video: Solving Equations Involving Roots**
> Visit mometrix.com/academy and enter code: 297670

Solving Equations with Exponents

To solve an equation involving an exponent, the first step is to isolate the variable with the exponent. We can then take the appropriate root of both sides to eliminate the exponent. For instance, for the equation $2x^3 + 17 = 5x^3 - 7$, we can subtract $5x^3$ from both sides to get $-3x^3 + 17 = -7$, and then subtract 17 from both sides to get $-3x^3 = -24$. Finally, we can divide both sides by -3 to get $x^3 = 8$. Finally, we can take the cube root of both sides to get $x = \sqrt[3]{8} = 2$.

One important but often overlooked point is that equations with an exponent greater than 1 may have more than one answer. The solution to $x^2 = 9$ isn't simply $x = 3$; it's $x = \pm 3$ (that is, $x = 3$ or $x = -3$). For a slightly more complicated example, consider the equation $(x - 1)^2 - 1 = 3$. Adding 1 to both sides yields $(x - 1)^2 = 4$; taking the square root of both sides yields $x - 1 = 2$. We can then add 1 to both sides to get $x = 3$. However, there's a second solution. We also have the possibility that $x - 1 = -2$, in which case $x = -1$. Both $x = 3$ and $x = -1$ are valid solutions, as can be verified by substituting them both into the original equation.

> **Review Video: Solving Equations with Exponents**
> Visit mometrix.com/academy and enter code: 514557

Solving Equations with Absolute Values

When solving an equation with an absolute value, the first step is to isolate the absolute value term. We then consider two possibilities: when the expression inside the absolute value is positive or when it is negative. In the former case, the expression in the absolute value equals the expression on the other side of the equation; in the latter, it equals the additive inverse of that expression—the expression times negative one. We consider each case separately and finally check for spurious solutions.

For instance, consider solving $|2x - 1| + x = 5$ for x. We can first isolate the absolute value by moving the x to the other side: $|2x - 1| = -x + 5$. Now, we have two possibilities. First, that $2x - 1$ is positive, and hence $2x - 1 = -x + 5$. Rearranging and combining like terms yields $3x = 6$, and hence $x = 2$. The other possibility is that $2x - 1$ is negative, and hence $2x - 1 = -(-x + 5) = x - 5$. In this case, rearranging and combining like terms yields $x = -4$. Substituting $x = 2$ and $x = -4$ back into the original equation, we see that they are both valid solutions.

Note that the absolute value of a sum or difference applies to the sum or difference as a whole, not to the individual terms; in general, $|2x - 1|$ is not equal to $|2x + 1|$ or to $|2x| - 1$.

Spurious Solutions

A **spurious solution** may arise when we square both sides of an equation as a step in solving it or under certain other operations on the equation. It is a solution to the squared or otherwise modified equation that is *not* a solution of the original equation. To identify a spurious solution, it's useful when you solve an equation involving roots or absolute values to plug the solution back into the original equation to make sure it's valid.

Choosing Which Variable to Isolate in Two-Variable Equations

Similar to methods for a one-variable equation, solving a two-variable equation involves isolating a variable: manipulating the equation so that a variable appears by itself on one side of the equation, and not at all on the other side. However, in a two-variable equation, you will usually only be able to isolate one of the variables; the other variable may appear on the other side along with constant terms, or with exponents or other functions.

Often one variable will be much more easily isolated than the other, and therefore that's the variable you should choose. If one variable appears with various exponents, and the other is only raised to the first power, the latter variable is the one to isolate: given the equation $a^2 + 2b = a^3 + b + 3$, the b only appears to the first power, whereas a appears squared and cubed, so b is the variable that can be solved for: combining like terms and isolating the b on the left side of the equation, we get $b = a^3 - a^2 + 3$. If both variables are equally easy to isolate, then it's best to isolate the dependent variable, if one is defined; if the two variables are x and y, the convention is that y is the dependent variable.

> **Review Video: Solving Equations with Variables on Both Sides**
> Visit mometrix.com/academy and enter code: 402497

Cross Multiplication

Finding an Unknown in Equivalent Expressions

It is often necessary to apply information given about a rate or proportion to a new scenario. For example, if you know that Jedha can run a marathon (26.2 miles) in 3 hours, how long would it take her to run 10 miles at the same pace? Start by setting up equivalent expressions:

$$\frac{26.2 \text{ mi}}{3 \text{ hr}} = \frac{10 \text{ mi}}{x \text{ hr}}$$

Now, cross multiply and solve for x:

$$\begin{aligned} 26.2x &= 30 \\ x &= \frac{30}{26.2} = \frac{15}{13.1} \\ x &\approx 1.15 \text{ hrs } or \text{ 1 hr 9 min} \end{aligned}$$

So, at this pace, Jedha could run 10 miles in about 1.15 hours or about 1 hour and 9 minutes.

> **Review Video: Cross Multiplying Fractions**
> Visit mometrix.com/academy and enter code: 893904

Graphing Equations

Graphical Solutions to Equations

When equations are shown graphically, they are usually shown on a **Cartesian coordinate plane**. The Cartesian coordinate plane consists of two number lines placed perpendicular to each other and intersecting at the zero point, also known as the origin. The horizontal number line is known as the x-axis, with positive values to the right of the origin, and negative values to the left of the origin. The vertical number line is known as the y-axis, with positive values above the origin, and negative values below the origin. Any point on the plane can be identified by an ordered pair in the form (x, y), called coordinates. The x-value of the coordinate is called the abscissa, and the y-value of the coordinate is called the ordinate. The two number lines divide the plane into **four quadrants**: I, II, III, and IV.

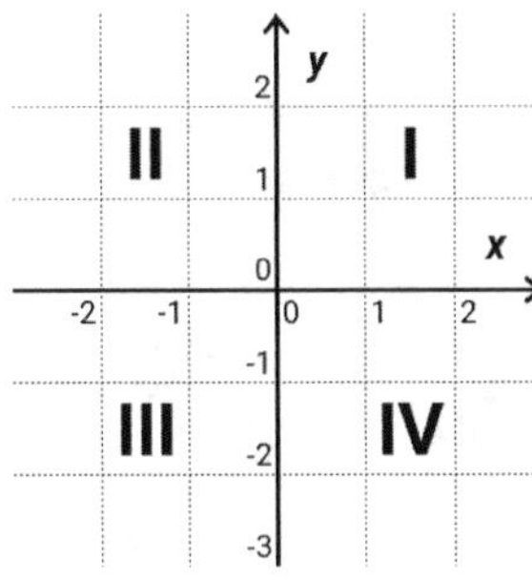

Note that in quadrant I $x > 0$ and $y > 0$, in quadrant II $x < 0$ and $y > 0$, in quadrant III $x < 0$ and $y < 0$, and in quadrant IV $x > 0$ and $y < 0$.

Recall that if the value of the slope of a line is positive, the line slopes upward from left to right. If the value of the slope is negative, the line slopes downward from left to right. If the y-coordinates are the same for two points on a line, the slope is 0 and the line is a **horizontal line**. If the x-coordinates are the same for two points on a line, there is no slope and the line is a **vertical line**. Two or more lines that have equivalent slopes are **parallel lines**. **Perpendicular lines** have slopes that are negative reciprocals of each other, such as $\frac{a}{b}$ and $\frac{-b}{a}$.

Review Video: Cartesian Coordinate Plane and Graphing
Visit mometrix.com/academy and enter code: 115173

Graphing Equations in Two Variables

One way of graphing an equation in two variables is to plot enough points to get an idea for its shape and then draw the appropriate curve through those points. A point can be plotted by substituting in a value for one variable and solving for the other. If the equation is linear, we only need two points and can then draw a straight line between them.

For example, consider the equation $y = 2x - 1$. This is a linear equation—both variables only appear raised to the first power—so we only need two points. When $x = 0$, $y = 2(0) - 1 = -1$. When $x = 2$, $y = 2(2) - 1 = 3$. We can therefore choose the points $(0, -1)$ and $(2, 3)$, and draw a line between them:

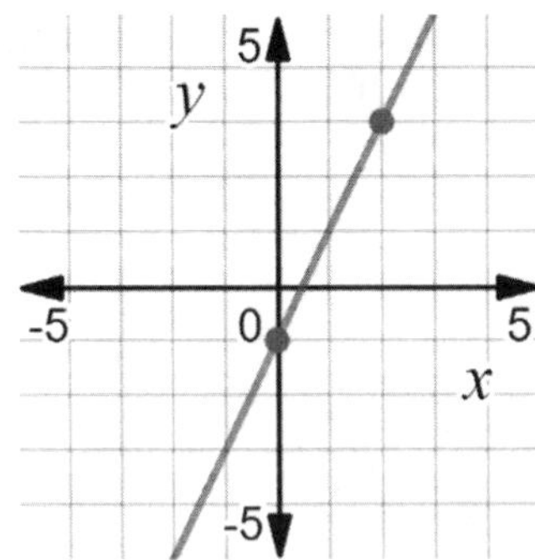

Inequalities

Working with Inequalities

Commonly in algebra and other upper-level fields of math you find yourself working with mathematical expressions that do not equal each other. The statement comparing such expressions with symbols such as $<$ (less than) or $>$ (greater than) is called an *inequality*. An example of an inequality is $7x > 5$. To solve for x, simply divide both sides by 7 and the solution is shown to be $x > \frac{5}{7}$. Graphs of the solution set of inequalities are represented on a number line. Open circles are used to show that an expression approaches a number but is never quite equal to that number.

Review Video: Solving Multi-Step Inequalities
Visit mometrix.com/academy and enter code: 347842

Review Video: Solving Inequalities Using All 4 Basic Operations
Visit mometrix.com/academy and enter code: 401111

Conditional inequalities are those with certain values for the variable that will make the condition true and other values for the variable where the condition will be false. **Absolute inequalities** can have any real number as the value for the variable to make the condition true, while there is no real number value for the variable that will make the condition false. Solving inequalities is done by following the same rules for solving equations with the exception that when multiplying or dividing by a negative number the direction of the inequality sign must be flipped or reversed. **Double inequalities** are situations where two inequality statements apply to the same variable expression. Example: $-c < ax + b < c$.

Review Video: Conditional and Absolute Inequalities
Visit mometrix.com/academy and enter code: 980164

Determining Solutions to Inequalities

To determine whether a coordinate is a solution of an inequality, you can substitute the values of the coordinate into the inequality, simplify, and check whether the resulting statement holds true. For instance, to determine whether $(-2,4)$ is a solution of the inequality $y \geq -2x + 3$, substitute the values into the inequality, $4 \geq -2(-2) + 3$. Simplify the right side of the inequality and the result is $4 \geq 7$, which is a false statement. Therefore, the coordinate is not a solution of the inequality. You can also use this method to determine which part of the graph of an inequality is shaded. The graph of $y \geq -2x + 3$ includes the solid line $y = -2x + 3$ and, since it excludes the point $(-2,4)$ to the left of the line, it is shaded to the right of the line.

Review Video: Graphing Linear Inequalities
Visit mometrix.com/academy and enter code: 439421

Flipping Inequality Signs

When given an inequality, we can always turn the entire inequality around, swapping the two sides of the inequality and changing the inequality sign. For instance, $x + 2 > 2x - 3$ is equivalent to $2x - 3 < x + 2$. Aside from that, normally the inequality does not change if we carry out the same operation on both sides of the inequality. There is, however, one principal exception: if we *multiply* or *divide* both sides of the inequality by a *negative number*, the inequality is flipped. For example, if we take the inequality $-2x < 6$ and divide both sides by -2, the inequality flips and we are left with $x > -3$. This *only* applies to multiplication and division, and only with negative numbers. Multiplying or dividing both sides by a positive number, or adding or subtracting any number regardless of sign, does not flip the inequality. Another special case that flips the inequality sign is when reciprocals are used. For instance, $3 > 2$ but the relation of the reciprocals is $\frac{1}{2} < \frac{1}{3}$.

Compound Inequalities

A **compound inequality** is an equality that consists of two inequalities combined with *and* or *or*. The two components of a proper compound inequality must be of opposite type: that is, one must be greater than (or greater than or equal to), the other less than (or less than or equal to). For instance, "$x + 1 < 2$ or $x + 1 > 3$" is a compound inequality, as is "$2x \geq 4$ and $2x \leq 6$." An *and* inequality can be written more compactly by having one inequality on each side of the common part: "$2x \geq 1$ and $2x \leq 6$," can also be written as $1 \leq 2x \leq 6$.

In order for the compound inequality to be meaningful, the two parts of an *and* inequality must overlap; otherwise, no numbers satisfy the inequality. On the other hand, if the two parts of an *or* inequality overlap, then *all* numbers satisfy the inequality and as such the inequality is usually not meaningful.

Solving a compound inequality requires solving each part separately. For example, given the compound inequality "$x + 1 < 2$ or $x + 1 > 3$," the first inequality, $x + 1 < 2$, reduces to $x < 1$, and the second part, $x + 1 > 3$, reduces to $x > 2$, so the whole compound inequality can be written as "$x < 1$ or $x > 2$." Similarly, $1 \leq 2x \leq 6$ can be solved by dividing each term by 2, yielding $\frac{1}{2} \leq x \leq 3$.

Review Video: Compound Inequalities
Visit mometrix.com/academy and enter code: 786318

Solving Inequalities Involving Absolute Values

To solve an inequality involving an absolute value, first isolate the term with the absolute value. Then proceed to treat the two cases separately as with an absolute value equation, but flipping the inequality in the case where the expression in the absolute value is negative (since that essentially involves multiplying both sides by −1.) The two cases are then combined into a compound inequality; if the absolute value is on the greater side of the inequality, then it is an *or* compound inequality, if on the lesser side, then it's an *and*.

Consider the inequality $2 + |x - 1| \geq 3$. We can isolate the absolute value term by subtracting 2 from both sides: $|x - 1| \geq 1$. Now, we're left with the two cases $x - 1 \geq 1$ or $x - 1 \leq -1$: note that in the latter, negative case, the inequality is flipped. $x - 1 \geq 1$ reduces to $x \geq 2$, and $x - 1 \leq -1$ reduces to $x \leq 0$. Since in the inequality $|x - 1| \geq 1$ the absolute value is on the greater side, the two cases combine into an *or* compound inequality, so the final, solved inequality is "$x \leq 0$ or $x \geq 2$."

Review Video: Solving Absolute Value Inequalities
Visit mometrix.com/academy and enter code: 997008

Solving Inequalities Involving Square Roots

Solving an inequality with a square root involves two parts. First, we solve the inequality as if it were an equation, isolating the square root and then squaring both sides of the equation. Second, we restrict the solution to the set of values of x for which the value inside the square root sign is non-negative.

For example, in the inequality, $\sqrt{x - 2} + 1 < 5$, we can isolate the square root by subtracting 1 from both sides, yielding $\sqrt{x - 2} < 4$. Squaring both sides of the inequality yields $x - 2 < 16$, so $x < 18$. Since we can't take the square root of a negative number, we also require the part inside the square root to be non-negative. In this case, that means $x - 2 \geq 0$. Adding 2 to both sides of the inequality yields $x \geq 2$. Our final answer is a compound inequality combining the two simple inequalities: $x \geq 2$ and $x < 18$, or $2 \leq x < 18$.

Note that we only get a compound inequality if the two simple inequalities are in opposite directions; otherwise, we take the one that is more restrictive.

The same technique can be used for other even roots, such as fourth roots. It is *not*, however, used for cube roots or other odd roots—negative numbers *do* have cube roots, so the condition that the quantity inside the root sign cannot be negative does not apply.

Review Video: Solving Inequalities Involving Square Roots
Visit mometrix.com/academy and enter code: 800288

Special Circumstances

Sometimes an inequality involving an absolute value or an even exponent is true for all values of x, and we don't need to do any further work to solve it. This is true if the inequality, once the absolute value or exponent term is isolated, says that term is greater than a negative number (or greater than or equal to zero). Since an absolute value or a number raised to an even exponent is *always* non-negative, this inequality is always true.

GRAPHICAL SOLUTIONS TO INEQUALITIES

GRAPHING SIMPLE INEQUALITIES

To graph a simple inequality, we first mark on the number line the value that signifies the end point of the inequality. If the inequality is strict (involves a less than or greater than), we use a hollow circle; if it is not strict (less than or equal to or greater than or equal to), we use a solid circle. We then fill in the part of the number line that satisfies the inequality: to the left of the marked point for less than (or less than or equal to), to the right for greater than (or greater than or equal to).

For example, we would graph the inequality $x < 5$ by putting a hollow circle at 5 and filling in the part of the line to the left:

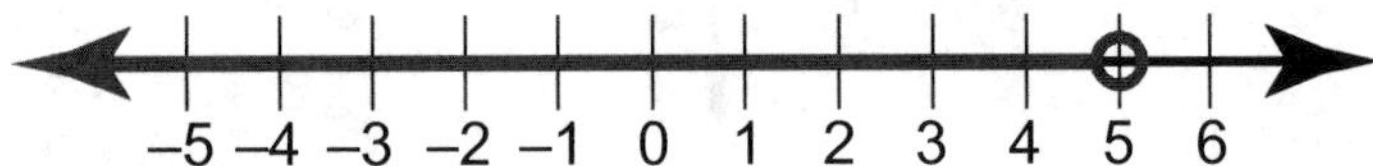

GRAPHING COMPOUND INEQUALITIES

To graph a compound inequality, we fill in both parts of the inequality for an *or* inequality, or the overlap between them for an *and* inequality. More specifically, we start by plotting the endpoints of each inequality on the number line. For an *or* inequality, we then fill in the appropriate side of the line for each inequality. Typically, the two component inequalities do not overlap, which means the shaded part is *outside* the two points. For an *and* inequality, we instead fill in the part of the line that meets both inequalities.

For the inequality "$x \leq -3$ or $x > 4$," we first put a solid circle at –3 and a hollow circle at 4. We then fill the parts of the line *outside* these circles:

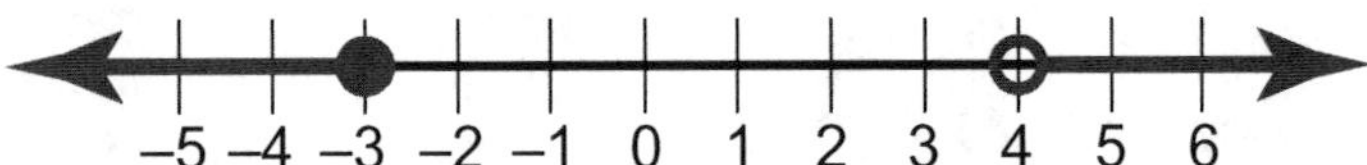

GRAPHING INEQUALITIES INCLUDING ABSOLUTE VALUES

An inequality with an absolute value can be converted to a compound inequality. To graph the inequality, first convert it to a compound inequality, and then graph that normally. If the absolute value is on the greater side of the inequality, we end up with an *or* inequality; we plot the endpoints of the inequality on the number line and fill in the part of the line *outside* those points. If the absolute value is on the smaller side of the inequality, we end up with an *and* inequality; we plot the endpoints of the inequality on the number line and fill in the part of the line *between* those points.

For example, the inequality $|x + 1| \geq 4$ can be rewritten as $x \geq 3$ or $x \leq -5$. We place solid circles at the points 3 and –5 and fill in the part of the line *outside* them:

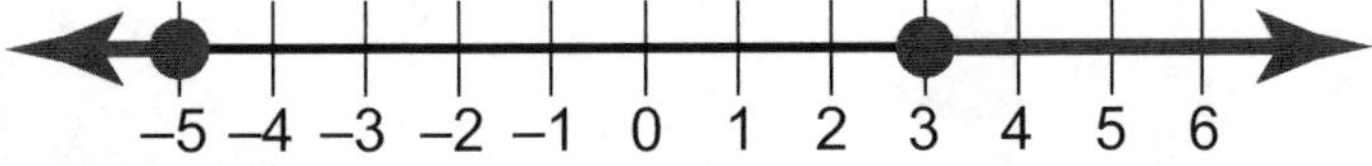

GRAPHING INEQUALITIES IN TWO VARIABLES

To graph an inequality in two variables, we first graph the border of the inequality. This means graphing the equation that we get if we replace the inequality sign with an equals sign. If the inequality is strict ($>$ or $<$), we graph the border with a dashed or dotted line; if it is not strict ($\geq$ or $\leq$), we use a solid line. We can then test any point not on the border to see if it satisfies the inequality. If it does, we shade in that side of the border; if not, we shade in the other side. As an example, consider $y > 2x + 2$. To graph this inequality, we first graph the border, $y = 2x + 2$. Since it is a strict inequality, we use a dashed line. Then, we choose a test point. This can be any point not on the border; in this case, we will choose the origin, (0,0). (This makes the calculation easy and is generally a good choice unless the border passes through the origin.) Putting this into the original inequality, we get $0 > 2(0) + 2$, i.e., $0 > 2$. This is *not* true, so we shade in the side of the border that does *not* include the point (0,0):

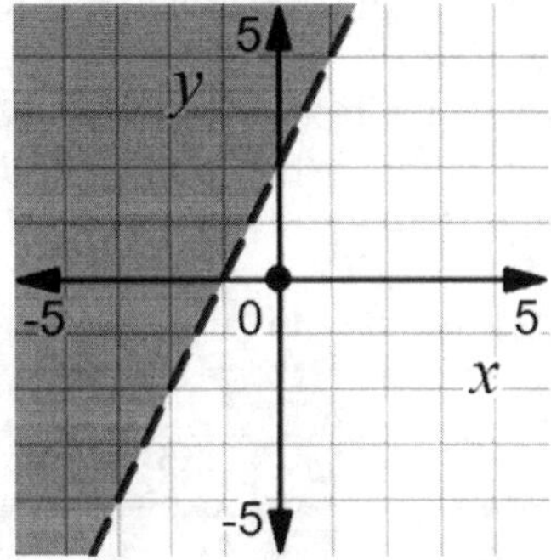

Graphing Compound Inequalities in Two Variables

One way to graph a compound inequality in two variables is to first graph each of the component inequalities. For an *and* inequality, we then shade in only the parts where the two graphs overlap; for an *or* inequality, we shade in any region that pertains to either of the individual inequalities.

Consider the graph of "$y \geq x - 1$ and $y \leq -x$":

We first shade in the individual inequalities:

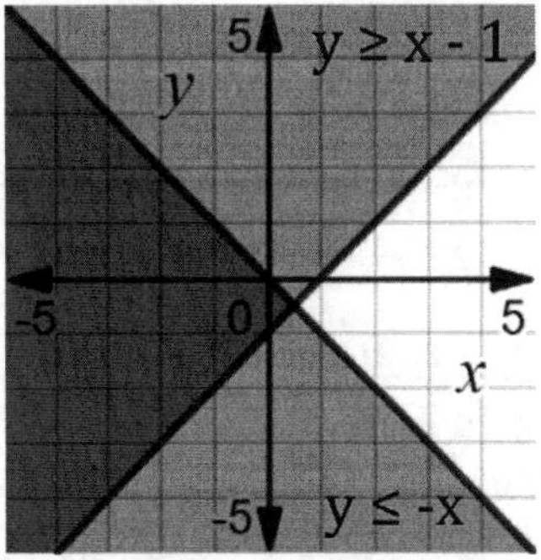

Now, since the compound inequality has an *and*, we only leave shaded the overlap—the part that pertains to *both* inequalities:

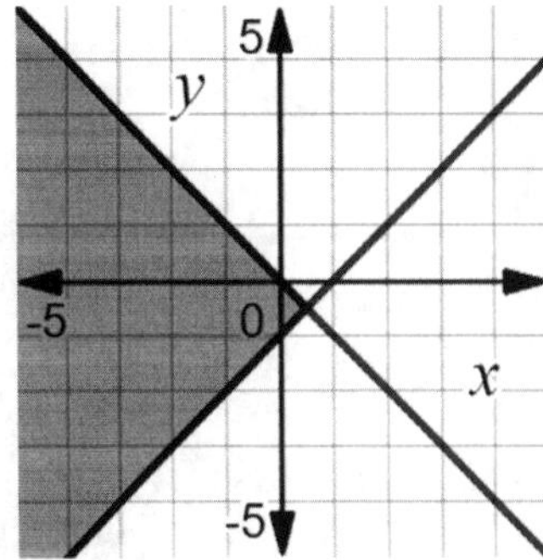

If instead the inequality had been "$y \geq x - 1$ or $y \leq -x$," our final graph would involve the *total* shaded area:

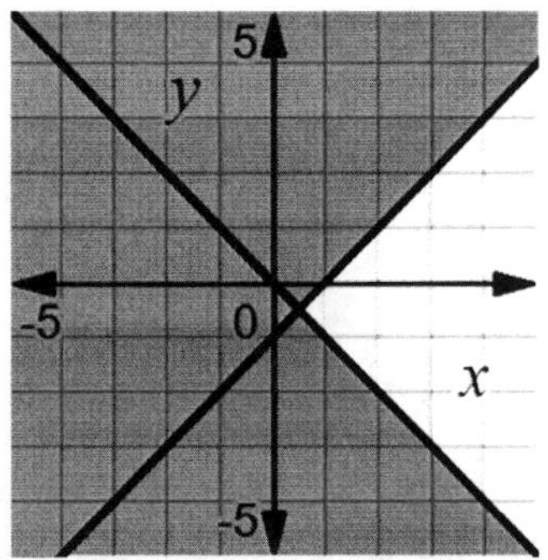

Review Video: Graphing Solutions to Inequalities
Visit mometrix.com/academy and enter code: 391281

SYSTEMS OF EQUATIONS

SOLVING SYSTEMS OF EQUATIONS

A **system of equations** is a set of simultaneous equations that all use the same variables. A solution to a system of equations must be true for each equation in the system. **Consistent systems** are those with at least one solution. **Inconsistent systems** are systems of equations that have no solution.

Review Video: Solving Systems of Linear Equations
Visit mometrix.com/academy and enter code: 746745

SUBSTITUTION

To solve a system of linear equations by **substitution**, start with the easier equation and solve for one of the variables. Express this variable in terms of the other variable. Substitute this expression in the other equation and solve for the other variable. The solution should be expressed in the form (x, y). Substitute the values into both of the original equations to check your answer. Consider the following system of equations:

$$x + 6y = 15$$
$$3x - 12y = 18$$

Solving the first equation for x: $x = 15 - 6y$

Substitute this value in place of x in the second equation, and solve for y:

$$3(15 - 6y) - 12y = 18$$
$$45 - 18y - 12y = 18$$
$$30y = 27$$
$$y = \frac{27}{30} = \frac{9}{10} = 0.9$$

Plug this value for y back into the first equation to solve for x:

$$x = 15 - 6(0.9) = 15 - 5.4 = 9.6$$

Check both equations if you have time:

$$\begin{aligned} 9.6 + 6(0.9) &= 15 \\ 9.6 + 5.4 &= 15 \\ 15 &= 15 \end{aligned} \qquad \begin{aligned} 3(9.6) - 12(0.9) &= 18 \\ 28.8 - 10.8 &= 18 \\ 18 &= 18 \end{aligned}$$

Therefore, the solution is (9.6,0.9).

Review Video: The Substitution Method
Visit mometrix.com/academy and enter code: 565151

Review Video: Substitution and Elimination
Visit mometrix.com/academy and enter code: 958611

Elimination

To solve a system of equations using **elimination**, begin by rewriting both equations in standard form $Ax + By = C$. Check to see if the coefficients of one pair of like variables add to zero. If not, multiply one or both of the equations by a non-zero number to make one set of like variables add to zero. Add the two equations to solve for one of the variables. Substitute this value into one of the original equations to solve for the other variable. Check your work by substituting into the other equation. Now, let's look at solving the following system using the elimination method:

$$\begin{aligned} 5x + 6y &= 4 \\ x + 2y &= 4 \end{aligned}$$

If we multiply the second equation by -3, we can eliminate the y-terms:

$$\begin{aligned} 5x + 6y &= 4 \\ -3x - 6y &= -12 \end{aligned}$$

Add the equations together and solve for x:

$$\begin{aligned} 2x &= -8 \\ x &= \frac{-8}{2} = -4 \end{aligned}$$

Plug the value for x back in to either of the original equations and solve for y:

$$\begin{aligned} -4 + 2y &= 4 \\ y &= \frac{4 + 4}{2} = 4 \end{aligned}$$

Check both equations if you have time:

$$\begin{aligned} 5(-4) + 6(4) &= 4 \\ -20 + 24 &= 4 \\ 4 &= 4 \end{aligned} \qquad \begin{aligned} -4 + 2(4) &= 4 \\ -4 + 8 &= 4 \\ 4 &= 4 \end{aligned}$$

Therefore, the solution is $(-4,4)$.

Review Video: The Elimination Method
Visit mometrix.com/academy and enter code: 449121

Graphically

To solve a system of linear equations **graphically**, plot both equations on the same graph. The solution of the equations is the point where both lines cross. If the lines do not cross (are parallel), then there is **no solution**.

For example, consider the following system of equations:

$$y = 2x + 7$$
$$y = -x + 1$$

Since these equations are given in slope-intercept form, they are easy to graph; the y-intercepts of the lines are $(0,7)$ and $(0,1)$. The respective slopes are 2 and –1, thus the graphs look like this:

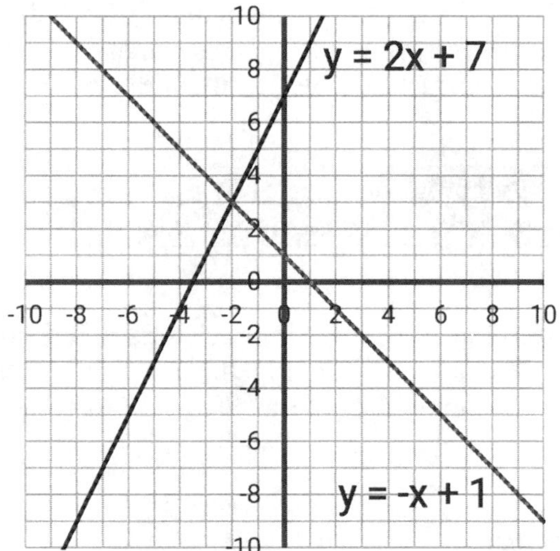

The two lines intersect at the point $(-2,3)$, thus this is the solution to the system of equations.

Solving a system graphically is generally only practical if both coordinates of the solution are integers; otherwise the intersection will lie between gridlines on the graph and the coordinates will be difficult or impossible to determine exactly. It also helps if, as in this example, the equations are in slope-intercept form or some other form that makes them easy to graph. Otherwise, another method of solution (by substitution or elimination) is likely to be more useful.

Review Video: Solving Systems by Graphing
Visit mometrix.com/academy and enter code: 634812

Solving Systems of Equations Using the Trace Feature

Using the trace feature on a calculator requires that you rewrite each equation, isolating the y-variable on one side of the equal sign. Enter both equations in the graphing calculator and plot the graphs simultaneously. Use the trace cursor to find where the two lines cross. Use the zoom feature if necessary to obtain more accurate results. Always check your answer by substituting into the original equations. The trace method is likely to be less accurate than other methods due to the resolution of graphing calculators but is a useful tool to provide an approximate answer.

Polynomials

Monomials and Polynomials

A **monomial** is a single constant, variable, or product of constants and variables, such as 7, x, $2x$, or x^3y. There will never be addition or subtraction symbols in a monomial. Like monomials have like variables, but they may have different coefficients. **Polynomials** are algebraic expressions that use addition and subtraction to combine two or more monomials. Two terms make a **binomial**, three terms make a **trinomial**, etc. The **degree of a monomial** is the sum of the exponents of the variables. The **degree of a polynomial** is the highest degree of any individual term.

Review Video: Polynomials
Visit mometrix.com/academy and enter code: 305005

Simplifying Polynomials

Simplifying polynomials requires combining like terms. The like terms in a polynomial expression are those that have the same variable raised to the same power. It is often helpful to connect the like terms with arrows or lines in order to separate them from the other monomials. Once you have determined the like terms, you can rearrange the polynomial by placing them together. Remember to include the sign that is in front of each term. Once the like terms are placed together, you can apply each operation and simplify. When adding and subtracting polynomials, only add and subtract the **coefficient**, or the number part; the variable and exponent stay the same.

Review Video: Adding and Subtracting Polynomials
Visit mometrix.com/academy and enter code: 124088

The FOIL Method

In general, multiplying polynomials is done by multiplying each term in one polynomial by each term in the other and adding the results. In the specific case for multiplying binomials, there is a useful acronym, FOIL, that can help you make sure to cover each combination of terms. The **FOIL method** for $(Ax + By)(Cx + Dy)$ would be:

F	Multiply the *first* terms of each binomial	$(\overset{first}{\widehat{Ax}} + By)(\overset{first}{\widehat{Cx}} + Dy)$	ACx^2
O	Multiply the *outer* terms	$(\overset{outer}{\widehat{Ax}} + By)(Cx + \overset{outer}{\widehat{Dy}})$	$ADxy$
I	Multiply the *inner* terms	$(Ax + \overset{inner}{\widehat{By}})(\overset{inner}{\widehat{Cx}} + Dy)$	$BCxy$
L	Multiply the *last* terms of each binomial	$(Ax + \overset{last}{\widehat{By}})(Cx + \overset{last}{\widehat{Dy}})$	BDy^2

Then, add up the result of each and combine like terms: $ACx^2 + (AD + BC)xy + BDy^2$.

For example, using the FOIL method on binomials $(x + 2)$ and $(x - 3)$:

$$\begin{aligned}
\text{First:}\quad & (\boxed{x} + 2)(\boxed{x} + (-3)) \rightarrow (x)(x) = x^2 \\
\text{Outer:}\quad & (\boxed{x} + 2)(x + \boxed{(-3)}) \rightarrow (x)(-3) = -3x \\
\text{Inner:}\quad & (x + \boxed{2})(\boxed{x} + (-3)) \rightarrow (2)(x) = 2x \\
\text{Last:}\quad & (x + \boxed{2})(x + \boxed{(-3)}) \rightarrow (2)(-3) = -6
\end{aligned}$$

This results in: $(x^2) + (-3x) + (2x) + (-6)$

Combine like terms: $x^2 + (-3 + 2)x + (-6) = x^2 - x - 6$

Review Video: Multiplying Terms Using the FOIL Method
Visit mometrix.com/academy and enter code: 854792

DIVIDING POLYNOMIALS

Use long division to divide a polynomial by either a monomial or another polynomial of equal or lesser degree.

When **dividing by a monomial**, divide each term of the polynomial by the monomial.

When **dividing by a polynomial**, begin by arranging the terms of each polynomial in order of one variable. You may arrange in ascending or descending order, but be consistent with both polynomials. To get the first term of the quotient, divide the first term of the dividend by the first term of the divisor. Multiply the first term of the quotient by the entire divisor and subtract that product from the dividend. Repeat for the second and successive terms until you either get a remainder of zero or a remainder whose degree is less than the degree of the divisor. If the quotient has a remainder, write the answer as a mixed expression in the form:

$$\text{quotient} + \frac{\text{remainder}}{\text{divisor}}$$

For example, we can evaluate the following expression in the same way as long division:

$$\frac{x^3 - 3x^2 - 2x + 5}{x - 5}$$

$$\begin{array}{r l}
 & x^2 \quad +2x \quad +8 \\
x - 5 \,\big) & x^3 - 3x^2 - 2x + 5 \\
 & -(x^3 - 5x^2) \\
 & 2x^2 - 2x \\
 & -(2x^2 - 10x) \\
 & 8x + 5 \\
 & -(8x - 40) \\
 & 45
\end{array}$$

$$\frac{x^3 - 3x^2 - 2x + 5}{x - 5} = x^2 + 2x + 8 + \frac{45}{x - 5}$$

When **factoring** a polynomial, first check for a common monomial factor, that is, look to see if each coefficient has a common factor or if each term has an x in it. If the factor is a trinomial but not a perfect trinomial square, look for a factorable form, such as one of these:

$$x^2 + (a + b)x + ab = (x + a)(x + b)$$
$$(ac)x^2 + (ad + bc)x + bd = (ax + b)(cx + d)$$

For factors with four terms, look for groups to factor. Once you have found the factors, write the original polynomial as the product of all the factors. Make sure all of the polynomial factors are prime. Monomial factors may be *prime* or *composite*. Check your work by multiplying the factors to make sure you get the original polynomial.

Below are patterns of some special products to remember to help make factoring easier:

- Perfect trinomial squares: $x^2 + 2xy + y^2 = (x + y)^2$ or $x^2 - 2xy + y^2 = (x - y)^2$
- Difference between two squares: $x^2 - y^2 = (x + y)(x - y)$
- Sum of two cubes: $x^3 + y^3 = (x + y)(x^2 - xy + y^2)$
    - Note: the second factor is *not* the same as a perfect trinomial square, so do not try to factor it further.
- Difference between two cubes: $x^3 - y^3 = (x - y)(x^2 + xy + y^2)$
    - Again, the second factor is *not* the same as a perfect trinomial square.
- Perfect cubes: $x^3 + 3x^2y + 3xy^2 + y^3 = (x + y)^3$ and $x^3 - 3x^2y + 3xy^2 - y^3 = (x - y)^3$

Rational Expressions

Rational expressions are fractions with polynomials in both the numerator and the denominator; the value of the polynomial in the denominator cannot be equal to zero. Be sure to keep track of values that make the denominator of the original expression zero as the final result inherits the same restrictions. For example, a denominator of $x - 3$ indicates that the expression is not defined when $x = 3$ and, as such, regardless of any operations done to the expression, it remains undefined there.

To **add or subtract** rational expressions, first find the common denominator, then rewrite each fraction as an equivalent fraction with the common denominator. Finally, add or subtract the numerators to get the numerator of the answer, and keep the common denominator as the denominator of the answer.

When **multiplying** rational expressions, factor each polynomial and cancel like factors (a factor which appears in both the numerator and the denominator). Then, multiply all remaining factors in the numerator to get the numerator of the product, and multiply the remaining factors in the denominator to get the denominator of the product. Remember: cancel entire factors, not individual terms.

To **divide** rational expressions, take the reciprocal of the divisor (the rational expression you are dividing by) and multiply by the dividend.

Review Video: Rational Expressions
Visit mometrix.com/academy and enter code: 415183

Simplifying Rational Expressions

To simplify a rational expression, factor the numerator and denominator completely. Factors that are the same and appear in the numerator and denominator have a ratio of 1. For example, look at the following expression:

$$\frac{x - 1}{1 - x^2}$$

The denominator, $(1 - x^2)$, is a difference of squares. It can be factored as $(1 - x)(1 + x)$. The factor $1 - x$ and the numerator $x - 1$ are opposites and have a ratio of -1. Rewrite the numerator as $-1(1 - x)$. So, the rational expression can be simplified as follows:

$$\frac{x - 1}{1 - x^2} = \frac{-1(1 - x)}{(1 - x)(1 + x)} = \frac{-1}{1 + x}$$

Note that since the original expression is only defined for $x \neq \{-1, 1\}$, the simplified expression has the same restrictions.

Review Video: Reducing Rational Expressions
Visit mometrix.com/academy and enter code: 788868

QUADRATICS

SOLVING QUADRATIC EQUATIONS

Quadratic equations are a special set of trinomials of the form $y = ax^2 + bx + c$ that occur commonly in math and real-world applications. The **roots** of a quadratic equation are the solutions that satisfy the equation when $y = 0$; in other words, where the graph touches the x-axis. There are several ways to determine these solutions including using the quadratic formula, factoring, completing the square, and graphing the function.

Review Video: Quadratic Equations Overview
Visit mometrix.com/academy and enter code: 476276

Review Video: Solutions of a Quadratic Equation on a Graph
Visit mometrix.com/academy and enter code: 328231

QUADRATIC FORMULA

The **quadratic formula** is used to solve quadratic equations when other methods are more difficult. To use the quadratic formula to solve a quadratic equation, begin by rewriting the equation in standard form $ax^2 + bx + c = 0$, where a, b, and c are coefficients. Once you have identified the values of the coefficients, substitute those values into the quadratic formula

$$x = \frac{-b \pm \sqrt{b^2 - 4ac}}{2a}$$

Evaluate the equation and simplify the expression. Again, check each root by substituting into the original equation. In the quadratic formula, the portion of the formula under the radical $(b^2 - 4ac)$ is called the **discriminant**. If the discriminant is zero, there is only one root: $-\frac{b}{2a}$. If the discriminant is positive, there are two different real roots. If the discriminant is negative, there are no real roots; you will instead find complex roots. Often these solutions don't make sense in context and are ignored.

Review Video: Using the Quadratic Formula
Visit mometrix.com/academy and enter code: 163102

FACTORING

To solve a quadratic equation by factoring, begin by rewriting the equation in standard form, $x^2 + bx + c = 0$. Remember that the goal of factoring is to find numbers f and g such that $(x + f)(x + g) = x^2 + (f + g)x + fg$, in other words $(f + g) = b$ and $fg = c$. This can be a really useful method when b and c are integers. Determine the factors of c and look for pairs that could sum to b.

For example, consider finding the roots of $x^2 + 6x - 16 = 0$. The factors of -16 include, -4 and 4, -8 and 2, -2 and 8, -1 and 16, and 1 and -16. The factors that sum to 6 are -2 and 8. Write these factors as the product of two binomials, $0 = (x - 2)(x + 8)$. Finally, since these binomials multiply together to equal zero, set them each equal to zero and solve each for x. This results in $x - 2 = 0$, which simplifies to $x = 2$ and $x + 8 = 0$, which simplifies to $x = -8$. Therefore, the roots of the equation are 2 and -8.

Review Video: Factoring Quadratic Equations
Visit mometrix.com/academy and enter code: 336566

Completing the Square

One way to find the roots of a quadratic equation is to find a way to manipulate it such that it follows the form of a perfect square $(x^2 + 2px + p^2)$ by adding and subtracting a constant. This process is called **completing the square**. In other words, if you are given a quadratic that is not a perfect square, $x^2 + bx + c = 0$, you can find a constant d that could be added in to make it a perfect square:

$$x^2 + bx + c + (d - d) = 0; \ \{\text{Let } b = 2p \text{ and } c + d = p^2\}$$

then:

$$x^2 + 2px + p^2 - d = 0 \text{ and } d = \frac{b^2}{4} - c$$

Once you have completed the square you can find the roots of the resulting equation:

$$\begin{aligned} x^2 + 2px + p^2 - d &= 0 \\ (x + p)^2 &= d \\ x + p &= \pm\sqrt{d} \\ x &= -p \pm \sqrt{d} \end{aligned}$$

It is worth noting that substituting the original expressions into this solution gives the same result as the quadratic formula where $a = 1$:

$$x = -p \pm \sqrt{d} = -\frac{b}{2} \pm \sqrt{\frac{b^2}{4} - c} = -\frac{b}{2} \pm \frac{\sqrt{b^2 - 4c}}{2} = \frac{-b \pm \sqrt{b^2 - 4c}}{2}$$

Completing the square can be seen as arranging block representations of each of the terms to be as close to a square as possible and then filling in the gaps. For example, consider the quadratic expression $x^2 + 6x + 2$:

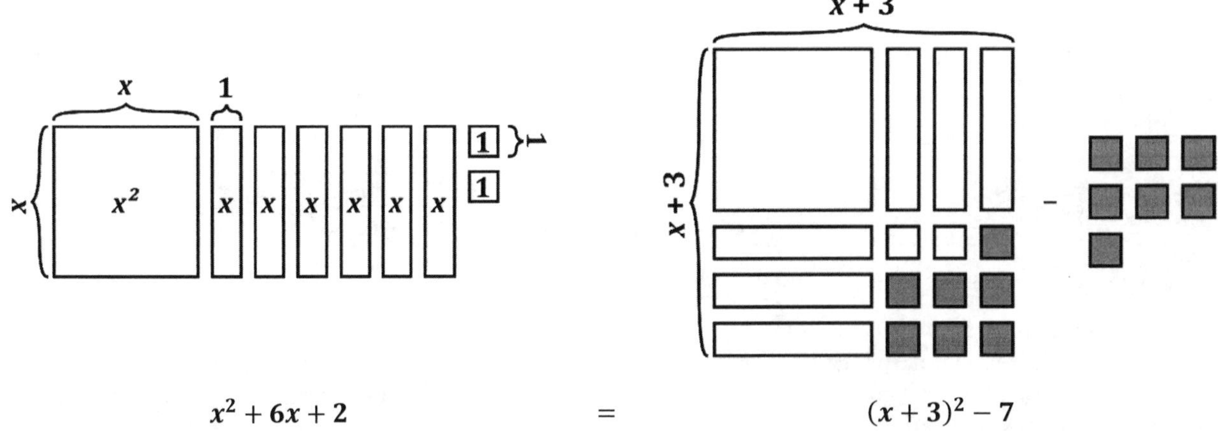

Review Video: Completing the Square
Visit mometrix.com/academy and enter code: 982479

Using Given Roots to Find Quadratic Equation

One way to find the roots of a quadratic equation is to factor the equation and use the **zero product property**, setting each factor of the equation equal to zero to find the corresponding root. We can use this technique in reverse to find an equation given its roots. Each root corresponds to a linear equation which in turn corresponds to a factor of the quadratic equation.

For example, we can find a quadratic equation whose roots are $x = 2$ and $x = -1$. The root $x = 2$ corresponds to the equation $x - 2 = 0$, and the root $x = -1$ corresponds to the equation $x + 1 = 0$.

These two equations correspond to the factors $(x - 2)$ and $(x + 1)$, from which we can derive the equation $(x - 2)(x + 1) = 0$, or $x^2 - x - 2 = 0$.

Any integer multiple of this entire equation will also yield the same roots, as the integer will simply cancel out when the equation is factored. For example, $2x^2 - 2x - 4 = 0$ factors as $2(x - 2)(x + 1) = 0$.

PARABOLAS

A **parabola** is the set of all points in a plane that are equidistant from a fixed line, called the **directrix**, and a fixed point not on the line, called the **focus**. The **axis** is the line perpendicular to the directrix that passes through the focus.

For parabolas that open up or down, the standard equation is $(x - h)^2 = 4c(y - k)$, where h, c, and k are coefficients. If c is positive, the parabola opens up. If c is negative, the parabola opens down. The vertex is the point (h, k). The directrix is the line having the equation $y = -c + k$, and the focus is the point $(h, c + k)$.

For parabolas that open left or right, the standard equation is $(y - k)^2 = 4c(x - h)$, where k, c, and h are coefficients. If c is positive, the parabola opens to the right. If c is negative, the parabola opens to the left. The vertex is the point (h, k). The directrix is the line having the equation $x = -c + h$, and the focus is the point $(c + h, k)$.

Review Video: Parabolas
Visit mometrix.com/academy and enter code: 129187

Review Video: Vertex of a Parabola
Visit mometrix.com/academy and enter code: 272300

Geometry

POINTS, LINES, AND PLANES

POINTS AND LINES

A **point** is a fixed location in space, has no size or dimensions, and is commonly represented by a dot. A **line** is a set of points that extends infinitely in two opposite directions. It has length, but no width or depth. A line can be defined by any two distinct points that it contains. A **line segment** is a portion of a line that has definite endpoints. A **ray** is a portion of a line that extends from a single point on that line in one direction along the line. It has a definite beginning, but no ending.

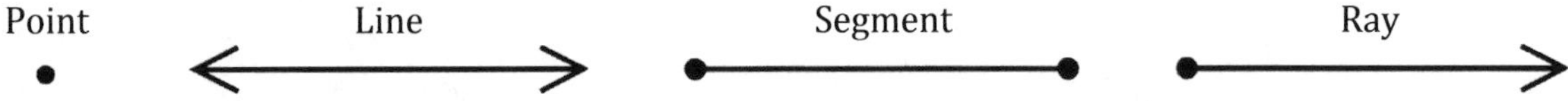

INTERACTIONS BETWEEN LINES

Intersecting lines are lines that have exactly one point in common. **Concurrent lines** are multiple lines that intersect at a single point. **Perpendicular lines** are lines that intersect at right angles. They are represented by the symbol $\perp$. The shortest distance from a line to a point not on the line is a perpendicular segment from the point to the line. **Parallel lines** are lines in the same plane that have no points in common and never meet. It is possible for lines to be in different planes, have no points in common, and never meet, but they are not parallel because they are in different planes.

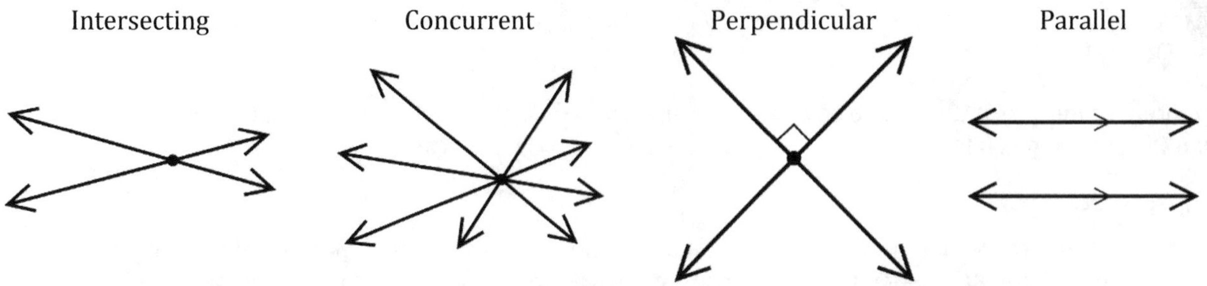

Review Video: Parallel and Perpendicular Lines
Visit mometrix.com/academy and enter code: 815923

A **transversal** is a line that intersects at least two other lines, which may or may not be parallel to one another. A transversal that intersects parallel lines is a common occurrence in geometry. A **bisector** is a line or line segment that divides another line segment into two equal lengths. A **perpendicular bisector** of a line segment is composed of points that are equidistant from the endpoints of the segment it is dividing.

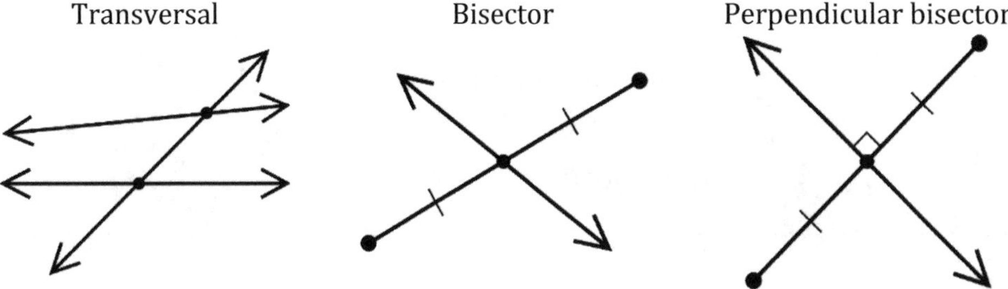

The **projection of a point on a line** is the point at which a perpendicular line drawn from the given point to the given line intersects the line. This is also the shortest distance from the given point to the line. The **projection of a segment on a line** is a segment whose endpoints are the points formed when perpendicular lines are drawn from the endpoints of the given segment to the given line. This is similar to the length a diagonal line appears to be when viewed from above.

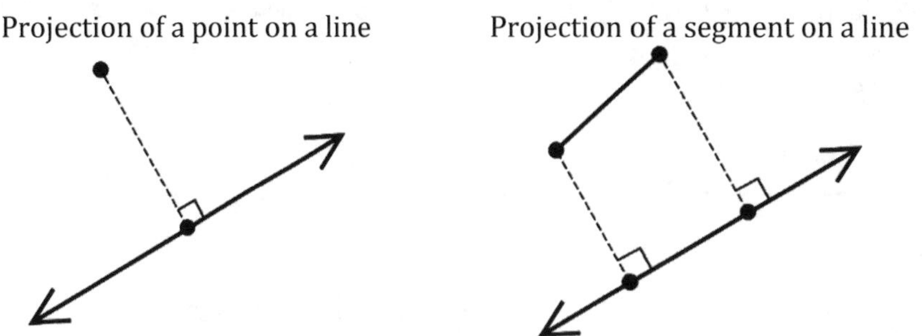

PLANES

A **plane** is a two-dimensional flat surface defined by three non-collinear points. A plane extends an infinite distance in all directions in those two dimensions. It contains an infinite number of points, parallel lines and segments, intersecting lines and segments, as well as parallel or intersecting rays. A plane will never contain a three-dimensional figure or skew lines, which are lines that don't intersect and are not parallel. Two given planes are either parallel or they intersect at a line. A plane may intersect a circular conic surface to form **conic sections**, such as a parabola, hyperbola, circle or ellipse.

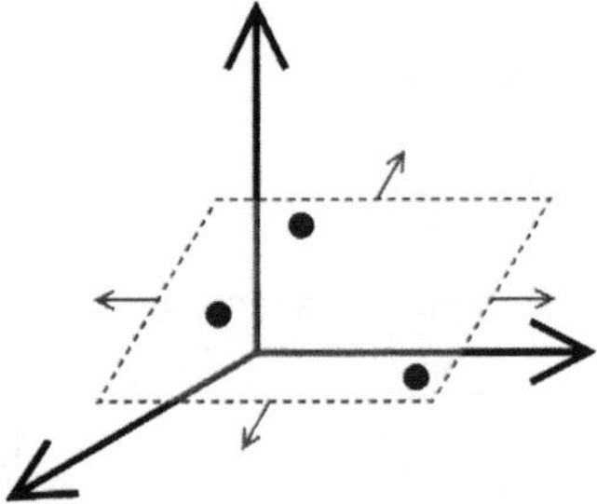

Review Video: Lines and Planes
Visit mometrix.com/academy and enter code: 554267

ANGLES

ANGLES AND VERTICES

An **angle** is formed when two lines or line segments meet at a common point. It may be a common starting point for a pair of segments or rays, or it may be the intersection of lines. Angles are represented by the symbol ∠.

The **vertex** is the point at which two segments or rays meet to form an angle. If the angle is formed by intersecting rays, lines, and/or line segments, the vertex is the point at which four angles are formed. The pairs of angles opposite one another are called vertical angles, and their measures are equal.

- An **acute** angle is an angle with a degree measure less than 90°.
- A **right** angle is an angle with a degree measure of exactly 90°.
- An **obtuse** angle is an angle with a degree measure greater than 90° but less than 180°.
- A **straight angle** is an angle with a degree measure of exactly 180°. This is also a semicircle.
- A **reflex angle** is an angle with a degree measure greater than 180° but less than 360°.
- A **full angle** is an angle with a degree measure of exactly 360°. This is also a circle.

Review Video: Angles
Visit mometrix.com/academy and enter code: 264624

RELATIONSHIPS BETWEEN ANGLES

Two angles whose sum is exactly 90° are said to be **complementary**. The two angles may or may not be adjacent. In a right triangle, the two acute angles are complementary.

Two angles whose sum is exactly 180° are said to be **supplementary**. The two angles may or may not be adjacent. Two intersecting lines always form two pairs of supplementary angles. Adjacent supplementary angles will always form a straight line.

Two angles that have the same vertex and share a side are said to be **adjacent**. Vertical angles are not adjacent because they share a vertex but no common side.

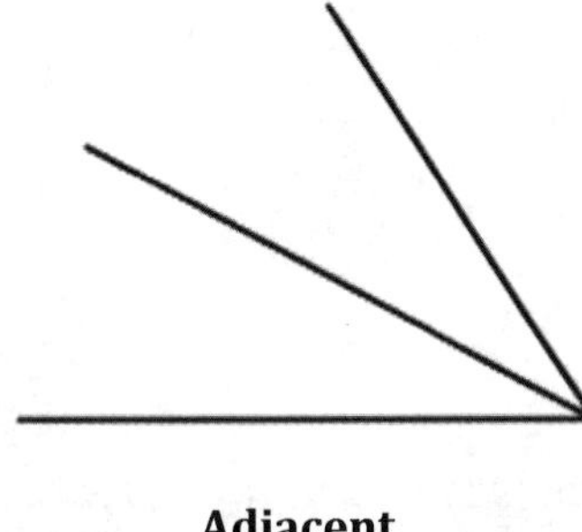

Adjacent
Share vertex and side

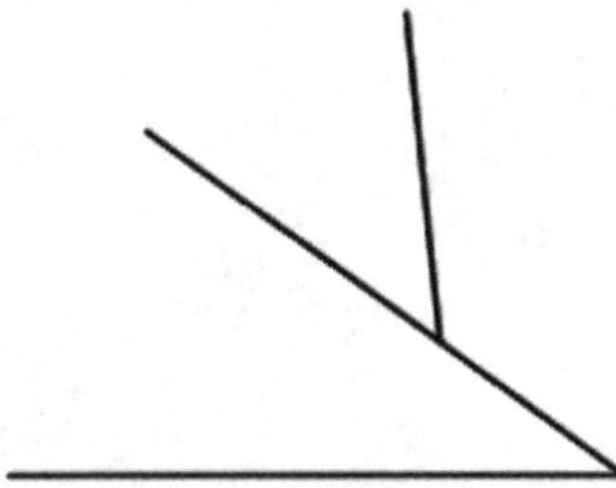

Not adjacent
Share part of a side, but not vertex

When two parallel lines are cut by a transversal, the angles that are between the two parallel lines are **interior angles**. In the diagram below, angles 3, 4, 5, and 6 are interior angles.

When two parallel lines are cut by a transversal, the angles that are outside the parallel lines are **exterior angles**. In the diagram below, angles 1, 2, 7, and 8 are exterior angles.

When two parallel lines are cut by a transversal, the angles that are in the same position relative to the transversal and a parallel line are **corresponding angles**. The diagram below has four pairs of corresponding angles: angles 1 and 5, angles 2 and 6, angles 3 and 7, and angles 4 and 8. Corresponding angles formed by parallel lines are congruent.

When two parallel lines are cut by a transversal, the two interior angles that are on opposite sides of the transversal are called **alternate interior angles**. In the diagram below, there are two pairs of alternate interior angles: angles 3 and 6, and angles 4 and 5. Alternate interior angles formed by parallel lines are congruent.

When two parallel lines are cut by a transversal, the two exterior angles that are on opposite sides of the transversal are called **alternate exterior angles**.

In the diagram below, there are two pairs of alternate exterior angles: angles 1 and 8, and angles 2 and 7. Alternate exterior angles formed by parallel lines are congruent.

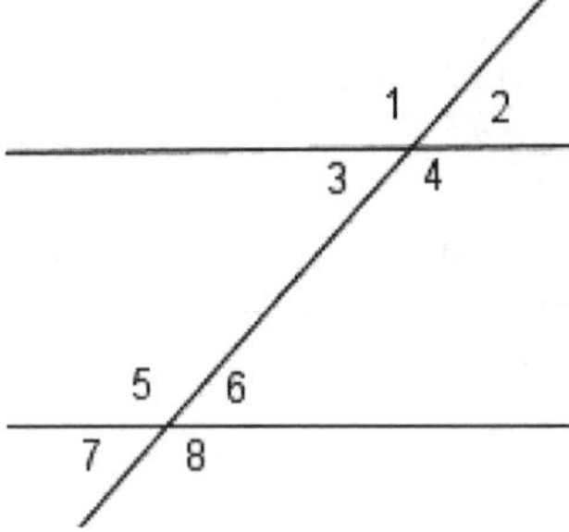

When two lines intersect, four angles are formed. The non-adjacent angles at this vertex are called vertical angles. Vertical angles are congruent. In the diagram, $\angle ABD \cong \angle CBE$ and $\angle ABC \cong \angle DBE$. The other pairs of angles, $(\angle ABC, \angle CBE)$ and $(\angle ABD, \angle DBE)$, are supplementary, meaning the pairs sum to 180°.

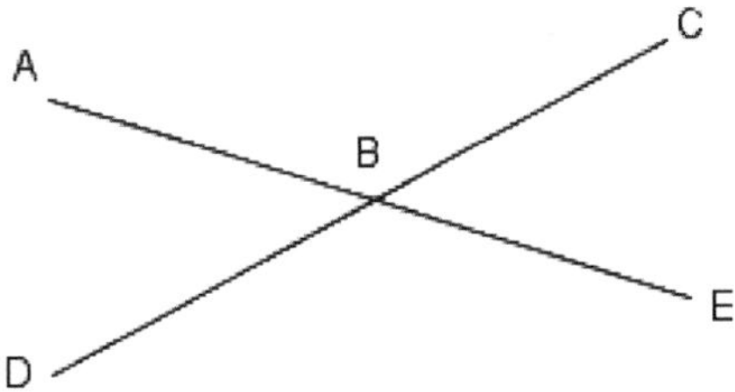

POLYGONS

A **polygon** is a closed, two-dimensional figure with three or more straight line segments called **sides**. The point at which two sides of a polygon intersect is called the **vertex**. In a polygon, the number of sides is always equal to the number of vertices. A polygon with all sides congruent and all angles equal is called a **regular polygon**. Common polygons are:

$$\begin{aligned} \text{Triangle} &= 3 \text{ sides} \\ \text{Quadrilateral} &= 4 \text{ sides} \\ \text{Pentagon} &= 5 \text{ sides} \\ \text{Hexagon} &= 6 \text{ sides} \\ \text{Heptagon} &= 7 \text{ sides} \\ \text{Octagon} &= 8 \text{ sides} \\ \text{Nonagon} &= 9 \text{ sides} \\ \text{Decagon} &= 10 \text{ sides} \\ \text{Dodecagon} &= 12 \text{ sides} \end{aligned}$$

More generally, an n-gon is a polygon that has n angles and n sides.

Review Video: Intro to Polygons
Visit mometrix.com/academy and enter code: 271869

The sum of the interior angles of an n-sided polygon is $(n - 2) \times 180°$. For example, in a triangle $n = 3$. So the sum of the interior angles is $(3 - 2) \times 180° = 180°$. In a quadrilateral, $n = 4$, and the sum of the angles is $(4 - 2) \times 180° = 360°$.

Review Video: Sum of Interior Angles
Visit mometrix.com/academy and enter code: 984991

CONVEX AND CONCAVE POLYGONS

A **convex polygon** is a polygon whose diagonals all lie within the interior of the polygon. A **concave polygon** is a polygon with a least one diagonal that is outside the polygon. In the diagram below, quadrilateral $ABCD$ is concave because diagonal $\overline{AC}$ lies outside the polygon and quadrilateral $EFGH$ is convex because both diagonals lie inside the polygon.

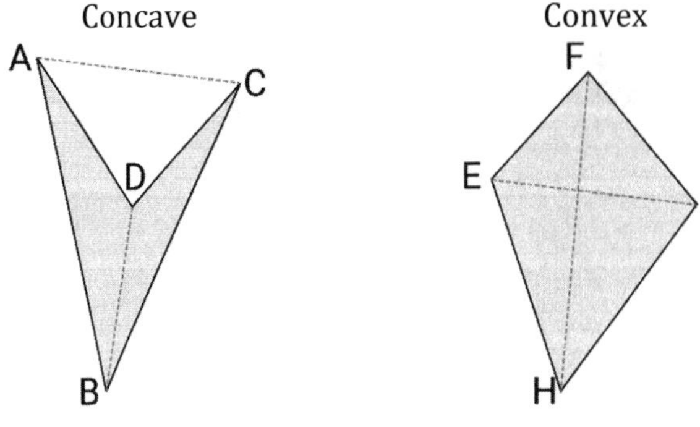

APOTHEM AND RADIUS

A line segment from the center of a polygon that is perpendicular to a side of the polygon is called the **apothem**. A line segment from the center of a polygon to a vertex of the polygon is called a **radius**. In a regular polygon, the apothem can be used to find the area of the polygon using the formula $A = \frac{1}{2}ap$, where a is the apothem, and p is the perimeter.

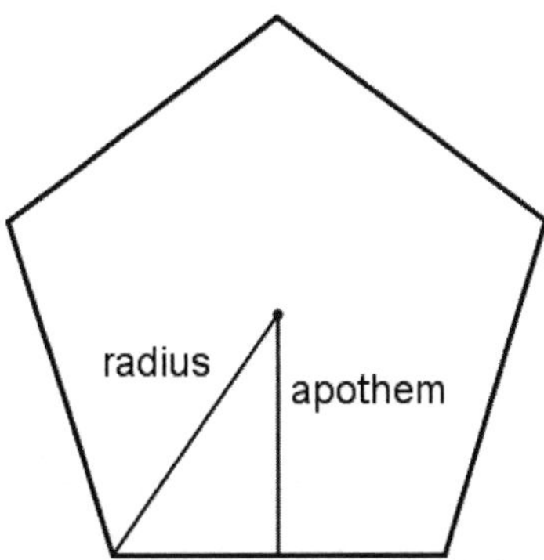

A **diagonal** is a line segment that joins two non-adjacent vertices of a polygon. The number of diagonals a polygon has can be found by using the formula:

$$\text{number of diagonals} = \frac{n(n-3)}{2}$$

Note that n is the number of sides in the polygon. This formula works for all polygons, not just regular polygons.

Congruence and Similarity

Congruent figures are geometric figures that have the same size and shape. All corresponding angles are equal, and all corresponding sides are equal. Congruence is indicated by the symbol $\cong$.

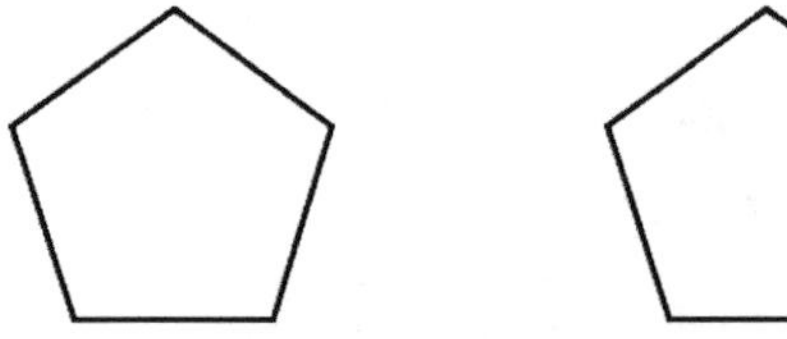

Congruent polygons

Similar figures are geometric figures that have the same shape, but do not necessarily have the same size. All corresponding angles are equal, and all corresponding sides are proportional, but they do not have to be equal. It is indicated by the symbol $\sim$.

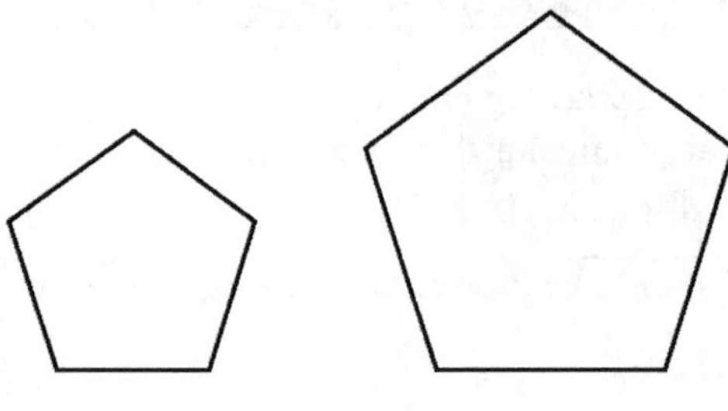

Similar polygons

Note that all congruent figures are also similar, but not all similar figures are congruent.

Review Video: Congruent Shapes
Visit mometrix.com/academy and enter code: 492281

Line of Symmetry

A line that divides a figure or object into congruent parts is called a **line of symmetry**. An object may have no lines of symmetry, one line of symmetry, or multiple (i.e., more than one) lines of symmetry.

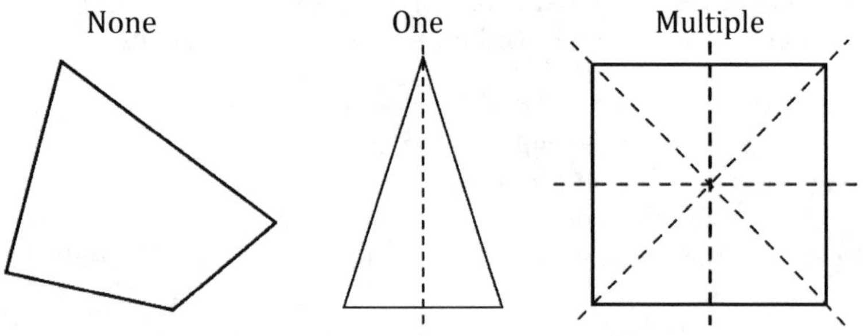

Review Video: Symmetry
Visit mometrix.com/academy and enter code: 528106

TRIANGLES

A triangle is a three-sided figure with the sum of its interior angles being 180°. The **perimeter of any triangle** is found by summing the three side lengths; $P = a + b + c$. For an equilateral triangle, this is the same as $P = 3a$, where a is any side length, since all three sides are the same length.

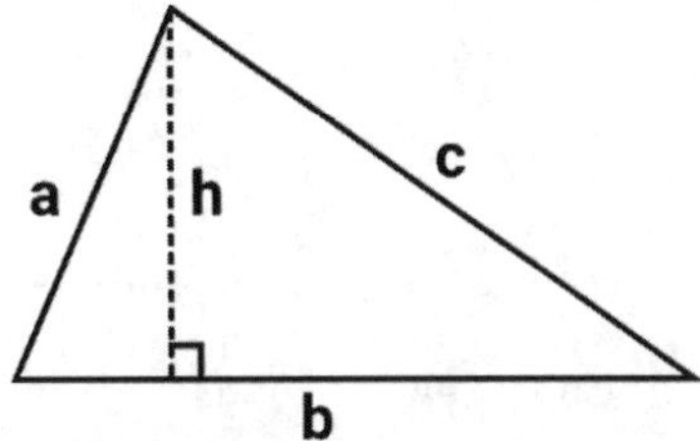

Review Video: Proof that a Triangle is 180 Degrees
Visit mometrix.com/academy and enter code: 687591

Review Video: Area and Perimeter of a Triangle
Visit mometrix.com/academy and enter code: 853779

The **area of any triangle** can be found by taking half the product of one side length referred to as the base, often given the variable b and the perpendicular distance from that side to the opposite vertex called the altitude or height and given the variable h. In equation form that is $A = \frac{1}{2}bh$. Another formula that works for any triangle is $A = \sqrt{s(s-a)(s-b)(s-c)}$, where s is the semiperimeter: $\frac{a+b+c}{2}$, and a, b, and c are the lengths of the three sides. Special cases include isosceles triangles, $A = \frac{1}{2}b\sqrt{a^2 - \frac{b^2}{4}}$, where b is the unique side and a is the length of one of the two congruent sides, and equilateral triangles, $A = \frac{\sqrt{3}}{4}a^2$, where a is the length of a side.

Review Video: Area of Any Triangle
Visit mometrix.com/academy and enter code: 138510

PARTS OF A TRIANGLE

An **altitude** of a triangle is a line segment drawn from one vertex perpendicular to the opposite side. In the diagram that follows, $\overline{BE}$, $\overline{AD}$, and $\overline{CF}$ are altitudes. The length of an altitude is also called the height of the triangle. The three altitudes in a triangle are always concurrent. The point of concurrency of the altitudes of a triangle, O, is called the **orthocenter**. Note that in an obtuse triangle, the orthocenter will be outside the triangle, and in a right triangle, the orthocenter is the vertex of the right angle.

A **median** of a triangle is a line segment drawn from one vertex to the midpoint of the opposite side. In the diagram that follows, $\overline{BH}$, $\overline{AG}$, and $\overline{CI}$ are medians. This is not the same as the altitude, except the altitude to the base of an isosceles triangle and all three altitudes of an equilateral triangle. The point of concurrency of the medians of a triangle, T, is called the **centroid**. This is the same point as the orthocenter only in an equilateral triangle. Unlike the orthocenter, the centroid is always inside the triangle. The centroid can also be considered the exact center of the triangle. Any shape triangle can be perfectly balanced on a tip placed at the centroid. The centroid is also the point that is two-thirds the distance from the vertex to the opposite side.

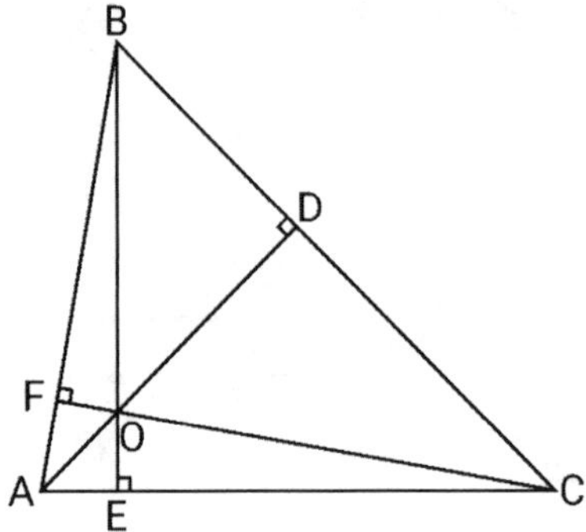

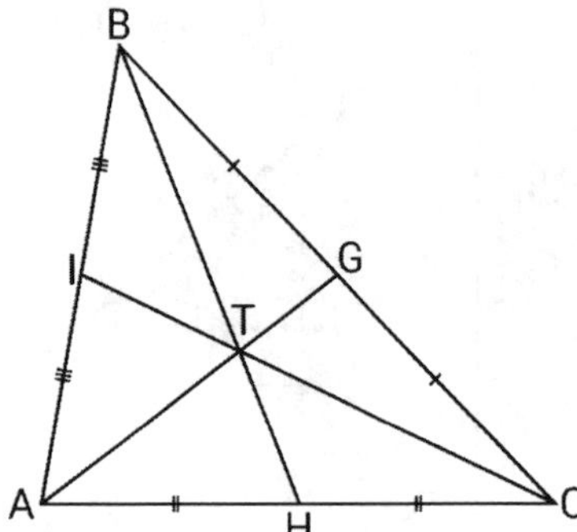

Review Video: Centroid, Incenter, Circumcenter, and Orthocenter
Visit mometrix.com/academy and enter code: 598260

Triangle Properties

Classifications of Triangles

A **scalene triangle** is a triangle with no congruent sides. A scalene triangle will also have three angles of different measures. The angle with the largest measure is opposite the longest side, and the angle with the smallest measure is opposite the shortest side. An **acute triangle** is a triangle whose three angles are all less than 90°. If two of the angles are equal, the acute triangle is also an **isosceles triangle**. An isosceles triangle will also have two congruent angles opposite the two congruent sides. If the three angles are all equal, the acute triangle is also an **equilateral triangle**. An equilateral triangle will also have three congruent angles, each 60°. All equilateral triangles are also acute triangles. An **obtuse triangle** is a triangle with exactly one angle greater than 90°. The other two angles may or may not be equal. If the two remaining angles are equal, the obtuse triangle is also an isosceles triangle. A **right triangle** is a triangle with exactly one angle equal to 90°. All right triangles follow the Pythagorean theorem. A right triangle can never be acute or obtuse.

The table below illustrates how each descriptor places a different restriction on the triangle:

Sides \ Angles	Acute: All angles < 90°	Obtuse: One angle > 90°	Right: One angle = 90°
Scalene: No equal side lengths	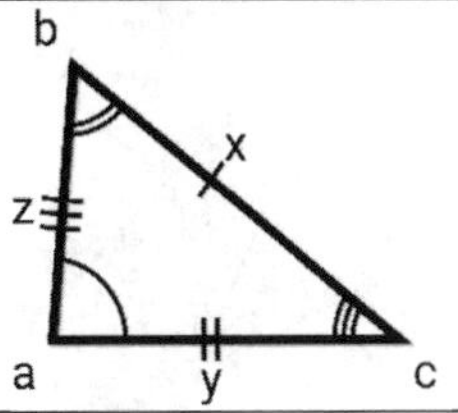 $90° > \angle a > \angle b > \angle c$ $x > y > z$	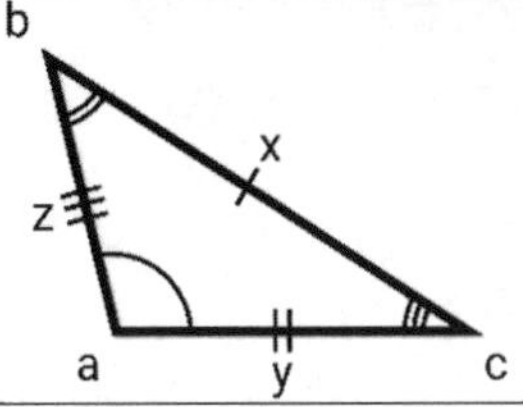 $\angle a > 90° > \angle b > \angle c$ $x > y > z$	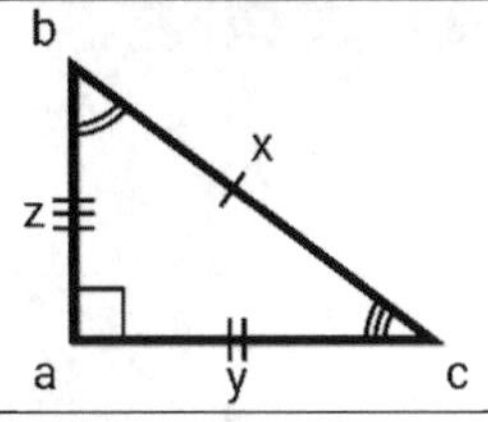 $90° = \angle a > \angle b > \angle c$ $x > y > z$
Isosceles: Two equal side lengths	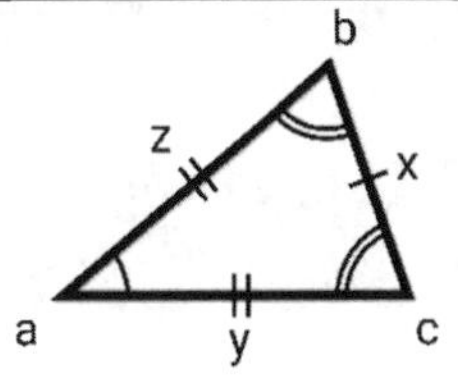 $90° > \angle a, \angle b, or\ \angle c$ $\angle b = \angle c, \quad y = z$	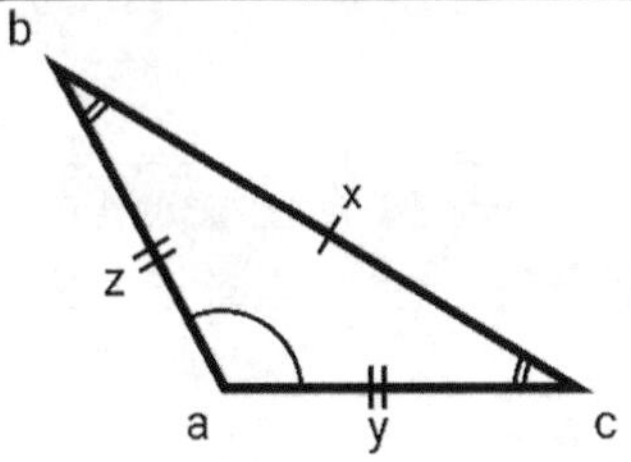 $\angle a > 90° > \angle b = \angle c$ $x > y = z$	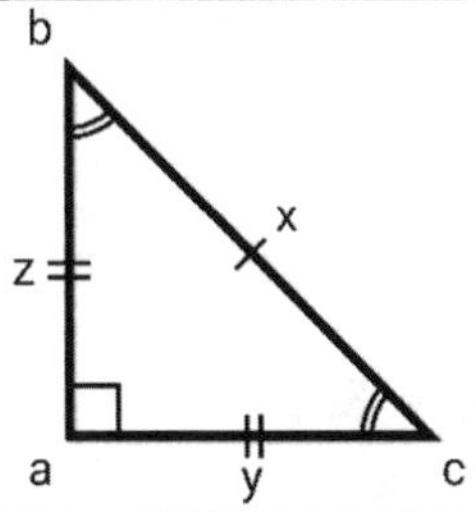 $\angle a = 90°$ $\angle b = \angle c = 45°$ $x > y = z$
Equilateral: Three equal side lengths	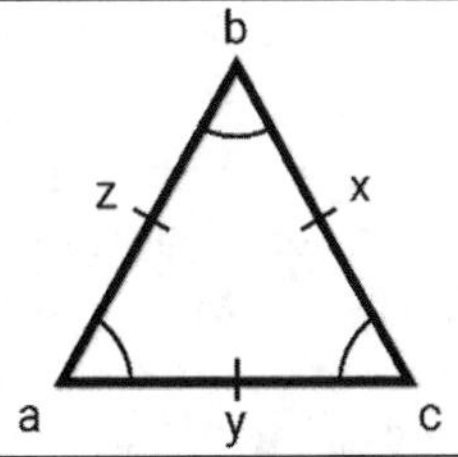 $60° = \angle a = \angle b = \angle c$ $x = y = z$		

Review Video: Introduction to Types of Triangles
Visit mometrix.com/academy and enter code: 511711

General Rules for Triangles

The **triangle inequality theorem** states that the sum of the measures of any two sides of a triangle is always greater than the measure of the third side. If the sum of the measures of two sides were equal to the third side, a triangle would be impossible because the two sides would lie flat across the third side and there would be no vertex. If the sum of the measures of two of the sides was less than the third side, a closed figure would be impossible because the two shortest sides would never meet. In other words, for a triangle with sides lengths A, B, and C: $A + B > C$, $B + C > A$, and $A + C > B$.

The sum of the measures of the interior angles of a triangle is always 180°. Therefore, a triangle can never have more than one angle greater than or equal to 90°.

In any triangle, the angles opposite congruent sides are congruent, and the sides opposite congruent angles are congruent. The largest angle is always opposite the longest side, and the smallest angle is always opposite the shortest side.

The line segment that joins the midpoints of any two sides of a triangle is always parallel to the third side and exactly half the length of the third side.

Review Video: General Rules (Triangle Inequality Theorem)
Visit mometrix.com/academy and enter code: 166488

Similarity and Congruence Rules

Similar triangles are triangles whose corresponding angles are equal and whose corresponding sides are proportional. Represented by AAA. Similar triangles whose corresponding sides are congruent are also congruent triangles.

Triangles can be shown to be **congruent** in 5 ways:

- **SSS**: Three sides of one triangle are congruent to the three corresponding sides of the second triangle.
- **SAS**: Two sides and the included angle (the angle formed by those two sides) of one triangle are congruent to the corresponding two sides and included angle of the second triangle.
- **ASA**: Two angles and the included side (the side that joins the two angles) of one triangle are congruent to the corresponding two angles and included side of the second triangle.
- **AAS**: Two angles and a non-included side of one triangle are congruent to the corresponding two angles and non-included side of the second triangle.
- **HL**: The hypotenuse and leg of one right triangle are congruent to the corresponding hypotenuse and leg of the second right triangle.

Review Video: Similar Triangles
Visit mometrix.com/academy and enter code: 398538

Transformations

Rotation

A **rotation** is a transformation that turns a figure around a point called the **center of rotation**, which can lie anywhere in the plane. If a line is drawn from a point on a figure to the center of rotation, and another line is drawn from the center to the rotated image of that point, the angle between the two lines is the **angle of rotation**. The vertex of the angle of rotation is the center of rotation.

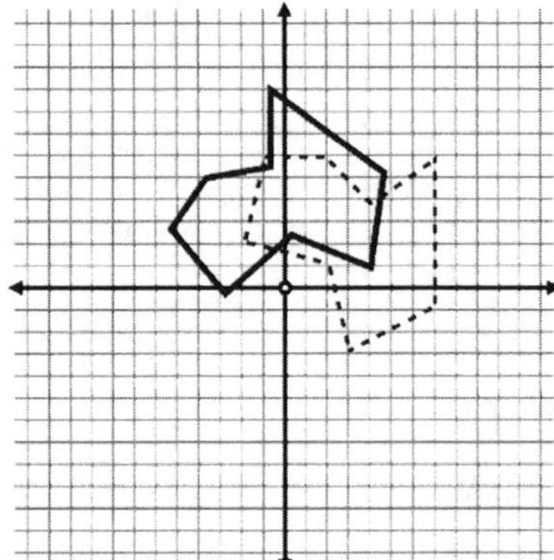

Review Video: Rotation
Visit mometrix.com/academy and enter code: 602600

Translation and Dilation

A **translation** is a transformation which slides a figure from one position in the plane to another position in the plane. The original figure and the translated figure have the same size, shape, and orientation. A **dilation** is a transformation which proportionally stretches or shrinks a figure by a **scale factor**. The dilated image is the same shape and orientation as the original image but a different size. A polygon and its dilated image are similar.

Translation

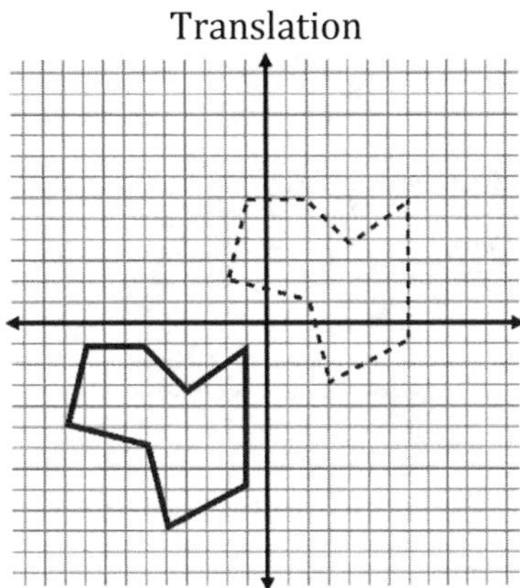

Dilation

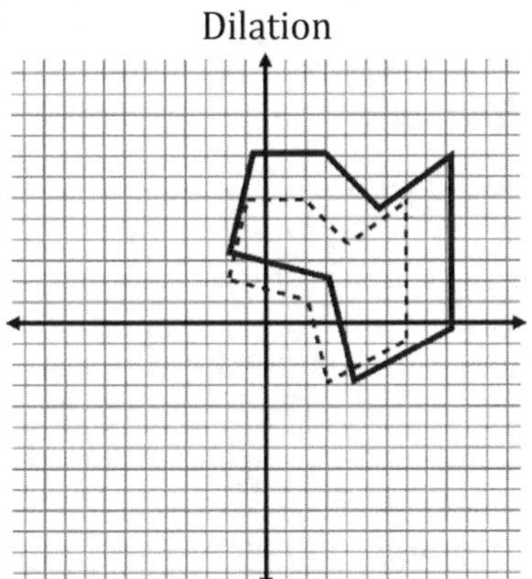

Review Video: Translation
Visit mometrix.com/academy and enter code: 718628

Review Video: Dilation
Visit mometrix.com/academy and enter code: 471630

A **reflection of a figure over a line** (a "flip") creates a congruent image that is the same distance from the line as the original figure but on the opposite side. The **line of reflection** is the perpendicular bisector of any line segment drawn from a point on the original figure to its reflected image (unless the point and its reflected image happen to be the same point, which happens when a figure is reflected over one of its own sides). A **reflection of a figure over a point** (an inversion) in two dimensions is the same as the rotation of the figure 180° about that point. The image of the figure is congruent to the original figure. The **point of reflection** is the midpoint of a line segment which connects a point in the figure to its image (unless the point and its reflected image happen to be the same point, which happens when a figure is reflected in one of its own points).

Reflection of a figure over a line

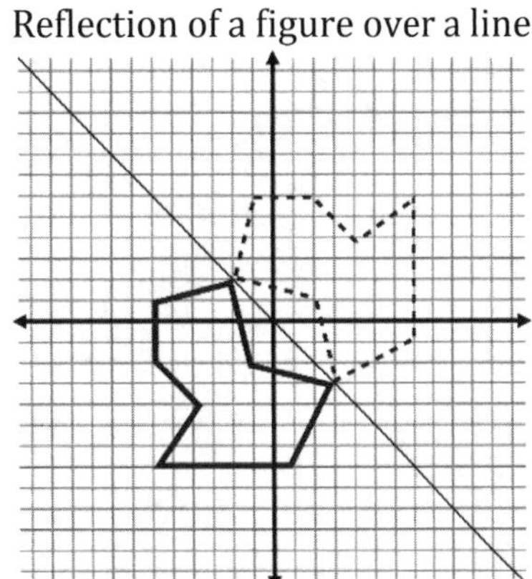

Reflection of a figure over a point

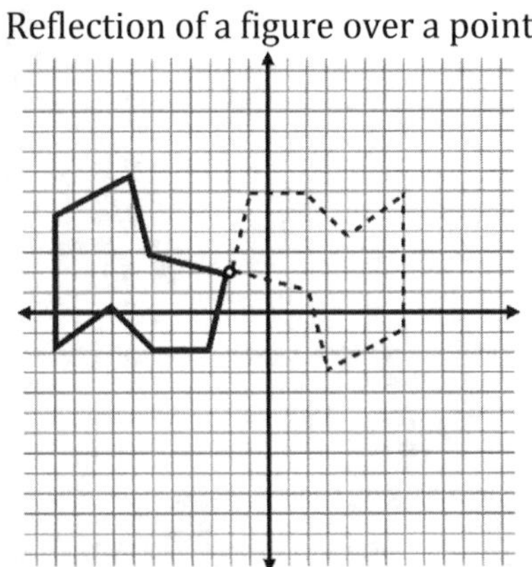

Review Video: Reflection
Visit mometrix.com/academy and enter code: 955068

PYTHAGOREAN THEOREM

The side of a triangle opposite the right angle is called the **hypotenuse**. The other two sides are called the legs. The Pythagorean theorem states a relationship among the legs and hypotenuse of a right triangle: $(a^2 + b^2 = c^2)$, where a and b are the lengths of the legs of a right triangle, and c is the length of the hypotenuse. Note that this formula will only work with right triangles.

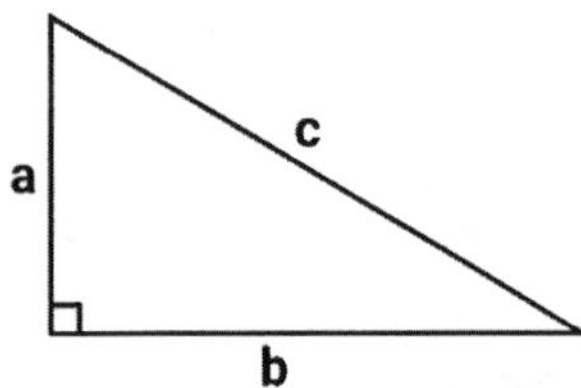

Review Video: Pythagorean Theorem
Visit mometrix.com/academy and enter code: 906576

TRIGONOMETRIC FORMULAS

In the diagram below, angle C is the right angle, and side c is the hypotenuse. Side a is the side opposite to angle A and side b is the side opposite to angle B. Using ratios of side lengths as a means to calculate the sine, cosine, and tangent of an acute angle only works for right triangles.

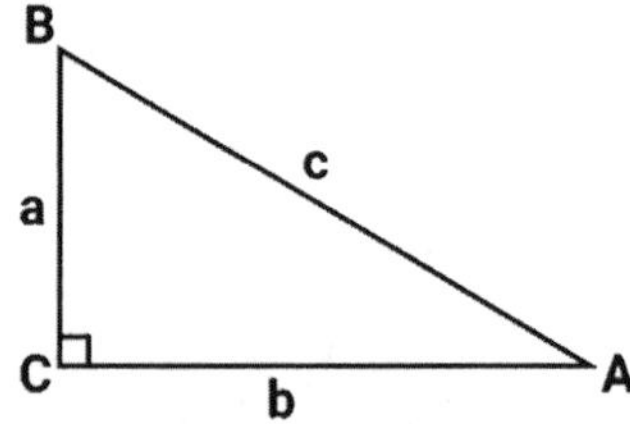

$$\sin A = \frac{\text{opposite side}}{\text{hypotenuse}} = \frac{a}{c} \qquad \csc A = \frac{1}{\sin A} = \frac{\text{hypotenuse}}{\text{opposite side}} = \frac{c}{a}$$

$$\cos A = \frac{\text{adjacent side}}{\text{hypotenuse}} = \frac{b}{c} \qquad \sec A = \frac{1}{\cos A} = \frac{\text{hypotenuse}}{\text{adjacent side}} = \frac{c}{b}$$

$$\tan A = \frac{\text{opposite side}}{\text{adjacent side}} = \frac{a}{b} \qquad \cot A = \frac{1}{\tan A} = \frac{\text{adjacent side}}{\text{opposite side}} = \frac{b}{a}$$

LAWS OF SINES AND COSINES

The **law of sines** states that $\frac{\sin A}{a} = \frac{\sin B}{b} = \frac{\sin C}{c}$, where A, B, and C are the angles of a triangle, and a, b, and c are the sides opposite their respective angles. This formula will work with all triangles, not just right triangles.

The **law of cosines** is given by the formula $c^2 = a^2 + b^2 - 2ab(\cos C)$, where a, b, and c are the sides of a triangle, and C is the angle opposite side c. This is a generalized form of the Pythagorean theorem that can be used on any triangle.

Review Video: Upper Level Trig: Law of Sines
Visit mometrix.com/academy and enter code: 206844

Review Video: Upper Level Trig: Law of Cosines
Visit mometrix.com/academy and enter code: 158911

QUADRILATERALS

A **quadrilateral** is a closed two-dimensional geometric figure that has four straight sides. The sum of the interior angles of any quadrilateral is 360°.

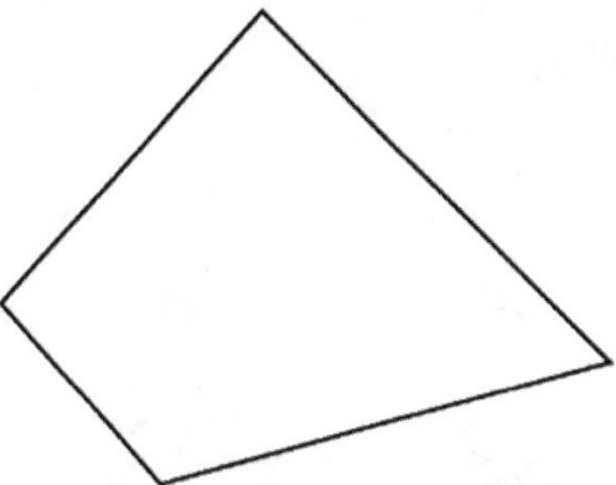

Review Video: Diagonals of Parallelograms, Rectangles, and Rhombi
Visit mometrix.com/academy and enter code: 320040

KITE

A **kite** is a quadrilateral with two pairs of adjacent sides that are congruent. A result of this is perpendicular diagonals. A kite can be concave or convex and has one line of symmetry.

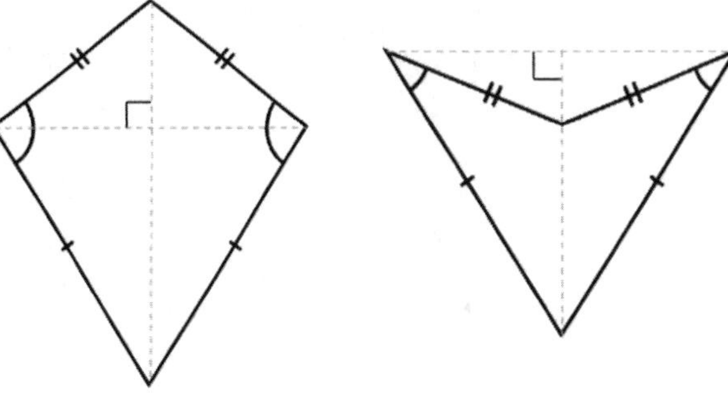

TRAPEZOID

Trapezoid: A trapezoid is defined as a quadrilateral that has at least one pair of parallel sides. There are no rules for the second pair of sides. So, there are no rules for the diagonals and no lines of symmetry for a trapezoid.

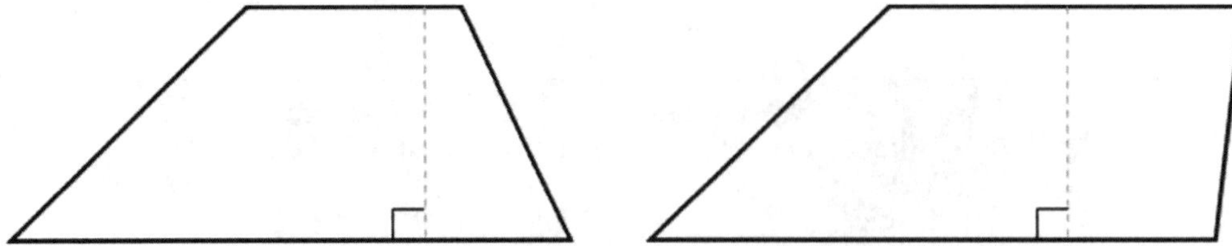

The **area of a trapezoid** is found by the formula $A = \frac{1}{2}h(b_1 + b_2)$, where h is the height (segment joining and perpendicular to the parallel bases), and b_1 and b_2 are the two parallel sides (bases). Do not use one of the other two sides as the height unless that side is also perpendicular to the parallel bases.

The **perimeter of a trapezoid** is found by the formula $P = a + b_1 + c + b_2$, where a, b_1, c, and b_2 are the four sides of the trapezoid.

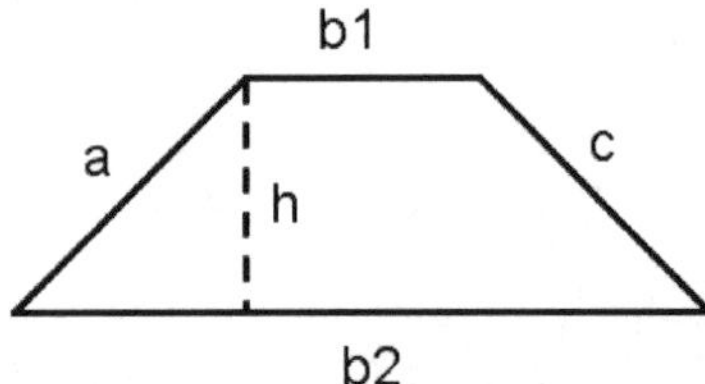

Review Video: Area and Perimeter of a Trapezoid
Visit mometrix.com/academy and enter code: 587523

Isosceles trapezoid: A trapezoid with equal base angles. This gives rise to other properties including: the two nonparallel sides have the same length, the two non-base angles are also equal, and there is one line of symmetry through the midpoints of the parallel sides.

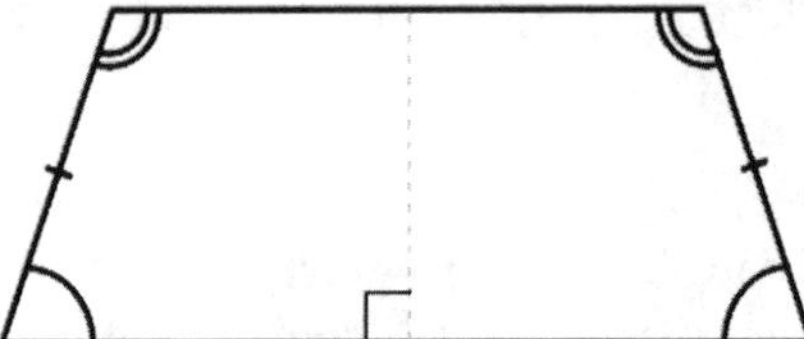

Parallelogram

A **parallelogram** is a quadrilateral that has two pairs of opposite parallel sides. As such it is a special type of trapezoid. The sides that are parallel are also congruent. The opposite interior angles are always congruent, and the consecutive interior angles are supplementary. The diagonals of a parallelogram divide each other. Each diagonal divides the parallelogram into two congruent triangles. A parallelogram has no line of symmetry, but does have 180-degree rotational symmetry about the midpoint.

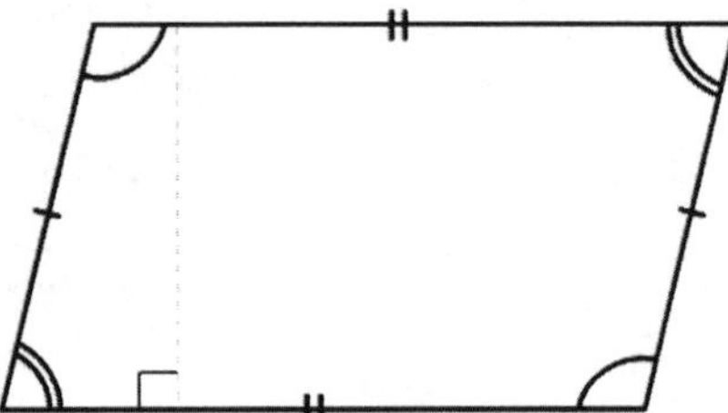

The **area of a parallelogram** is found by the formula $A = bh$, where b is the length of the base, and h is the height. Note that the base and height correspond to the length and width in a rectangle, so this formula would apply to rectangles as well. Do not confuse the height of a parallelogram with the length of the second side. The two are only the same measure in the case of a rectangle.

The **perimeter of a parallelogram** is found by the formula $P = 2a + 2b$ or $P = 2(a + b)$, where a and b are the lengths of the two sides.

Review Video: How to Find the Area and Perimeter of a Parallelogram
Visit mometrix.com/academy and enter code: 718313

Rectangle

A **rectangle** is a quadrilateral with four right angles. All rectangles are parallelograms and trapezoids, but not all parallelograms or trapezoids are rectangles. The diagonals of a rectangle are congruent. Rectangles have two lines of symmetry (through each pair of opposing midpoints) and 180-degree rotational symmetry about the midpoint.

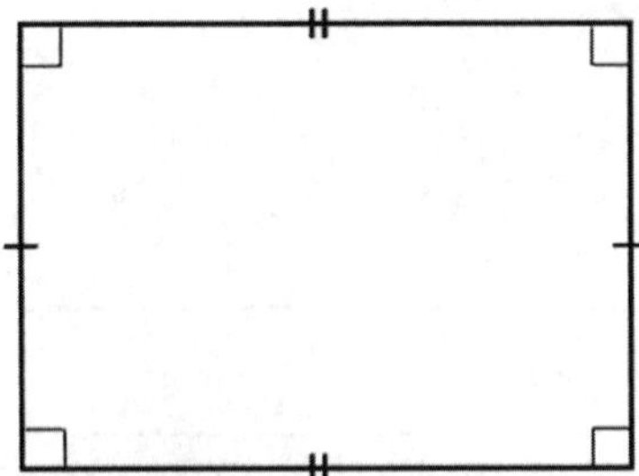

The **area of a rectangle** is found by the formula $A = lw$, where A is the area of the rectangle, l is the length (usually considered to be the longer side) and w is the width (usually considered to be the shorter side). The numbers for l and w are interchangeable.

The **perimeter of a rectangle** is found by the formula $P = 2l + 2w$ or $P = 2(l + w)$, where l is the length, and w is the width. It may be easier to add the length and width first and then double the result, as in the second formula.

Rhombus

A **rhombus** is a quadrilateral with four congruent sides. All rhombuses are parallelograms and kites; thus, they inherit all the properties of both types of quadrilaterals. The diagonals of a rhombus are perpendicular to each other. Rhombi have two lines of symmetry (along each of the diagonals) and 180° rotational symmetry. The **area of a rhombus** is half the product of the diagonals: $A = \frac{d_1 d_2}{2}$ and the perimeter of a rhombus is: $P = 2\sqrt{(d_1)^2 + (d_2)^2}$.

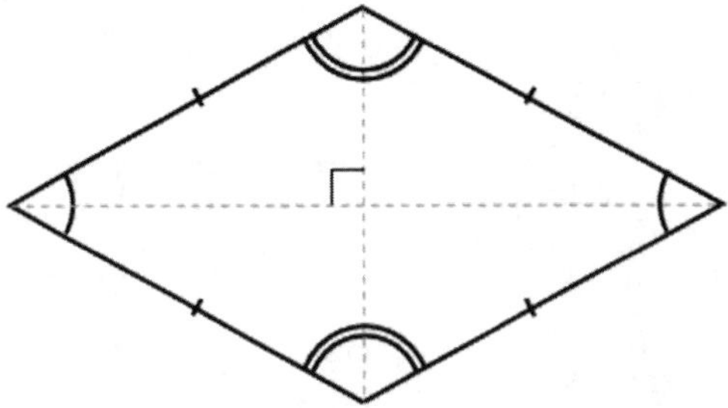

Square

A **square** is a quadrilateral with four right angles and four congruent sides. Squares satisfy the criteria of all other types of quadrilaterals. The diagonals of a square are congruent and perpendicular to each other. Squares have four lines of symmetry (through each pair of opposing midpoints and along each of the diagonals) as well as 90° rotational symmetry about the midpoint.

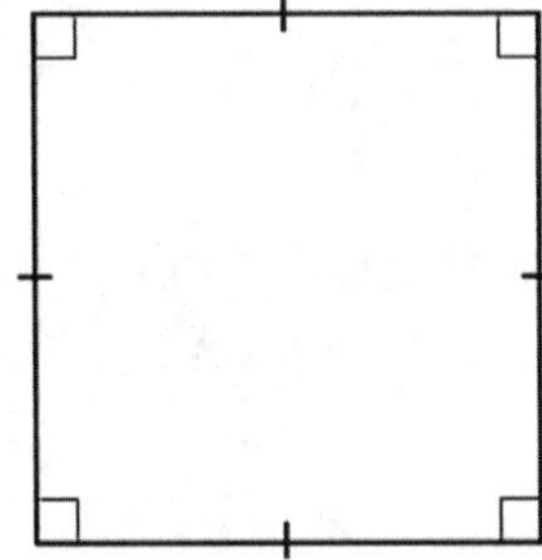

The **area of a square** is found by using the formula $A = s^2$, where s is the length of one side. The **perimeter of a square** is found by using the formula $P = 4s$, where s is the length of one side. Because all four sides are equal in a square, it is faster to multiply the length of one side by 4 than to add the same number four times. You could use the formulas for rectangles and get the same answer.

Review Video: <u>Area and Perimeter of Rectangles and Squares</u>
Visit mometrix.com/academy and enter code: 428109

Hierarchy of Quadrilaterals

The hierarchy of quadrilaterals is as follows:

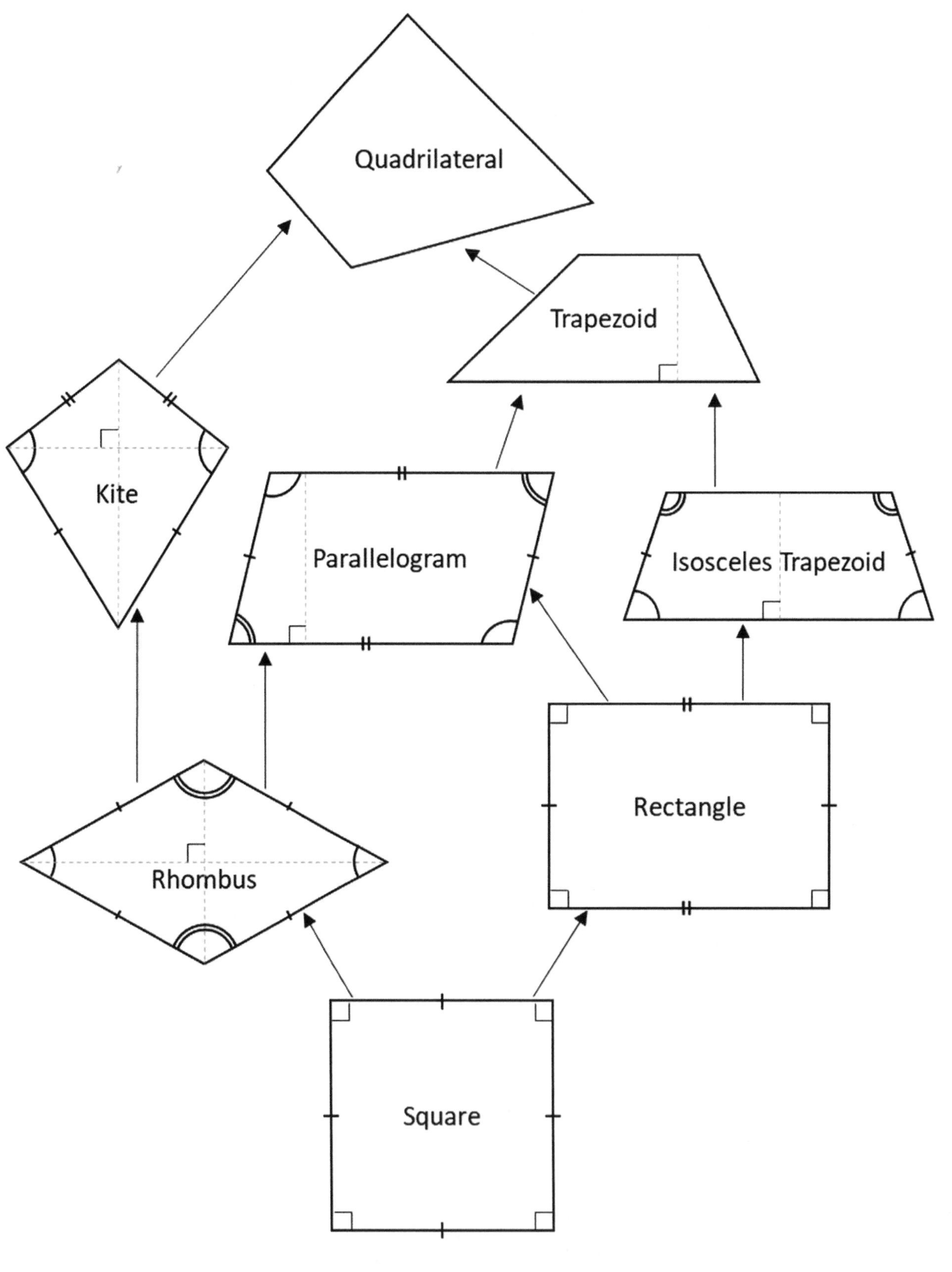

CIRCLES

The **center** of a circle is the single point from which every point on the circle is **equidistant**. The **radius** is a line segment that joins the center of the circle and any one point on the circle. All radii of a circle are equal. Circles that have the same center but not the same length of radii are **concentric**. The **diameter** is a line segment that passes through the center of the circle and has both endpoints on the circle. The length of the diameter is exactly twice the length of the radius. Point O in the diagram below is the center of the circle, segments $\overline{OX}$, $\overline{OY}$, and $\overline{OZ}$ are radii; and segment $\overline{XZ}$ is a diameter.

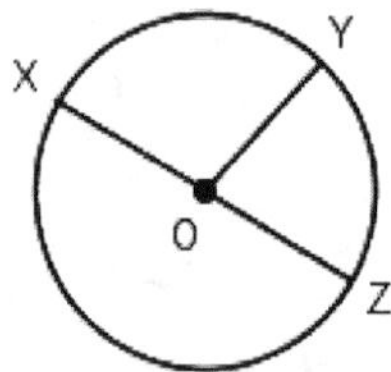

Review Video: Points of a Circle
Visit mometrix.com/academy and enter code: 420746

Review Video: The Diameter, Radius, and Circumference of Circles
Visit mometrix.com/academy and enter code: 448988

The **area of a circle** is found by the formula $A = \pi r^2$, where r is the length of the radius. If the diameter of the circle is given, remember to divide it in half to get the length of the radius before proceeding.

The **circumference** of a circle is found by the formula $C = 2\pi r$, where r is the radius. Again, remember to convert the diameter if you are given that measure rather than the radius.

Review Video: Area and Circumference of a Circle
Visit mometrix.com/academy and enter code: 243015

INSCRIBED AND CIRCUMSCRIBED FIGURES

These terms can both be used to describe a given arrangement of figures, depending on perspective. If each of the vertices of figure A lie on figure B, then it can be said that figure A is **inscribed** in figure B, but it can also be said that figure B is **circumscribed** about figure A. The following table and examples help to illustrate the concept. Note that the figures cannot both be circles, as they would be completely overlapping and neither would be inscribed or circumscribed.

Given	Description	Equivalent Description	Figures
Each of the sides of a pentagon is tangent to a circle	The circle is inscribed in the pentagon	The pentagon is circumscribed about the circle	
Each of the vertices of a pentagon lie on a circle	The pentagon is inscribed in the circle	The circle is circumscribed about the pentagon	

3D SHAPES

SOLIDS

The **surface area of a solid object** is the area of all sides or exterior surfaces. For objects such as prisms and pyramids, a further distinction is made between base surface area (B) and lateral surface area (LA). For a prism, the total surface area (SA) is $SA = LA + 2B$. For a pyramid or cone, the total surface area is $SA = LA + B$.

The **surface area of a sphere** can be found by the formula $A = 4\pi r^2$, where r is the radius. The volume is given by the formula $V = \frac{4}{3}\pi r^3$, where r is the radius. Both quantities are generally given in terms of π.

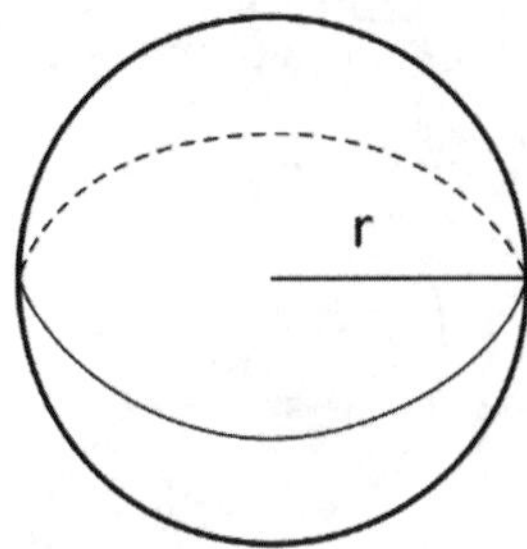

Review Video: Volume and Surface Area of a Sphere
Visit mometrix.com/academy and enter code: 786928

Review Video: How to Calculate the Volume of 3D Objects
Visit mometrix.com/academy and enter code: 163343

The **volume of any prism** is found by the formula $V = Bh$, where B is the area of the base, and h is the height (perpendicular distance between the bases). The surface area of any prism is the sum of the areas of both bases and all sides. It can be calculated as $SA = 2B + Ph$, where P is the perimeter of the base.

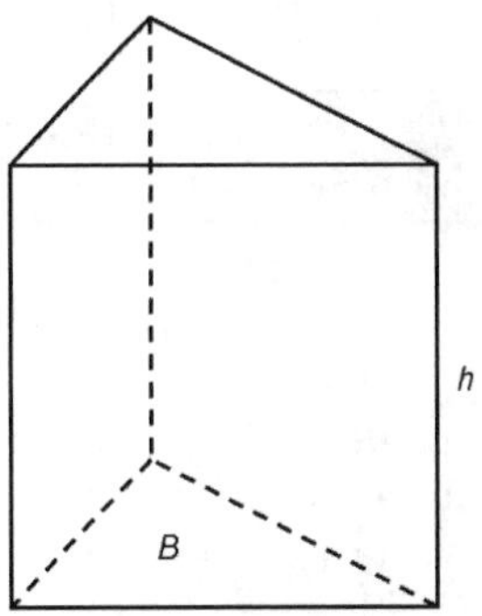

Review Video: Volume and Surface Area of a Prism
Visit mometrix.com/academy and enter code: 420158

For a **rectangular prism**, the volume can be found by the formula $V = lwh$, where V is the volume, l is the length, w is the width, and h is the height. The surface area can be calculated as $SA = 2lw + 2hl + 2wh$ or $SA = 2(lw + hl + wh)$.

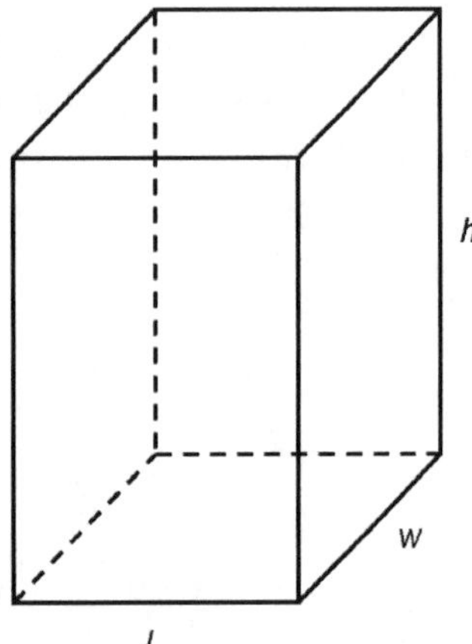

Review Video: Volume and Surface Area of a Rectangular Prism
Visit mometrix.com/academy and enter code: 282814

The **volume of a cube** can be found by the formula $V = s^3$, where s is the length of a side. The surface area of a cube is calculated as $SA = 6s^2$, where SA is the total surface area and s is the length of a side. These formulas are the same as the ones used for the volume and surface area of a rectangular prism, but simplified since all three quantities (length, width, and height) are the same.

Review Video: Volume and Surface Area of a Cube
Visit mometrix.com/academy and enter code: 664455

The **volume of a cylinder** can be calculated by the formula $V = \pi r^2 h$, where r is the radius, and h is the height. The surface area of a cylinder can be found by the formula $SA = 2\pi r^2 + 2\pi rh$. The first term is the base area multiplied by two, and the second term is the perimeter of the base multiplied by the height.

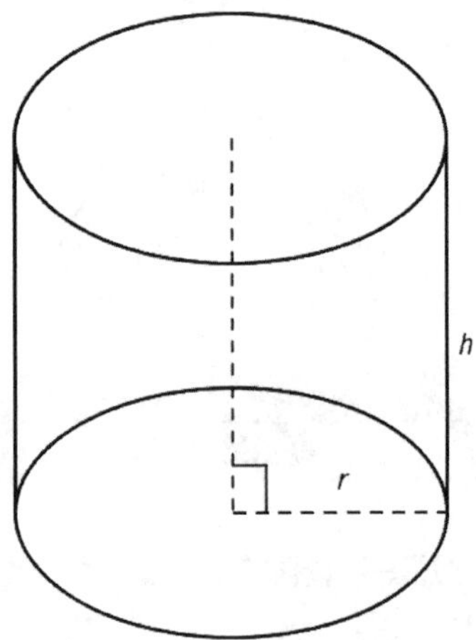

Review Video: Finding the Volume and Surface Area of a Right Circular Cylinder
Visit mometrix.com/academy and enter code: 226463

The **volume of a pyramid** is found by the formula $V = \frac{1}{3}Bh$, where B is the area of the base, and h is the height (perpendicular distance from the vertex to the base). Notice this formula is the same as $\frac{1}{3}$ times the volume of a prism. Like a prism, the base of a pyramid can be any shape.

Finding the **surface area of a pyramid** is not as simple as the other shapes we've looked at thus far. If the pyramid is a right pyramid, meaning the base is a regular polygon and the vertex is directly over the center of that polygon, the surface area can be calculated as $SA = B + \frac{1}{2}Ph_s$, where P is the perimeter of the base, and h_s is the slant height (distance from the vertex to the midpoint of one side of the base). If the pyramid is irregular, the area of each triangle side must be calculated individually and then summed, along with the base.

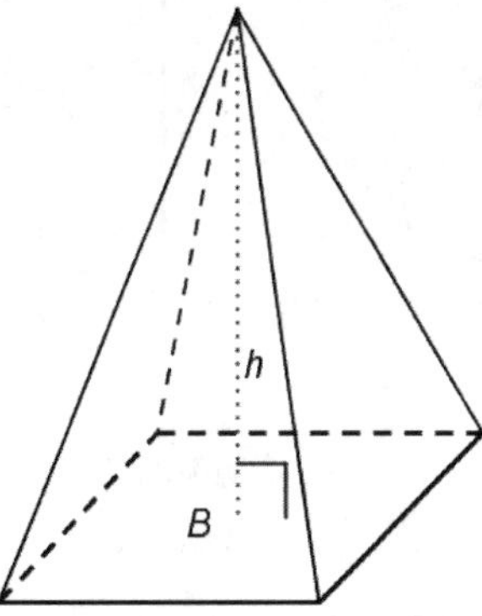

Review Video: Finding the Volume and Surface Area of a Pyramid
Visit mometrix.com/academy and enter code: 621932

The **volume of a cone** is found by the formula $V = \frac{1}{3}\pi r^2 h$, where r is the radius, and h is the height. Notice this is the same as $\frac{1}{3}$ times the volume of a cylinder. The surface area can be calculated as $SA = \pi r^2 + \pi rs$, where s is the slant height. The slant height can be calculated using the Pythagorean theorem to be $\sqrt{r^2 + h^2}$, so the surface area formula can also be written as $SA = \pi r^2 + \pi r\sqrt{r^2 + h^2}$.

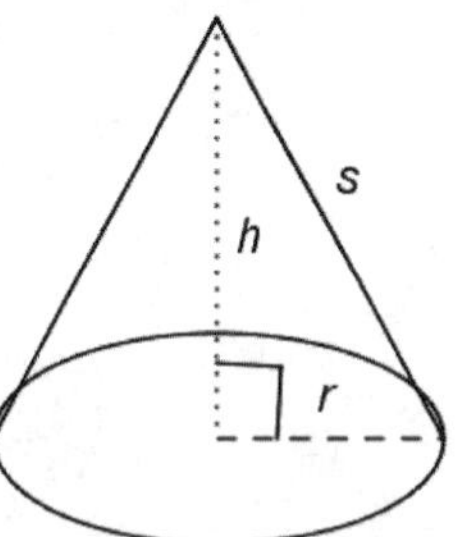

Review Video: Volume and Surface Area of a Right Circular Cone
Visit mometrix.com/academy and enter code: 573574

Mathematical Concepts

Number Basics

Classifications of Numbers

Numbers are the basic building blocks of mathematics. Specific features of numbers are identified by the following terms:

Integer – any positive or negative whole number, including zero. Integers do not include fractions $\left(\frac{1}{3}\right)$, decimals (0.56), or mixed numbers $\left(7\frac{3}{4}\right)$.

Prime number – any whole number greater than 1 that has only two factors, itself and 1; that is, a number that can be divided evenly only by 1 and itself.

Composite number – any whole number greater than 1 that has more than two different factors; in other words, any whole number that is not a prime number. For example: The composite number 8 has the factors of 1, 2, 4, and 8.

Even number – any integer that can be divided by 2 without leaving a remainder. For example: 2, 4, 6, 8, and so on.

Odd number – any integer that cannot be divided evenly by 2. For example: 3, 5, 7, 9, and so on.

Decimal number – any number that uses a decimal point to show the part of the number that is less than one. Example: 1.234.

Decimal point – a symbol used to separate the ones place from the tenths place in decimals or dollars from cents in currency.

Decimal place – the position of a number to the right of the decimal point. In the decimal 0.123, the 1 is in the first place to the right of the decimal point, indicating tenths; the 2 is in the second place, indicating hundredths; and the 3 is in the third place, indicating thousandths.

The **decimal**, or base 10, system is a number system that uses ten different digits (0, 1, 2, 3, 4, 5, 6, 7, 8, 9). An example of a number system that uses something other than ten digits is the **binary**, or base 2, number system, used by computers, which uses only the numbers 0 and 1. It is thought that the decimal system originated because people had only their 10 fingers for counting.

Rational numbers include all integers, decimals, and fractions. Any terminating or repeating decimal number is a rational number.

Irrational numbers cannot be written as fractions or decimals because the number of decimal places is infinite and there is no recurring pattern of digits within the number. For example, pi (π) begins with 3.141592 and continues without terminating or repeating, so pi is an irrational number.

Real numbers are the set of all rational and irrational numbers.

Review Video: Classification of Numbers
Visit mometrix.com/academy and enter code: 461071

Review Video: Prime and Composite Numbers
Visit mometrix.com/academy and enter code: 565581

Numbers in Word Form and Place Value

When writing numbers out in word form or translating word form to numbers, it is essential to understand how a place value system works. In the decimal or base-10 system, each digit of a number represents how many of the corresponding place value—a specific factor of 10—are contained in the number being represented. To make reading numbers easier, every three digits to the left of the decimal place is preceded by a comma. The following table demonstrates some of the place values:

Power of 10	10^3	10^2	10^1	10^0	10^{-1}	10^{-2}	10^{-3}
Value	1,000	100	10	1	0.1	0.01	0.001
Place	thousands	hundreds	tens	ones	tenths	hundredths	thousandths

For example, consider the number 4,546.09, which can be separated into each place value like this:

4: thousands
5: hundreds
4: tens
6: ones
0: tenths
9: hundredths

This number in word form would be *four thousand five hundred forty-six and nine hundredths.*

Review Video: Place Value
Visit mometrix.com/academy and enter code: 205433

Rational Numbers

The term **rational** means that the number can be expressed as a ratio or fraction. That is, a number, r, is rational if and only if it can be represented by a fraction $\frac{a}{b}$ where a and b are integers and b does not equal 0. The set of rational numbers includes integers and decimals. If there is no finite way to represent a value with a fraction of integers, then the number is **irrational**. Common examples of irrational numbers include: $\sqrt{5}$, $(1+\sqrt{2})$, and π.

Review Video: Rational and Irrational Numbers
Visit mometrix.com/academy and enter code: 280645

Review Video: Ordering Rational Numbers
Visit mometrix.com/academy and enter code: 419578

Number Lines

A number line is a graph to see the distance between numbers. Basically, this graph shows the relationship between numbers. So a number line may have a point for zero and may show negative numbers on the left side of the line. Any positive numbers are placed on the right side of the line. For example, consider the points labeled on the following number line:

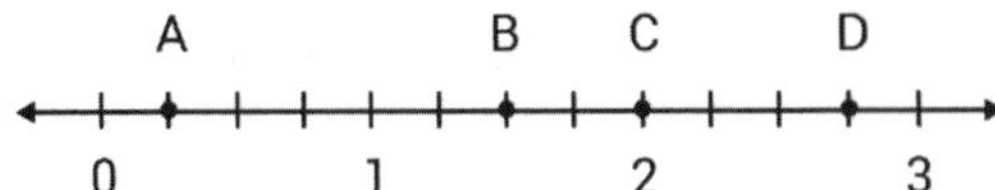

We can use the dashed lines on the number line to identify each point. Each dashed line between two whole numbers is $\frac{1}{4}$. The line halfway between two numbers is $\frac{1}{2}$.

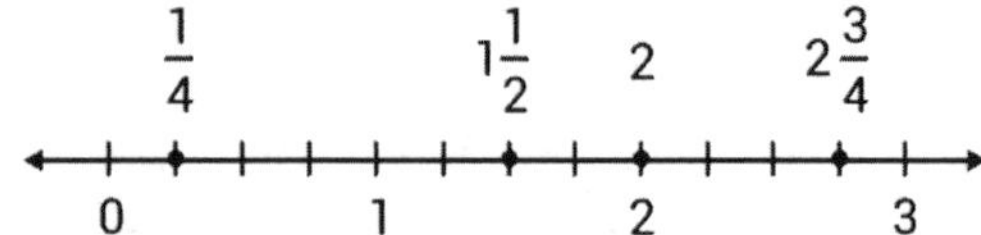

> **Review Video: The Number Line**
> Visit mometrix.com/academy and enter code: 816439

Rounding and Estimation

Rounding is reducing the digits in a number while still trying to keep the value similar. The result will be less accurate but in a simpler form and easier to use. Whole numbers can be rounded to the nearest ten, hundred, or thousand.

When you are asked to estimate the solution to a problem, you will need to provide only an approximate figure or **estimation** for your answer. In this situation, you will need to round each number in the calculation to the level indicated (nearest hundred, nearest thousand, etc.) or to a level that makes sense for the numbers involved. When estimating a sum **all numbers must be rounded to the same level**. You cannot round one number to the nearest thousand while rounding another to the nearest hundred.

> **Review Video: Rounding and Estimation**
> Visit mometrix.com/academy and enter code: 126243

Absolute Value

A precursor to working with negative numbers is understanding what **absolute values** are. A number's absolute value is simply the distance away from zero a number is on the number line. The absolute value of a number is always positive and is written $|x|$. For example, the absolute value of 3, written as $|3|$, is 3 because the distance between 0 and 3 on a number line is three units. Likewise, the absolute value of –3, written as $|-3|$, is 3 because the distance between 0 and –3 on a number line is three units. So $|3| = |-3|$.

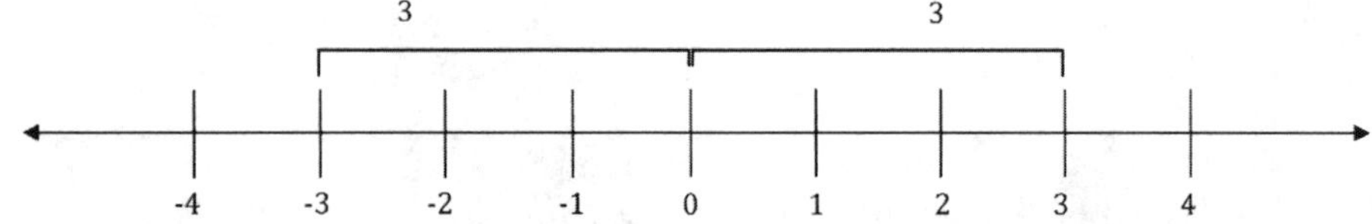

> **Review Video: Absolute Value**
> Visit mometrix.com/academy and enter code: 314669

Operations

An **operation** is simply a mathematical process that takes some value(s) as input(s) and produces an output. Elementary operations are often written in the following form: *value operation value*. For instance, in the expression $1 + 2$ the values are 1 and 2 and the operation is addition. Performing the operation gives the output of 3. In this way we can say that $1 + 2$ and 3 are equal, or $1 + 2 = 3$.

Addition

Addition increases the value of one quantity by the value of another quantity (both called **addends**). Example: $2 + 4 = 6$ or $8 + 9 = 17$. The result is called the **sum**. With addition, the order does not matter, $4 + 2 = 2 + 4$.

When adding signed numbers, if the signs are the same simply add the absolute values of the addends and apply the original sign to the sum. For example, $(+4) + (+8) = +12$ and $(-4) + (-8) = -12$. When the original signs are different, take the absolute values of the addends and subtract the smaller value from the larger value, then apply the original sign of the larger value to the difference. Example: $(+4) + (-8) = -4$ and $(-4) + (+8) = +4$.

Subtraction

Subtraction is the opposite operation to addition; it decreases the value of one quantity (the **minuend**) by the value of another quantity (the **subtrahend**). For example, $6 - 4 = 2$ or $17 - 8 = 9$. The result is called the **difference**. Note that with subtraction, the order does matter, $6 - 4 \neq 4 - 6$.

For subtracting signed numbers, change the sign of the subtrahend and then follow the same rules used for addition. Example: $(+4) - (+8) = (+4) + (-8) = -4$

Multiplication

Multiplication can be thought of as repeated addition. One number (the **multiplier**) indicates how many times to add the other number (the **multiplicand**) to itself. Example: $3 \times 2 = 2 + 2 + 2 = 6$. With multiplication, the order does not matter, $2 \times 3 = 3 \times 2$ or $3 + 3 = 2 + 2 + 2$, either way the result (the **product**) is the same.

If the signs are the same, the product is positive when multiplying signed numbers. Example: $(+4) \times (+8) = +32$ and $(-4) \times (-8) = +32$. If the signs are opposite, the product is negative. Example: $(+4) \times (-8) = -32$ and $(-4) \times (+8) = -32$. When more than two factors are multiplied together, the sign of the product is determined by how many negative factors are present. If there are an odd number of negative factors then the product is negative, whereas an even number of negative factors indicates a positive product. Example: $(+4) \times (-8) \times (-2) = +64$ and $(-4) \times (-8) \times (-2) = -64$.

Division

Division is the opposite operation to multiplication; one number (the **divisor**) tells us how many parts to divide the other number (the **dividend**) into. The result of division is called the **quotient**. Example: $20 \div 4 = 5$. If 20 is split into 4 equal parts, each part is 5. With division, the order of the numbers does matter, $20 \div 4 \neq 4 \div 20$.

The rules for dividing signed numbers are similar to multiplying signed numbers. If the dividend and divisor have the same sign, the quotient is positive. If the dividend and divisor have opposite signs, the quotient is negative. Example: $(-4) \div (+8) = -0.5$.

Review Video: Mathematical Operations
Visit mometrix.com/academy and enter code: 208095

Parentheses

Parentheses are used to designate which operations should be done first when there are multiple operations. Example: $4 - (2 + 1) = 1$; the parentheses tell us that we must add 2 and 1, and then subtract the sum from 4, rather than subtracting 2 from 4 and then adding 1 (this would give us an answer of 3).

Review Video: Mathematical Parentheses
Visit mometrix.com/academy and enter code: 978600

Exponents

An **exponent** is a superscript number placed next to another number at the top right. It indicates how many times the base number is to be multiplied by itself. Exponents provide a shorthand way to write what would be a longer mathematical expression, Example: $2^4 = 2 \times 2 \times 2 \times 2$. A number with an exponent of 2 is said to be "squared," while a number with an exponent of 3 is said to be "cubed." The value of a number raised to an exponent is called its power. So 8^4 is read as "8 to the 4th power," or "8 raised to the power of 4."

Review Video: What is an Exponent?
Visit mometrix.com/academy and enter code: 600998

Roots

A **root**, such as a square root, is another way of writing a fractional exponent. Instead of using a superscript, roots use the radical symbol ($\sqrt{\ }$) to indicate the operation. A radical will have a number underneath the bar, and may sometimes have a number in the upper left: $\sqrt[n]{a}$, read as "the nth root of a." The relationship between radical notation and exponent notation can be described by this equation:

$$\sqrt[n]{a} = a^{\frac{1}{n}}$$

The two special cases of $n = 2$ and $n = 3$ are called square roots and cube roots. If there is no number to the upper left, the radical is understood to be a square root ($n = 2$). Nearly all of the roots you encounter will be square roots. A square root is the same as a number raised to the one-half power. When we say that a is the square root of b ($a = \sqrt{b}$), we mean that a multiplied by itself equals b: ($a \times a = b$).

A **perfect square** is a number that has an integer for its square root. There are 10 perfect squares from 1 to 100: 1, 4, 9, 16, 25, 36, 49, 64, 81, 100 (the squares of integers 1 through 10).

Review Video: Roots
Visit mometrix.com/academy and enter code: 795655

Review Video: Perfect Squares and Square Roots
Visit mometrix.com/academy and enter code: 648063

Word Problems and Mathematical Symbols

When working on word problems, you must be able to translate verbal expressions or "math words" into math symbols. This chart contains several "math words" and their appropriate symbols:

Phrase	Symbol
equal, is, was, will be, has, costs, gets to, is the same as, becomes	=
times, of, multiplied by, product of, twice, doubles, halves, triples	×
divided by, per, ratio of/to, out of	÷
plus, added to, sum, combined, and, more than, totals of	+
subtracted from, less than, decreased by, minus, difference between	−
what, how much, original value, how many, a number, a variable	x, n, etc.

Examples of Translated Mathematical Phrases

- The phrase four more than twice a number can be written algebraically as $2x + 4$.
- The phrase half a number decreased by six can be written algebraically as $\frac{1}{2}x - 6$.
- The phrase the sum of a number and the product of five and that number can be written algebraically as $x + 5x$.
- You may see a test question that says, "Olivia is constructing a bookcase from seven boards. Two of them are for vertical supports and five are for shelves. The height of the bookcase is twice the width of the bookcase. If the seven boards total 36 feet in length, what will be the height of Olivia's bookcase?" You would need to make a sketch and then create the equation to determine the width of the shelves. The height can be represented as double the width. (If x represents the width of the shelves in feet, then the height of the bookcase is $2x$. Since the seven boards total 36 feet, $2x + 2x + x + x + x + x + x = 36$ or $9x = 36$; $x = 4$. The height is twice the width, or 8 feet.)

Properties of Exponents

The properties of exponents are as follows:

Property	Description
$a^1 = a$	Any number to the power of 1 is equal to itself
$1^n = 1$	The number 1 raised to any power is equal to 1
$a^0 = 1$	Any number raised to the power of 0 is equal to 1
$a^n \times a^m = a^{n+m}$	Add exponents to multiply powers of the same base number
$a^n \div a^m = a^{n-m}$	Subtract exponents to divide powers of the same base number
$(a^n)^m = a^{n \times m}$	When a power is raised to a power, the exponents are multiplied
$(a \times b)^n = a^n \times b^n$ $(a \div b)^n = a^n \div b^n$	Multiplication and division operations inside parentheses can be raised to a power. This is the same as each term being raised to that power.
$a^{-n} = \frac{1}{a^n}$	A negative exponent is the same as the reciprocal of a positive exponent

Note that exponents do not have to be integers. Fractional or decimal exponents follow all the rules above as well. Example: $5^{\frac{1}{4}} \times 5^{\frac{3}{4}} = 5^{\frac{1}{4}+\frac{3}{4}} = 5^1 = 5$.

Review Video: Properties of Exponents
Visit mometrix.com/academy and enter code: 532558

Scientific Notation

Scientific notation is a way of writing large numbers in a shorter form. The form $a \times 10^n$ is used in scientific notation, where a is greater than or equal to 1 but less than 10, and n is the number of places the decimal must move to get from the original number to a. Example: The number 230,400,000 is cumbersome to write. To write the value in scientific notation, place a decimal point between the first and second numbers, and include all digits through the last non-zero digit ($a = 2.304$). To find the appropriate power of 10, count the number of places the decimal point had to move ($n = 8$). The number is positive if the decimal moved to the left, and negative if it moved to the right. We can then write 230,400,000 as 2.304×10^8. If we look instead at the number 0.00002304, we have the same value for a, but this time the decimal moved 5 places to the right ($n = -5$). Thus, 0.00002304 can be written as 2.304×10^{-5}. Using this notation makes it simple to compare very large or very small numbers. By comparing exponents, it is easy to see that 3.28×10^4 is smaller than 1.51×10^5, because 4 is less than 5.

Review Video: Scientific Notation
Visit mometrix.com/academy and enter code: 976454

Factors and Multiples

Factors and Greatest Common Factor

Factors are numbers that are multiplied together to obtain a **product**. For example, in the equation $2 \times 3 = 6$, the numbers 2 and 3 are factors. A **prime number** has only two factors (1 and itself), but other numbers can have many factors.

A **common factor** is a number that divides exactly into two or more other numbers. For example, the factors of 12 are 1, 2, 3, 4, 6, and 12, while the factors of 15 are 1, 3, 5, and 15. The common factors of 12 and 15 are 1 and 3.

A **prime factor** is also a prime number. Therefore, the prime factors of 12 are 2 and 3. For 15, the prime factors are 3 and 5.

The **greatest common factor** (**GCF**) is the largest number that is a factor of two or more numbers. For example, the factors of 15 are 1, 3, 5, and 15; the factors of 35 are 1, 5, 7, and 35. Therefore, the greatest common factor of 15 and 35 is 5.

Review Video: Factors
Visit mometrix.com/academy and enter code: 920086

Review Video: Prime Numbers and Factorization
Visit mometrix.com/academy and enter code: 760669

Review Video: Greatest Common Factor and Least Common Multiple
Visit mometrix.com/academy and enter code: 838699

Multiples and Least Common Multiple

Often listed out in multiplication tables, **multiples** are integer increments of a given factor. In other words, dividing a multiple by the factor will result in an integer. For example, the multiples of 7 include: $1 \times 7 = 7$, $2 \times 7 = 14, 3 \times 7 = 21, 4 \times 7 = 28, 5 \times 7 = 35$. Dividing 7, 14, 21, 28, or 35 by 7 will result in the integers 1, 2, 3, 4, and 5, respectively.

The least common multiple (**LCM**) is the smallest number that is a multiple of two or more numbers. For example, the multiples of 3 include 3, 6, 9, 12, 15, etc.; the multiples of 5 include 5, 10, 15, 20, etc. Therefore, the least common multiple of 3 and 5 is 15.

Review Video: Multiples
Visit mometrix.com/academy and enter code: 626738

Calculations Using Points

Sometimes you need to perform calculations using only points on a graph as input data. Using points, you can determine what the **midpoint** and **distance** are. If you know the equation for a line, you can calculate the distance between the line and the point.

To find the **midpoint** of two points (x_1, y_1) and (x_2, y_2), average the x-coordinates to get the x-coordinate of the midpoint, and average the y-coordinates to get the y-coordinate of the midpoint. The formula is: $\left(\frac{x_1+x_2}{2}, \frac{y_1+y_2}{2}\right)$.

The **distance** between two points is the same as the length of the hypotenuse of a right triangle with the two given points as endpoints, and the two sides of the right triangle parallel to the x-axis and y-axis, respectively. The length of the segment parallel to the x-axis is the difference between the x-coordinates of the two points. The length of the segment parallel to the y-axis is the difference between the y-coordinates of the two points. Use the Pythagorean theorem $a^2 + b^2 = c^2$ or $c = \sqrt{a^2 + b^2}$ to find the distance. The formula is $d = \sqrt{(x_2 - x_1)^2 + (y_2 - y_1)^2}$.

When a line is in the format $Ax + By + C = 0$, where A, B, and C are coefficients, you can use a point (x_1, y_1) not on the line and apply the formula $d = \frac{|Ax_1+By_1+C|}{\sqrt{A^2+B^2}}$ to find the distance between the line and the point (x_1, y_1).

Review Video: Calculations Using Points on a Graph
Visit mometrix.com/academy and enter code: 883228

Basic Functions

Function and Relation

When expressing functional relationships, the **variables** x and y are typically used. These values are often written as the **coordinates** (x, y). The x-value is the independent variable and the y-value is the dependent variable. A **relation** is a set of data in which there is not a unique y-value for each x-value in the dataset. This means that there can be two of the same x-values assigned to different y-values. A relation is simply a relationship between the x- and y-values in each coordinate but does not apply to the relationship between the values of x and y in the data set. A **function** is a relation where one quantity depends on the other. For example, the amount of money that you make depends on the number of hours that you work. In a function, each x-value in the data set has one unique y-value because the y-value depends on the x-value.

Functions

A function has exactly one value of **output variable** (dependent variable) for each value of the **input variable** (independent variable). The set of all values for the input variable (here assumed to be x) is the domain of the function, and the set of all corresponding values of the output variable (here assumed to be y) is the range of the function. When looking at a graph of an equation, the easiest way to determine if the equation is a function or not is to conduct the vertical line test. If a vertical line drawn through any value of x crosses the graph in more than one place, the equation is not a function.

Determining a Function

You can determine whether an equation is a **function** by substituting different values into the equation for x. You can display and organize these numbers in a data table. A **data table** contains the values for x and y, which you can also list as coordinates. In order for a function to exist, the table cannot contain any repeating x-values that correspond with different y-values. If each x-coordinate has a unique y-coordinate, the table contains a function. However, there can be repeating y-values that correspond with different x-values. An example of this is when the function contains an exponent. Example: if $x^2 = y$, $2^2 = 4$, and $(-2)^2 = 4$.

Review Video: Definition of a Function
Visit mometrix.com/academy and enter code: 784611

Finding the Domain and Range of a Function

The **domain** of a function $f(x)$ is the set of all input values for which the function is defined. The **range** of a function $f(x)$ is the set of all possible output values of the function—that is, of every possible value of $f(x)$, for any value of x in the function's domain. For a function expressed in a table, every input-output pair is given explicitly. To find the domain, we just list all the x-values and to find the range, we just list all the values of $f(x)$. Consider the following example:

x	-1	4	2	1	0	3	8	6
$f(x)$	3	0	3	-1	-1	2	4	6

In this case, the domain would be $\{-1, 4, 2, 1, 0, 3, 8, 6\}$ or, putting them in ascending order, $\{-1, 0, 1, 2, 3, 4, 6, 8\}$. (Putting the values in ascending order isn't strictly necessary, but generally makes the set easier to read.) The range would be $\{3, 0, 3, -1, -1, 2, 4, 6\}$. Note that some of these values appear more than once. This is entirely permissible for a function; while each value of x must be matched to a unique value of $f(x)$, the converse is not true. We don't need to list each value more than once, so eliminating duplicates, the range is $\{3, 0, -1, 2, 4, 6\}$, or, putting them in ascending order, $\{-1, 0, 2, 3, 4, 6\}$.

Note that by definition of a function, no input value can be matched to more than one output value. It is good to double-check to make sure that the data given follows this and is therefore actually a function.

Review Video: Domain and Range
Visit mometrix.com/academy and enter code: 778133

Review Video: Domain and Range of Quadratic Functions
Visit mometrix.com/academy and enter code: 331768

Writing a Function Rule Using a Table

If given a set of data, place the corresponding x- and y-values into a table and analyze the relationship between them. Consider what you can do to each x-value to obtain the corresponding y-value. Try adding or subtracting different numbers to and from x and then try multiplying or dividing different numbers to and from x. If none of these **operations** give you the y-value, try combining the operations. Once you find a rule that works for one pair, make sure to try it with each additional set of ordered pairs in the table. If the same operation or combination of operations satisfies each set of coordinates, then the table contains a function. The rule is then used to write the equation of the function in "$y = f(x)$" form.

Direct and Inverse Variations of Variables

Variables that vary directly are those that either both increase at the same rate or both decrease at the same rate. For example, in the functions $y = kx$ or $y = kx^n$, where k and n are positive, the value of y increases as the value of x increases and decreases as the value of x decreases.

Variables that vary inversely are those where one increases while the other decreases. For example, in the functions $y = \frac{k}{x}$ or $y = \frac{k}{x^n}$ where k and n are positive, the value of y increases as the value of x decreases and decreases as the value of x increases.

In both cases, k is the constant of variation.

Properties of Functions

There are many different ways to classify functions based on their structure or behavior. Important features of functions include:

- **End behavior**: the behavior of the function at extreme values ($f(x)$ as $x \to \pm\infty$)
- **y-intercept**: the value of the function at $f(0)$
- **Roots**: the values of x where the function equals zero ($f(x) = 0$)
- **Extrema**: minimum or maximum values of the function or where the function changes direction ($f(x) \geq k$ or $f(x) \leq k$)

Classification of Functions

An **invertible function** is defined as a function, $f(x)$, for which there is another function, $f^{-1}(x)$, such that $f^{-1}(f(x)) = x$. For example, if $f(x) = 3x - 2$ the inverse function, $f^{-1}(x)$, can be found:

$$x = 3(f^{-1}(x)) - 2$$
$$\frac{x+2}{3} = f^{-1}(x)$$

$$f^{-1}(f(x)) = \frac{3x - 2 + 2}{3}$$
$$= \frac{3x}{3}$$
$$= x$$

Note that $f^{-1}(x)$ is a valid function over all values of x.

In a **one-to-one function**, each value of x has exactly one value for y on the coordinate plane (this is the definition of a function) and each value of y has exactly one value for x. While the vertical line test will determine if a graph is that of a function, the horizontal line test will determine if a function is a one-to-one function. If a horizontal line drawn at any value of y intersects the graph in more than one place, the graph is not that of a one-to-one function. Do not make the mistake of using the horizontal line test exclusively in determining if a graph is that of a one-to-one function. A one-to-one function must pass both the vertical line test and the horizontal line test. As such, one-to-one functions are invertible functions.

A **many-to-one function** is a function whereby the relation is a function, but the inverse of the function is not a function. In other words, each element in the domain is mapped to one and only one element in the range. However, one or more elements in the range may be mapped to the same element in the domain. A graph of a many-to-one function would pass the vertical line test, but not the horizontal line test. This is why many-to-one functions are not invertible.

A **monotone function** is a function whose graph either constantly increases or constantly decreases. Examples include the functions $f(x) = x$, $f(x) = -x$, or $f(x) = x^3$.

An **even function** has a graph that is symmetric with respect to the y-axis and satisfies the equation $f(x) = f(-x)$. Examples include the functions $f(x) = x^2$ and $f(x) = ax^n$, where a is any real number and n is a positive even integer.

An **odd function** has a graph that is symmetric with respect to the origin and satisfies the equation $f(x) = -f(-x)$. Examples include the functions $f(x) = x^3$ and $f(x) = ax^n$, where a is any real number and n is a positive odd integer.

Review Video: Even and Odd Functions
Visit mometrix.com/academy and enter code: 278985

Constant functions are given by the equation $f(x) = b$, where b is a real number. There is no independent variable present in the equation, so the function has a constant value for all x. The graph of a constant function is a horizontal line of slope 0 that is positioned b units from the x-axis. If b is positive, the line is above the x-axis; if b is negative, the line is below the x-axis.

Identity functions are identified by the equation $f(x) = x$, where every value of the function is equal to its corresponding value of x. The only zero is the point (0,0). The graph is a line with a slope of 1.

In **linear functions**, the value of the function changes in direct proportion to x. The rate of change, represented by the slope on its graph, is constant throughout. The standard form of a linear equation is $ax + cy = d$, where a, c, and d are real numbers. As a function, this equation is commonly in the form $y = mx + b$ or $f(x) = mx + b$ where $m = -\frac{a}{c}$ and $b = \frac{d}{c}$. This is known as the slope-intercept form, because the coefficients give the slope of the graphed function (m) and its y-intercept (b). Solve the equation $mx + b = 0$ for x to get $x = -\frac{b}{m}$, which is the only zero of the function. The domain and range are both the set of all real numbers.

Review Video: Graphing Linear Functions
Visit mometrix.com/academy and enter code: 699478

Algebraic functions are those that exclusively use polynomials and roots. These would include polynomial functions, rational functions, square root functions, and all combinations of these functions, such as polynomials as the radicand. These combinations may be joined by addition, subtraction, multiplication, or division, but may not include variables as exponents.

Review Video: Common Functions
Visit mometrix.com/academy and enter code: 629798

Absolute Value Functions

An **absolute value function** is in the format $f(x) = |ax + b|$. Like other functions, the domain is the set of all real numbers. However, because absolute value indicates positive numbers, the range is limited to positive real numbers. To find the zero of an absolute value function, set the portion inside the absolute value sign equal to zero and solve for x. An absolute value function is also known as a piecewise function because it must be solved in pieces—one for if the value inside the absolute value sign is positive, and one for if the value is negative. The function can be expressed as:

$$f(x) = \begin{cases} ax + b \text{ if } ax + b \geq 0 \\ -(ax + b) \text{ if } ax + b < 0 \end{cases}$$

This will allow for an accurate statement of the range. The graph of an example absolute value function, $f(x) = |2x - 1|$, is below:

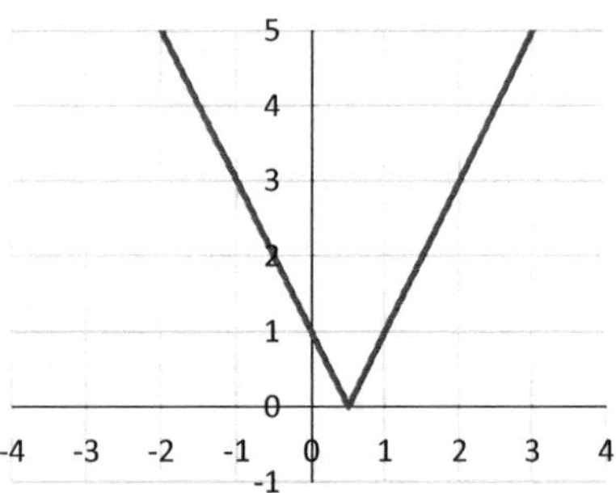

Piecewise Functions

A **piecewise function** is a function that has different definitions on two or more different intervals. The following, for instance, is one example of a piecewise-defined function:

$$f(x) = \begin{cases} x^2, & x < 0 \\ x, & 0 \leq x \leq 2 \\ (x-2)^2, & x > 2 \end{cases}$$

To graph this function, you would simply graph each part separately in the appropriate domain. The final graph would look like this:

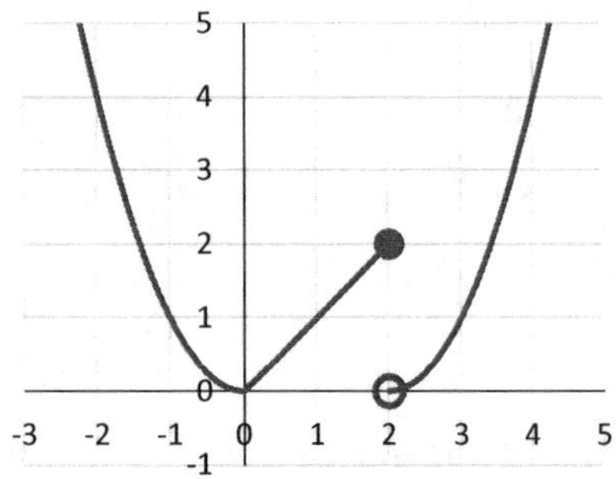

Note the filled and hollow dots at the discontinuity at $x = 2$. This is important to show which side of the graph that point corresponds to. Because $f(x) = x$ on the closed interval $0 \leq x \leq 2$, $f(2) = 2$. The point $(2, 2)$ is therefore marked with a filled circle, and the point (2,0), which is the endpoint of the rightmost $(x - 2)^2$ part of the graph but *not actually part of the function*, is marked with a hollow dot to indicate this.

Review Video: Piecewise Functions
Visit mometrix.com/academy and enter code: 707921

Quadratic Functions

A **quadratic function** is a function in the form $y = ax^2 + bx + c$, where a does not equal 0. While a linear function forms a line, a quadratic function forms a **parabola**, which is a u-shaped figure that either opens upward or downward. A parabola that opens upward is said to be a **positive quadratic function,** and a parabola that opens downward is said to be a **negative quadratic function**. The shape of a parabola can differ, depending on the values of a, b, and c. All parabolas contain a **vertex**, which is the highest possible point, the **maximum**, or the lowest possible point, the **minimum**. This is the point where the graph begins moving in the opposite direction. A quadratic function can have zero, one, or two solutions, and therefore zero, one, or two x-intercepts. Recall that the x-intercepts are referred to as the zeros, or roots, of a function. A quadratic function will have only one y-intercept. Understanding the basic components of a quadratic function can give you an idea of the shape of its graph.

Example graph of a positive quadratic function, $x^2 + 2x - 3$:

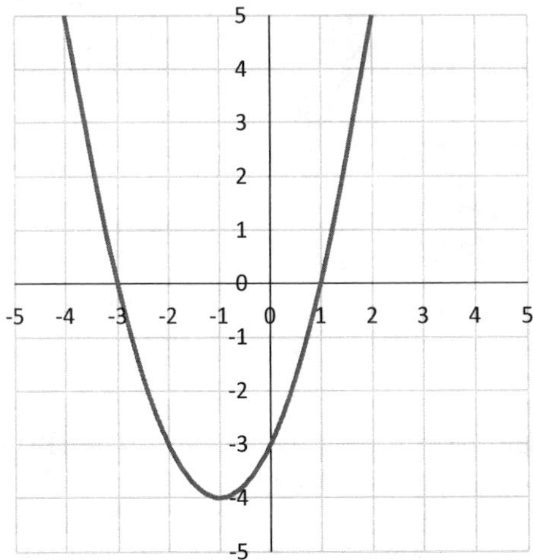

Polynomial Functions

A **polynomial function** is a function with multiple terms and multiple powers of x, such as:

$$f(x) = a_n x^n + a_{n-1}x^{n-1} + a_{n-2}x^{n-2} + \cdots + a_1 x + a_0$$

where n is a non-negative integer that is the highest exponent in the polynomial and $a_n \neq 0$. The domain of a polynomial function is the set of all real numbers. If the greatest exponent in the polynomial is even, the polynomial is said to be of even degree and the range is the set of real numbers that satisfy the function. If the greatest exponent in the polynomial is odd, the polynomial is said to be odd and the range, like the domain, is the set of all real numbers.

Rational Functions

A **rational function** is a function that can be constructed as a ratio of two polynomial expressions: $f(x) = \frac{p(x)}{q(x)}$, where $p(x)$ and $q(x)$ are both polynomial expressions and $q(x) \neq 0$. The domain is the set of all real numbers, except any values for which $q(x) = 0$. The range is the set of real numbers that satisfies the function when the domain is applied. When you graph a rational function, you will have vertical asymptotes wherever $q(x) = 0$. If the polynomial in the numerator is of lesser degree than the polynomial in the denominator, the x-axis will also be a horizontal asymptote. If the numerator and denominator have equal degrees, there will be a horizontal asymptote not on the x-axis. If the degree of the numerator is exactly one greater than the degree of the denominator, the graph will have an oblique, or diagonal, asymptote. The asymptote will be along the line $y = \frac{p_n}{q_{n-1}}x + \frac{p_{n-1}}{q_{n-1}}$, where p_n and q_{n-1} are the coefficients of the highest degree terms in their respective polynomials.

Square Root Functions

A **square root function** is a function that contains a radical and is in the format $f(x) = \sqrt{ax + b}$. The domain is the set of all real numbers that yields a positive radicand or a radicand equal to zero. Because square root values are assumed to be positive unless otherwise identified, the range is all real numbers from zero to infinity. To find the zero of a square root function, set the radicand equal to zero and solve for x. The graph of a square root function is always to the right of the zero and always above the x-axis.

Example graph of a square root function, $f(x) = \sqrt{2x+1}$:

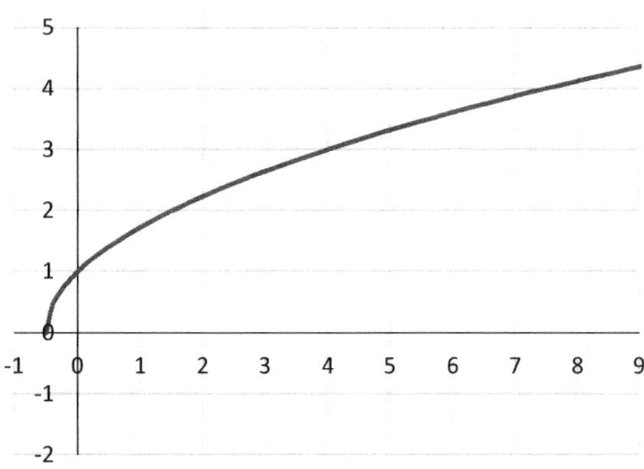

Basic Trigonometric Functions

Sine

The **sine** (sin) function has a period of 360° or 2π radians. This means that its graph makes one complete cycle every 360° or 2π. Because $\sin 0 = 0$, the graph of $y = \sin x$ begins at the origin, with the x-axis representing the angle measure, and the y-axis representing the sine of the angle. The graph of the sine function is a smooth curve that begins at the origin, peaks at the point $\left(\frac{\pi}{2}, 1\right)$, crosses the x-axis at $(\pi, 0)$, has its lowest point at $\left(\frac{3\pi}{2}, -1\right)$, and returns to the x-axis to complete one cycle at $(2\pi, 0)$.

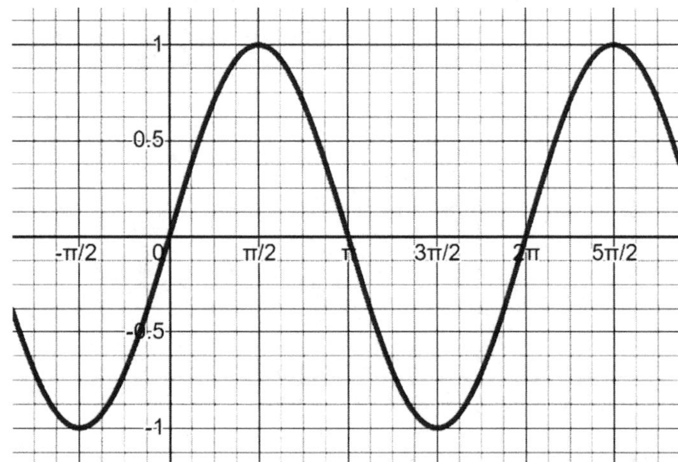

Review Video: Upper Level Trig: Sine
Visit mometrix.com/academy and enter code: 193339

Cosine

The **cosine** (cos) function also has a period of 360° or 2π radians, which means that its graph also makes one complete cycle every 360° or 2π. Because $\cos 0° = 1$, the graph of $y = \cos x$ begins at the point $(0, 1)$, with the x-axis representing the angle measure, and the y-axis representing the cosine of the angle. The graph of the cosine function is a smooth curve that begins at the point (0,1), crosses the x-axis at the point $\left(\frac{\pi}{2}, 0\right)$, has its lowest point at $(\pi, -1)$, crosses the x-axis again at the point $\left(\frac{3\pi}{2}, 0\right)$, and returns to a peak at the point $(2\pi, 1)$ to complete one cycle.

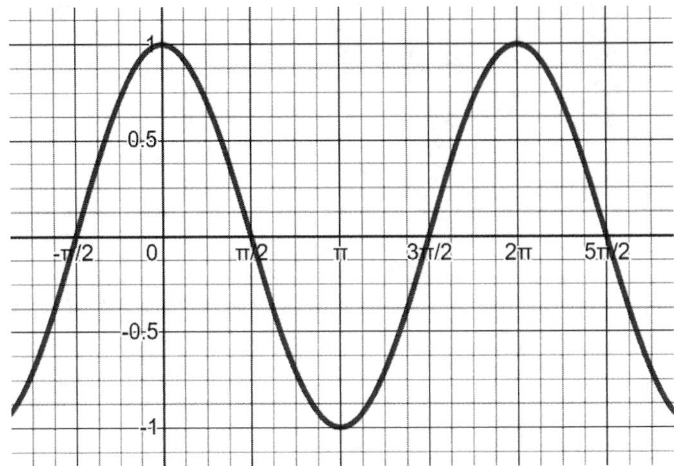

Review Video: Upper Level Trig: Cosine
Visit mometrix.com/academy and enter code: 361120

Tangent

The **tangent** (tan) function has a period of 180° or π radians, which means that its graph makes one complete cycle every 180° or π radians. The x-axis represents the angle measure, and the y-axis represents the tangent of the angle. The graph of the tangent function is a series of smooth curves that cross the x-axis at every 180° or π radians and have an asymptote every $k \times 90°$ or $\frac{k\pi}{2}$ radians, where k is an odd integer. This can be explained by the fact that the tangent is calculated by dividing the sine by the cosine, since the cosine equals zero at those asymptote points.

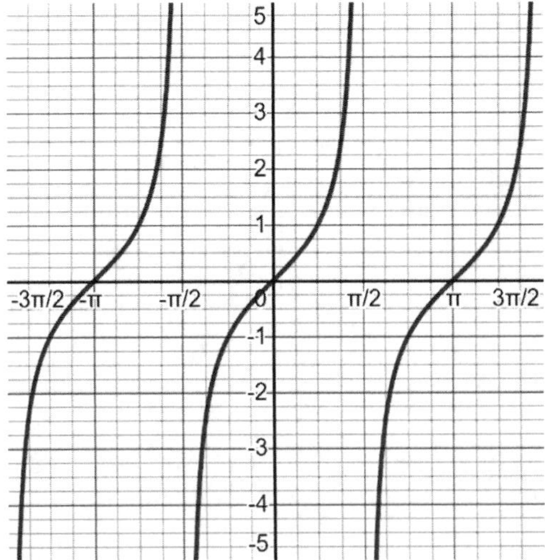

Review Video: Upper Level Trig: Tangent
Visit mometrix.com/academy and enter code: 947639

Measures of Central Tendency

A **measure of central tendency** is a statistical value that gives a reasonable estimate for the center of a group of data. There are several different ways of describing the measure of central tendency. Each one has a unique way it is calculated, and each one gives a slightly different perspective on the data set. Whenever you give a measure of central tendency, always make sure the units are the same. If the data has different units, such as hours, minutes, and seconds, convert all the data to the same unit, and use the same unit in the measure of central tendency. If no units are given in the data, do not give units for the measure of central tendency.

MEAN

The **statistical mean** of a group of data is the same as the arithmetic average of that group. To find the mean of a set of data, first convert each value to the same units, if necessary. Then find the sum of all the values, and count the total number of data values, making sure you take into consideration each individual value. If a value appears more than once, count it more than once. Divide the sum of the values by the total number of values and apply the units, if any. Note that the mean does not have to be one of the data values in the set, and may not divide evenly.

$$\text{mean} = \frac{\text{sum of the data values}}{\text{quantity of data values}}$$

For instance, the mean of the data set {88, 72, 61, 90, 97, 68, 88, 79, 86, 93, 97, 71, 80, 84, 89} would be the sum of the fifteen numbers divided by 15:

$$\frac{88 + 72 + 61 + 90 + 97 + 68 + 88 + 79 + 86 + 93 + 97 + 71 + 80 + 84 + 89}{15} = \frac{1242}{15} = 82.8$$

While the mean is relatively easy to calculate and averages are understood by most people, the mean can be very misleading if it is used as the sole measure of central tendency. If the data set has outliers (data values that are unusually high or unusually low compared to the rest of the data values), the mean can be very distorted, especially if the data set has a small number of values. If unusually high values are countered with unusually low values, the mean is not affected as much. For example, if five of twenty students in a class get a 100 on a test, but the other 15 students have an average of 60 on the same test, the class average would appear as 70. Whenever the mean is skewed by outliers, it is always a good idea to include the median as an alternate measure of central tendency.

A **weighted mean**, or weighted average, is a mean that uses "weighted" values. The formula is weighted mean $= \frac{w_1x_1+w_2x_2+w_3x_3...+w_nx_n}{w_1+w_2+w_3+\cdots+w_n}$. Weighted values, such as $w_1, w_2, w_3, ... w_n$ are assigned to each member of the set $x_1, x_2, x_3, ... x_n$. When calculating the weighted mean, make sure a weight value for each member of the set is used.

Review Video: All About Averages
Visit mometrix.com/academy and enter code: 176521

MEDIAN

The **statistical median** is the value in the middle of the set of data. To find the median, list all data values in order from smallest to largest or from largest to smallest. Any value that is repeated in the set must be listed the number of times it appears. If there are an odd number of data values, the median is the value in the middle of the list. If there is an even number of data values, the median is the arithmetic mean of the two middle values.

For example, the median of the data set {88, 72, 61, 90, 97, 68, 88, 79, 86, 93, 97, 71, 80, 84, 88} is 86 since the ordered set is {61, 68, 71, 72, 79, 80, 84, **86**, 88, 88, 88, 90, 93, 97, 97}.

The big disadvantage of using the median as a measure of central tendency is that is relies solely on a value's relative size as compared to the other values in the set. When the individual values in a set of data are evenly dispersed, the median can be an accurate tool. However, if there is a group of rather large values or a group of rather small values that are not offset by a different group of values, the information that can be inferred from the median may not be accurate because the distribution of values is skewed.

MODE

The **statistical mode** is the data value that occurs the greatest number of times in the data set. It is possible to have exactly one mode, more than one mode, or no mode. To find the mode of a set of data, arrange the data like you do to find the median (all values in order, listing all multiples of data values). Count the number of times each value appears in the data set. If all values appear an equal number of times, there is no mode. If one value appears more than any other value, that value is the mode. If two or more values appear the same number of times, but there are other values that appear fewer times and no values that appear more times, all of those values are the modes.

For example, the mode of the data set {**88**, 72, 61, 90, 97, 68, **88**, 79, 86, 93, 97, 71, 80, 84, **88**} is 88.

The main disadvantage of the mode is that the values of the other data in the set have no bearing on the mode. The mode may be the largest value, the smallest value, or a value anywhere in between in the set. The mode only tells which value or values, if any, occurred the greatest number of times. It does not give any suggestions about the remaining values in the set.

Review Video: Mean, Median, and Mode
Visit mometrix.com/academy and enter code: 286207

DISPLAYING INFORMATION

FREQUENCY TABLES

Frequency tables show how frequently each unique value appears in a set. A **relative frequency table** is one that shows the proportions of each unique value compared to the entire set. Relative frequencies are given as percentages; however, the total percent for a relative frequency table will not necessarily equal 100 percent due to rounding. An example of a frequency table with relative frequencies is below.

Favorite Color	Frequency	Relative Frequency
Blue	4	13%
Red	7	22%
Green	3	9%
Purple	6	19%
Cyan	12	38%

Review Video: Data Interpretation of Graphs
Visit mometrix.com/academy and enter code: 200439

CIRCLE GRAPHS

Circle graphs, also known as *pie charts*, provide a visual depiction of the relationship of each type of data compared to the whole set of data. The circle graph is divided into sections by drawing radii to create central angles whose percentage of the circle is equal to the individual data's percentage of the whole set. Each 1% of data is equal to 3.6° in the circle graph. Therefore, data represented by a 90° section of the circle graph makes up 25% of the whole. When complete, a circle graph often looks like a pie cut into uneven wedges. The pie chart below shows the data from the frequency table referenced earlier where people were asked their favorite color.

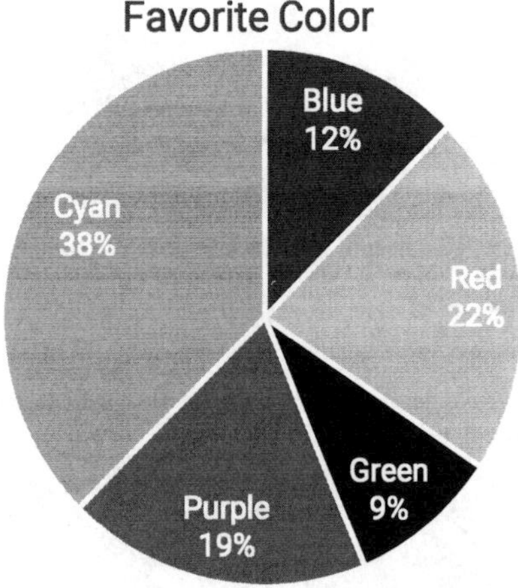

Pictographs

A **pictograph** is a graph, generally in the horizontal orientation, that uses pictures or symbols to represent the data. Each pictograph must have a key that defines the picture or symbol and gives the quantity each picture or symbol represents. Pictures or symbols on a pictograph are not always shown as whole elements. In this case, the fraction of the picture or symbol shown represents the same fraction of the quantity a whole picture or symbol stands for. For example, a row with $3\frac{1}{2}$ ears of corn, where each ear of corn represents 100 stalks of corn in a field, would equal $3\frac{1}{2} \times 100 = 350$ stalks of corn in the field.

Review Video: Pictographs Visit mometrix.com/academy and enter code: 147860

Line Graphs

Line graphs have one or more lines of varying styles (solid or broken) to show the different values for a set of data. The individual data are represented as ordered pairs, much like on a Cartesian plane. In this case, the x- and y-axes are defined in terms of their units, such as dollars or time. The individual plotted points are joined by line segments to show whether the value of the data is increasing (line sloping upward), decreasing (line sloping downward), or staying the same (horizontal line). Multiple sets of data can be graphed on the same line graph to give an easy visual comparison. An example of this would be graphing achievement test scores for different groups of students over the same time period to see which group had the greatest increase or decrease in performance from year to year (as shown below).

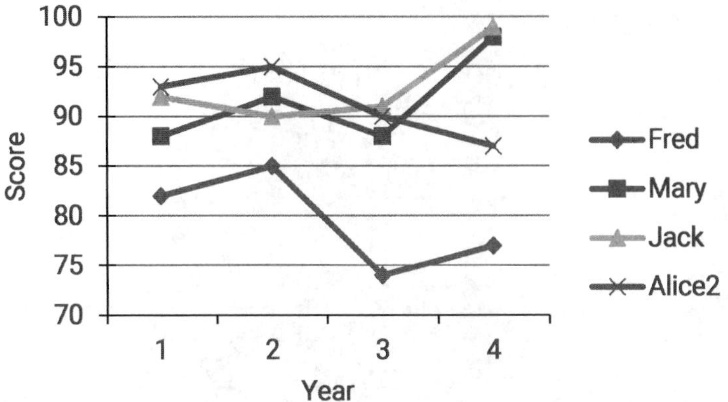

Review Video: How to Create a Line Graph
Visit mometrix.com/academy and enter code: 480147

Line Plots

A **line plot**, also known as a *dot plot*, has plotted points that are not connected by line segments. In this graph, the horizontal axis lists the different possible values for the data, and the vertical axis lists the number of times the individual value occurs. A single dot is graphed for each value to show the number of times it occurs. This graph is more closely related to a bar graph than a line graph. Do not connect the dots in a line plot or it will misrepresent the data.

Review Video: Line Plot
Visit mometrix.com/academy and enter code: 754610

Stem and Leaf Plots

A **stem and leaf plot** is useful for depicting groups of data that fall into a range of values. Each piece of data is separated into two parts: the first, or left, part is called the stem; the second, or right, part is called the leaf. Each stem is listed in a column from smallest to largest. Each leaf that has the common stem is listed in that stem's row from smallest to largest. For example, in a set of two-digit numbers, the digit in the tens place is the stem, and the digit in the ones place is the leaf. With a stem and leaf plot, you can easily see which subset of numbers (10s, 20s, 30s, etc.) is the largest. This information is also readily available by looking at a histogram, but a stem and leaf plot also allows you to look closer and see exactly which values fall in that range. Using a sample set of test scores (82, 88, 92, 93, 85, 90, 92, 95, 74, 88, 90, 91, 78, 87, 98, 99), we can assemble a stem and leaf plot like the one below.

Test Scores

7	4	8							
8	2	5	7	8	8				
9	0	0	1	2	2	3	5	8	9

Review Video: Stem and Leaf Plots
Visit mometrix.com/academy and enter code: 302339

BAR GRAPHS

A **bar graph** is one of the few graphs that can be drawn correctly in two different configurations – both horizontally and vertically. A bar graph is similar to a line plot in the way the data is organized on the graph. Both axes must have their categories defined for the graph to be useful. Rather than placing a single dot to mark the point of the data's value, a bar, or thick line, is drawn from zero to the exact value of the data, whether it is a number, percentage, or other numerical value. Longer bar lengths correspond to greater data values. To read a bar graph, read the labels for the axes to find the units being reported. Then, look where the bars end in relation to the scale given on the corresponding axis and determine the associated value.

The bar chart below represents the responses from our favorite-color survey.

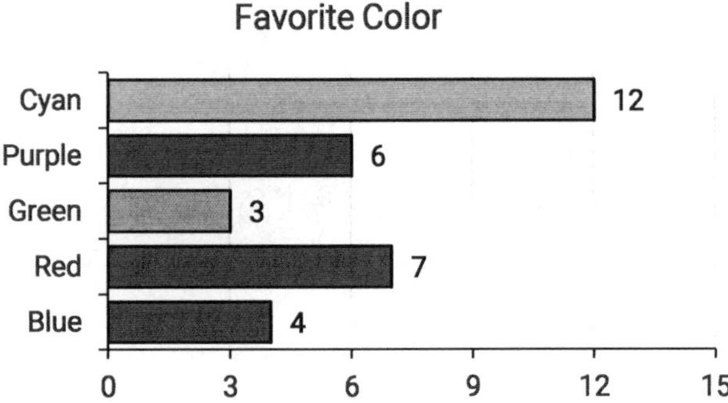

HISTOGRAMS

At first glance, a **histogram** looks like a vertical bar graph. The difference is that a bar graph has a separate bar for each piece of data and a histogram has one continuous bar for each *range* of data. For example, a histogram may have one bar for the range 0–9, one bar for 10–19, etc. While a bar graph has numerical values on one axis, a histogram has numerical values on both axes. Each range is of equal size, and they are ordered left to right from lowest to highest. The height of each column on a histogram represents the number of data values within that range. Like a stem and leaf plot, a histogram makes it easy to glance at the graph and quickly determine which range has the greatest quantity of values. A simple example of a histogram is below.

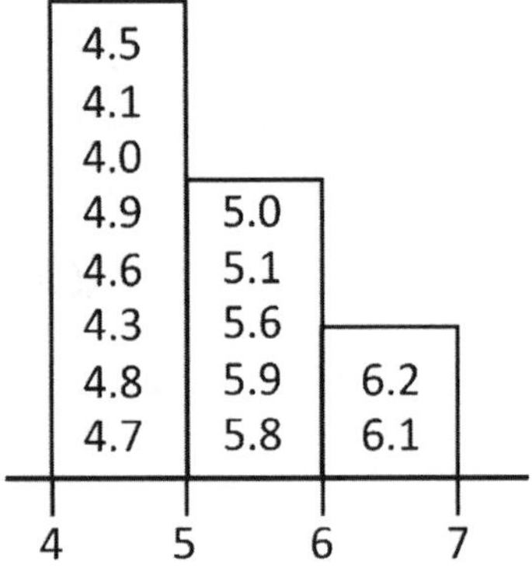

5-NUMBER SUMMARY

The **5-number summary** of a set of data gives a very informative picture of the set. The five numbers in the summary include the minimum value, maximum value, and the three quartiles. This information gives the reader the range and median of the set, as well as an indication of how the data is spread about the median.

BOX AND WHISKER PLOTS

A **box-and-whiskers plot** is a graphical representation of the 5-number summary. To draw a box-and-whiskers plot, plot the points of the 5-number summary on a number line. Draw a box whose ends are through the points for the first and third quartiles. Draw a vertical line in the box through the median to divide the box in half. Draw a line segment from the first quartile point to the minimum value, and from the third quartile point to the maximum value.

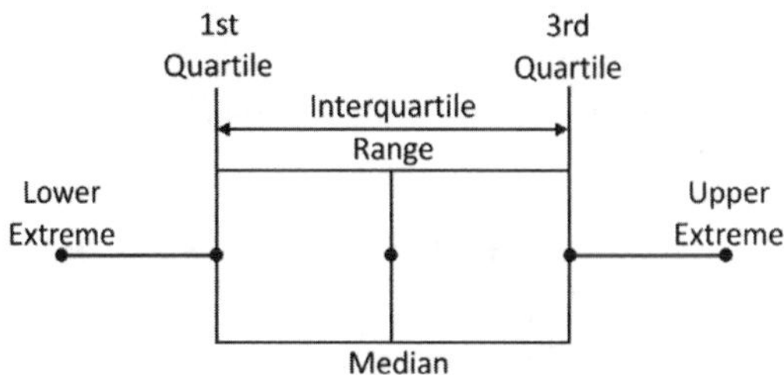

Review Video: Box and Whisker Plots
Visit mometrix.com/academy and enter code: 810817

EXAMPLE

Given the following data (32, 28, 29, 26, 35, 27, 30, 31, 27, 32), we first sort it into numerical order: 26, 27, 27, 28, 29, 30, 31, 32, 32, 35. We can then find the median. Since there are ten values, we take the average of the 5th and 6th values to get 29.5. We find the lower quartile by taking the median of the data smaller than the median. Since there are five values, we take the 3rd value, which is 27. We find the upper quartile by taking the median of the data larger than the overall median, which is 32. Finally, we note our minimum and maximum, which are simply the smallest and largest values in the set: 26 and 35, respectively. Now we can create our box plot:

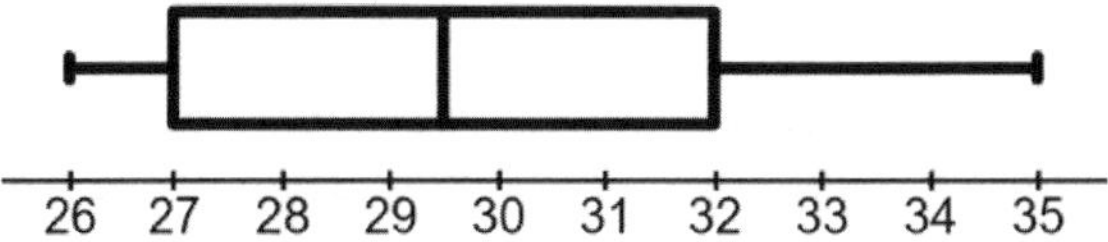

This plot is fairly "long" on the right whisker, showing one or more unusually high values (but not quite outliers). The other quartiles are similar in length, showing a fairly even distribution of data.

INTERQUARTILE RANGE

The **interquartile range, or IQR**, is the difference between the upper and lower quartiles. It measures how the data is dispersed: a high IQR means that the data is more spread out, while a low IQR means that the data is clustered more tightly around the median. To find the IQR, subtract the lower quartile value (Q_1) from the upper quartile value (Q_3).

EXAMPLE

To find the upper and lower quartiles, we first find the median and then take the median of all values above it and all values below it. In the following data set (16, 18, 13, 24, 16, 51, 32, 21, 27, 39), we first rearrange the values in numerical order: 13, 16, 16, 18, 21, 24, 27, 32, 39, 51. There are 10 values, so the median is the average of the 5th and 6th: $\frac{21+24}{2} = \frac{45}{2} = 22.5$. We do not actually need this value to find the upper and lower quartiles. We look at the set of numbers below the median: 13, 16, 16, 18, 21. There are five values, so the 3rd is the median (16), or the value of the lower quartile (Q_1). Then we look at the numbers above the median: 24, 27, 32, 39, 51. Again there are five values, so the 3rd is the median (32), or the value of the upper quartile (Q_3). We find the IQR by subtracting Q_1 from Q_3: $32 - 16 = 16$.

68-95-99.7 Rule

The **68–95–99.7 rule** describes how a normal distribution of data should appear when compared to the mean. This is also a description of a normal bell curve. According to this rule, 68 percent of the data values in a normally distributed set should fall within one standard deviation of the mean (34 percent above and 34 percent below the mean), 95 percent of the data values should fall within two standard deviations of the mean (47.5 percent above and 47.5 percent below the mean), and 99.7 percent of the data values should fall within three standard deviations of the mean, again, equally distributed on either side of the mean. This means that only 0.3 percent of all data values should fall more than three standard deviations from the mean. On the graph below, the normal curve is centered on the y-axis. The x-axis labels are how many standard deviations away from the center you are. Therefore, it is easy to see how the 68-95-99.7 rule can apply.

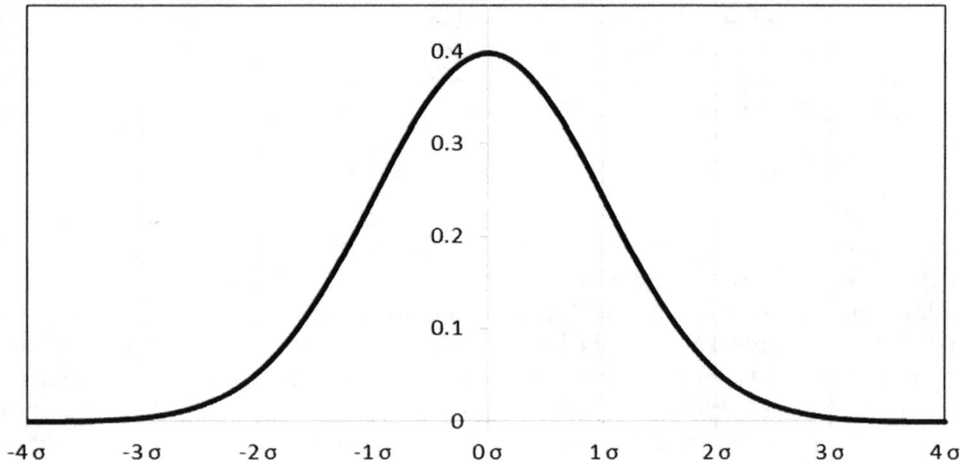

Science

Science Cognitive Skills

Safety and Equipment

Laboratory Accidents

Any spills or accidents should be **reported** to the teacher so that the teacher can determine the safest clean-up method. The student should start to wash off a **chemical** spilled on the skin while reporting the incident. Some spills may require removal of contaminated clothing and use of the **safety shower**. Broken glass should be disposed of in a designated container. If someone's clothing catches fire they should walk to the safety shower and use it to extinguish the flames. A fire blanket may be used to smother a **lab fire**. A fire extinguisher, phone, spill neutralizers, and a first aid box are other types of **safety equipment** found in the lab. Students should be familiar with **routes** out of the room and the building in case of fire. Students should use the **eye wash station** if a chemical gets in the eyes.

Safety Procedures

Students should wear a **lab apron** and **safety goggles**. Loose or dangling clothing and jewelry, necklaces, and earrings should not be worn. Those with long hair should tie it back. Care should always be taken not to splash chemicals. Open-toed shoes such as sandals and flip-flops should not be worn, nor should wrist watches. Glasses are preferable to contact lenses since the latter carries a risk of chemicals getting caught between the lens and the eye. Students should always be supervised. The area where the experiment is taking place and the surrounding floor should be free of clutter. Only the lab book and the items necessary for the experiment should be present. Smoking, eating, and chewing gum are not permitted in the lab. Cords should not be allowed to dangle from work stations. There should be no rough-housing in the lab. Hands should be washed after the lab is complete.

Fume Hoods

Because of the potential safety hazards associated with chemistry lab experiments, such as fire from vapors and the inhalation of toxic fumes, a **fume hood** should be used in many instances. A fume hood carries away vapors from reagents or reactions. Equipment or reactions are placed as far back in the hood as practical to help enhance the collection of the fumes. The **glass safety shield** automatically closes to the appropriate height, and should be low enough to protect the face and body. The safety shield should only be raised to move equipment in and out of the hood. One should not climb inside a hood or stick one's head inside. All spills should be wiped up immediately and the glass should be cleaned if a splash occurs.

Common Safety Hazards

Some specific safety hazards possible in a chemistry lab include:

- **Fire**: Fire can be caused by volatile solvents such as ether, acetone, and benzene being kept in an open beaker or Erlenmeyer flask. Vapors can creep along the table and ignite if they reach a flame or spark. Solvents should be heated in a hood with a steam bath, not on a hot plate.
- **Explosion**: Heating or creating a reaction in a closed system can cause an explosion, resulting in flying glass and chemical splashes. The system should be vented to prevent this.
- **Chemical and thermal burns**: Many chemicals are corrosive to the skin and eyes.
- **Inhalation of toxic fumes**: Some compounds severely irritate membranes in the eyes, nose, throat, and lungs.
- **Absorption** of toxic chemicals such as dimethyl sulfoxide (DMSO) and nitrobenzene through the skin.
- **Ingestion** of toxic chemicals.

Safety Gloves

There are many types of **gloves** available to help protect the skin from cuts, burns, and chemical splashes. There are many considerations to take into account when choosing a glove. For example, gloves that are highly protective may limit dexterity. Some gloves may not offer appropriate protection against a specific chemical. Other considerations include degradation rating, which indicates how effective a glove is when exposed to chemicals; breakthrough time, which indicates how quickly a chemical can break through the surface of the glove; and permeation rate, which indicates how quickly chemicals seep through after the initial breakthrough. Disposable latex, vinyl, or nitrile gloves are usually appropriate for most circumstances, and offer protection from incidental splashes and contact. Other types of gloves include butyl, neoprene, PVC, PVA, viton, silver shield, and natural rubber. Each offers its own type of protection, but may have drawbacks as well. **Double-gloving** can improve resistance or dexterity in some instances.

Proper Handling and Storage of Chemicals

Students should take care when **carrying chemicals** from one place to another. Chemicals should never be taken from the room, tasted, or touched with bare hands. **Safety gloves** should be worn when appropriate and glove/chemical interactions and glove deterioration should be considered. Hands should always be **washed** thoroughly after a lab. Potentially hazardous materials intended for use in chemistry, biology, or other science labs should be secured in a safe area where relevant **Safety Data Sheets (SDS)** can be accessed. Chemicals and solutions should be used as directed and labels should be read before handling solutions and chemicals. Extra chemicals should not be returned to their original containers, but should be disposed of as directed by the school district's rules or local ordinances. Local municipalities often have hazardous waste disposal programs. Acids should be stored separately from other chemicals. Flammable liquids should be stored away from acids, bases, and oxidizers.

Bunsen Burners

When using a **Bunsen burner**, loose clothing should be tucked in, long hair should be tied back, and safety goggles and aprons should be worn. Students should know what to do in case of a fire or accident. When lighting the burner, strikers should always be used instead of matches. Do not touch the hot barrel. Tongs (never fingers) should be used to hold the material in the flame. To heat liquid, a flask may be set upon wire gauze on a tripod and secured with an iron ring or clamp on a stand. The flame is extinguished by turning off the gas at the source.

Safety Procedures Related to Animals

Animals to be used for **dissections** should be obtained from a company that provides animals for this purpose. Road kill or decaying animals that a student brings in should not be used. It is possible that such an animal may have a pathogen or a virus, such as rabies, which can be transmitted via the saliva of even a dead animal. Students should use gloves and should not participate if they have open sores or moral objections to dissections. It is generally accepted that biological experiments may be performed on lower-order life forms and invertebrates, but not on mammalian vertebrates and birds. No animals should be harmed physiologically. Experimental animals should be kept, cared for, and handled in a safe manner and with compassion. Pathogenic (anything able to cause a disease) substances should not be used in lab experiments.

Lab Notebooks

A **lab notebook** is a record of all pre-lab work and lab work. It differs from a lab report, which is prepared after lab work is completed. A lab notebook is a formal record of lab preparations and what was done. **Observational recordings** should not be altered, erased, or whited-out to make corrections. Drawing a single line through an entry is sufficient to make changes. Pages should be numbered and should not be torn out. Entries should be made neatly, but don't necessarily have to be complete sentences. **Entries** should provide detailed information and be recorded in such a way that another person could use them to replicate the experiment. **Quantitative data** may be recorded in tabular form, and may include calculations made during an experiment. Lab book entries can also include references and research performed before the experiment.

Entries may also consist of information about a lab experiment, including the objective or purpose, the procedures, data collected, and the results.

Lab Reports

A **lab report** is an item developed after an experiment that is intended to present the results of a lab experiment. Generally, it should be prepared using a word processor, not hand-written or recorded in a notebook. A lab report should be formally presented. It is intended to persuade others to accept or reject a hypothesis. It should include a brief but descriptive **title** and an **abstract**. The abstract is a summary of the report. It should include a purpose that states the problem that was explored or the question that was answered. It should also include a **hypothesis** that describes the anticipated results of the experiment. The experiment should include a **control** and one **variable** to ensure that the results can be interpreted correctly. Observations and results can be presented using written narratives, tables, graphs, and illustrations. The report should also include a **summation** or **conclusion** explaining whether the results supported the hypothesis.

Types of Laboratory Glassware

Two types of flasks are Erlenmeyer flasks and volumetric flasks. **Volumetric flasks** are used to accurately prepare a specific volume and concentration of solution. **Erlenmeyer flasks** can be used for mixing, transporting, and reacting, but are not appropriate for accurate measurements.

A **pipette** can be used to accurately measure small amounts of liquid. Liquid is drawn into the pipette through a bulb. The liquid measurement is read at the **meniscus**. There are also plastic disposable pipettes. A **repipette** is a hand-operated pump that dispenses solutions.

Beakers can be used to measure mass or dissolve a solvent into a solute. They do not measure volume as accurately as a volumetric flask, pipette, graduated cylinder, or burette.

Graduated cylinders are used for precise measurements and are considered more accurate than Erlenmeyer flasks or beakers. To read a graduated cylinder, it should be placed on a flat surface and read at eye level. The surface of a liquid in a graduated cylinder forms a lens-shaped curve. The measurement should be taken from the bottom of the curve. A ring may be placed at the top of tall, narrow cylinders to help avoid breakage if they are tipped over.

A **burette**, or buret, is a piece of lab glassware used to accurately dispense liquid. It looks similar to a narrow graduated cylinder, but includes a stopcock and tip. It may be filled with a funnel or pipette.

Microscopes

There are different kinds of microscopes, but **optical** or **light microscopes** are the most commonly used in lab settings. Light and lenses are used to magnify and view samples. A specimen or sample is placed on a slide and the slide is placed on a stage with a hole in it. Light passes through the hole and illuminates the sample. The sample is magnified by lenses and viewed through the eyepiece. A simple microscope has one lens, while a typical compound microscope has three lenses. The light source can be room light redirected by a mirror or the microscope can have its own independent light source that passes through a condenser. In this case, there are diaphragms and filters to allow light intensity to be controlled. Optical microscopes also have coarse and fine adjustment knobs.

Other types of microscopes include **digital microscopes**, which use a camera and a monitor to allow viewing of the sample. **Scanning electron microscopes (SEMs)** provide greater detail of a sample in terms of the surface topography and can produce magnifications much greater than those possible with optical microscopes. The technology of an SEM is quite different from an optical microscope in that it does not rely on lenses to magnify objects, but uses samples placed in a chamber. In one type of SEM, a beam of electrons from an electron gun scans and actually interacts with the sample to produce an image.

Wet mount slides designed for use with a light microscope typically require a thin portion of the specimen to be placed on a standard glass slide. A drop of water is added and a cover slip or cover glass is placed on top. Air bubbles and fingerprints can make viewing difficult. Placing the cover slip at a 45-degree angle and allowing it to drop into place can help avoid the problem of air bubbles. A **cover slip** should always be used when viewing wet mount slides. The viewer should start with the objective in its lowest position and then fine focus. The microscope should be carried with two hands and stored with the low-power objective in the down position. **Lenses** should be cleaned with lens paper only. A **graticule slide** is marked with a grid line, and is useful for counting or estimating a quantity.

Balances

Balances such as triple-beam balances, spring balances, and electronic balances measure mass and force. An **electronic balance** is the most accurate, followed by a **triple-beam balance** and then a **spring balance**. One part of a **triple-beam balance** is the plate, which is where the item to be weighed is placed. There are also three beams that have hatch marks indicating amounts and hold the weights that rest in the notches. The front beam measures weights between 0 and 10 grams, the middle beam measures weights in 100 gram increments, and the far beam measures weights in 10 gram increments. The sum of the weight of each beam is the total weight of the object. A triple beam balance also includes a set screw to calibrate the equipment and a mark indicating the object and counterweights are in balance.

Chromatography

Chromatography refers to a set of laboratory techniques used to separate or analyze **mixtures**. Mixtures are dissolved in their mobile phases. In the stationary or bonded phase, the desired component is separated from other molecules in the mixture. In chromatography, the analyte is the substance to be separated. **Preparative chromatography** refers to the type of chromatography that involves purifying a substance for further use rather than further analysis. **Analytical chromatography** involves analyzing the isolated substance. Other types of chromatography include column, planar, paper, thin layer, displacement, supercritical fluid, affinity, ion exchange, and size exclusion chromatography. Reversed phase, two-dimensional, simulated moving bed, pyrolysis, fast protein, counter current, and chiral are also types of chromatography. **Gas chromatography** refers to the separation technique in which the mobile phase of a substance is in gas form.

Review Video: Paper Chromatography
Visit mometrix.com/academy and enter code: 543963

Reagents and Reactants

A **reagent** or **reactant** is a chemical agent for use in chemical reactions. When preparing for a lab, it should be confirmed that glassware and other equipment has been cleaned and/or sterilized. There should be enough materials, reagents, or other solutions needed for the lab for every group of students completing the experiment. Distilled water should be used instead of tap water when performing lab experiments because distilled water has most of its impurities removed. Other needed apparatus such as funnels, filter paper, balances, Bunsen burners, ring stands, and/or microscopes should also be set up. After the lab, it should be confirmed that sinks, workstations, and any equipment used have been cleaned. If chemicals or specimens need to be kept at a certain temperature by refrigerating them or using another storage method, the temperature should be checked periodically to ensure the sample does not spoil.

Diluting Acids

When preparing a solution of **dilute acid**, always add the concentrated acid solution to water, not water to concentrated acid. Start by adding approximately $\frac{2}{3}$ of the total volume of water to the graduated cylinder or volumetric flask. Next, add the concentrated acid to the water. Add additional water to the diluted acid to bring the solution to the final desired volume.

Cleaning After Acid Spills

In the event of an **acid spill**, any clothes that have come into contact with the acid should be removed and any skin contacted with acid must be rinsed with clean water. To the extent a window can be opened or a fume hood can be turned on, do so. Do not try force circulation, such as by adding a fan, as acid fumes can be harmful if spread.

Next, pour one of the following over the spill area: sodium bicarbonate, baking soda, soda ash, or cat litter. Start from the outside of the spill and then move towards the center, in order to prevent splashing. When the clumps have thoroughly dried, sweep up the clumps and dispose of them as chemical waste.

Centrifuges

A **centrifuge** is used to separate the components of a heterogeneous mixture (consisting of two or more compounds) by spinning it. The solid precipitate settles in the bottom of the container and the liquid component of the solution, called the **centrifugate**, is at the top. A well-known application of this process is using a centrifuge to separate blood cells and plasma. The heavier cells settle on the bottom of the test tube and the lighter plasma stays on top. Another example is using a salad spinner to help dry lettuce.

Electrophoresis, Calorimetry, and Titration

- **Electrophoresis** is the separation of molecules based on electrical charge. This is possible because particles disbursed in a fluid usually carry electric charges on their surfaces. Molecules are pulled through the fluid toward the positive end if the molecules have a negative charge and are pulled through the fluid toward the negative end if the molecules have a positive charge.
- **Calorimetry** is used to determine the heat released or absorbed in a chemical reaction.
- **Titration** helps determine the precise endpoint of a reaction. With this information, the precise quantity of reactant in the titration flask can be determined. A burette is used to deliver the second reactant to the flask and an indicator or pH meter is used to detect the endpoint of the reaction.

Field Studies and Research Projects

Field studies may facilitate scientific inquiry in a manner similar to indoor lab experiments. Field studies can be interdisciplinary in nature and can help students learn and apply scientific concepts and processes. **Research projects** can be conducted in any number of locations, including school campuses, local parks, national parks, beaches, or mountains. Students can practice the general techniques of observation, data collection, collaborative planning, and analysis of experiments. Field studies give students the chance to learn through hands-on applications of scientific processes, such as map making in geography, observation of stratification in geology, observation of life cycles of plants and animals, and analysis of water quality.

Students should watch out for obvious outdoor **hazards**. These include poisonous flora and fauna such as poison ivy, poison oak, and sumac. Depending on the region of the United States in which the field study is being conducted, hazards may also include rattlesnakes and black widow or brown recluse spiders. Students should also be made aware of potentially hazardous situations specific to **geographic locales** and the possibility of coming into contact with **pathogens**.

Field studies allow for great flexibility in the use of traditional and technological methods for **making observations** and **collecting data**. For example, a nature study could consist of a simple survey of bird species within a given area. Information could be recorded using still photography or a video camera. This type of activity gives students the chance to use technologies other than computers. Computers could still be used to create a slide show of transferred images or a digital lab report. If a quantitative study of birds was being performed, the simple technique of using a pencil and paper to tabulate the number of birds counted in the field could also be used. Other techniques used during field studies could include collecting specimens for lab study, observing coastal ecosystems and tides, and collecting weather data such as temperature, precipitation amounts, and air pressure in a particular locale.

Scientific Inquiry and Reasoning

Scientific Inquiry

The concept of **scientific inquiry** refers to the idea of how one thinks and asks questions in a logical way to gain trustworthy information. The underlying motivation of science is to try to understand the natural world. Much of human thought is based on assumptions about how things work that may or may not be true. The goal of scientific inquiry is to test those assumptions to gain a greater understanding of the world with good questions and objective tests, and then re-use what was learned to ask better questions. The more we understand about the natural world, the better the questions we can ask, and that is the general idea behind scientific inquiry. The applied practice of scientific inquiry is to ask questions in a systematic method, called the scientific method.

Scientific Knowledge

Scientific knowledge refers to any topic that is studied **empirically**, meaning that it is based on observation of a **phenomenon** in an objective way. The body of **scientific knowledge** is often broken down into several domains including biology, ecology, Earth science, space science, physics, and chemistry. These each have further subdomains and are overlapping in many ways. For instance, ecology is the study of ecosystems, which are made up of biological factors and geological factors, so it contains elements of both biology and Earth science. Each of these domains is subject to the concepts of scientific inquiry, such as the scientific method, scientific facts, hypotheses, and scientific laws.

Important Terminology

- A **phenomenon** is an event or effect that is observed.
- A **scientific fact** is considered an objective and verifiable observation. Usually, a fact can be repeated or demonstrated to others.
- A **scientific theory** is a proposition explaining why or how something happens and is built on scientific facts and laws. Scientific theories can be tested, but are not fully proven. If new evidence is found that disproves the theory, it is no longer considered true.
- A **hypothesis** is an educated guess that is not yet proven. It is used to predict the outcome of an experiment in an attempt to solve a problem or answer a question.
- A **law** is an explanation of events that always leads to the same outcome. It is a fact that an object falls. The law of gravity explains why an object falls. The theory of relativity, although generally accepted, has been neither proven nor disproved.
- A **model** is used to explain something on a smaller scale or in simpler terms to provide an example. It is a representation of an idea that can be used to explain events or applied to new situations to predict outcomes or determine results.

Review Video: Science Process Skills
Visit mometrix.com/academy and enter code: 601624

History of Scientific Knowledge

When one examines the history of **scientific knowledge**, it is clear that it is constantly **evolving**. The body of facts, models, theories, and laws grows and changes over time. In other words, one scientific discovery leads to the next. Some advances in science and technology have important and long-lasting effects on science and society. Some discoveries were so alien to the accepted beliefs of the time that not only were they rejected as wrong, but were also considered outright blasphemy. Today, however, many beliefs once considered incorrect have become an ingrained part of scientific knowledge, and have also been the basis of new advances. Examples of advances include: Copernicus's heliocentric view of the universe, Newton's laws of motion and planetary orbits, relativity, geologic time scale, plate tectonics, atomic theory, nuclear physics, biological evolution, germ theory, industrial revolution, molecular biology, information and communication, quantum theory, galactic universe, and medical and health technology.

SCIENTIFIC INQUIRY AND SCIENTIFIC METHOD

Scientists use a number of generally accepted techniques collectively known as the **scientific method**. The scientific method generally involves carrying out the following steps:

- Identifying a problem or posing a question
- Formulating a hypothesis or an educated guess
- Conducting experiments or tests that will provide a basis to solve the problem or answer the question
- Observing the results of the test
- Drawing conclusions

An important part of the scientific method is using acceptable experimental techniques. Objectivity is also important if valid results are to be obtained. Another important part of the scientific method is peer review. It is essential that experiments be performed and data be recorded in such a way that experiments can be reproduced to verify results. Historically, the scientific method has been taught with a more linear approach, but it is important to recognize that the scientific method should be a cyclical or **recursive process**. This means that as hypotheses are tested and more is learned, the questions should continue to change to reflect the changing body of knowledge. One cycle of experimentation is not enough.

Review Video: The Scientific Method
Visit mometrix.com/academy and enter code: 191386

METRIC AND INTERNATIONAL SYSTEM OF UNITS

The **metric system** is the accepted standard of measurement in the scientific community. The **International System of Units (SI)** is a set of measurements (including the metric system) that is almost globally accepted. The United States, Liberia, and Myanmar have not accepted this system. **Standardization** is important because it allows the results of experiments to be compared and reproduced without the need to laboriously convert measurements. The SI is based partially on the **meter-kilogram-second (MKS) system** rather than the **centimeter-gram-second (CGS) system**. The MKS system considers meters, kilograms, and seconds to be the basic units of measurement, while the CGS system considers centimeters, grams, and seconds to be the basic units of measurement. Under the MKS system, the length of an object would be expressed as 1 meter instead of 100 centimeters, which is how it would be described under the CGS system.

Review Video: Metric System Conversions
Visit mometrix.com/academy and enter code: 163709

BASIC UNITS OF MEASUREMENT

Using the **metric system** is generally accepted as the preferred method for taking measurements. Having a **universal standard** allows individuals to interpret measurements more easily, regardless of where they are located. The basic units of measurement are: the **meter**, which measures length; the **liter**, which measures volume; and the **gram**, which measures mass. The metric system starts with a base unit and increases or decreases in units of 10. The prefix and the base unit combined are used to indicate an amount. For example, deka- is 10 times the base unit. A dekameter is 10 meters; a dekaliter is 10 liters; and a dekagram is 10 grams. The prefix hecto- refers to 100 times the base amount; kilo- is 1,000 times the base amount. The prefixes that indicate a fraction of the base unit are deci-, which is $\frac{1}{10}$ of the base unit; centi-, which is $\frac{1}{100}$ of the base unit; and milli-, which is $\frac{1}{1,000}$ of the base unit.

COMMON PREFIXES

The prefixes for multiples are as follows:

Deka	(da)	**10^1** (deka is the American spelling, but deca is also used)
Hecto	(h)	10^2

Kilo	(k)	10^3
Mega	(M)	10^6
Giga	(G)	10^9
Tera	(T)	10^{12}

The prefixes for subdivisions are as follows:

Deci	(d)	10^{-1}
Centi	(c)	10^{-2}
Milli	(m)	10^{-3}
Micro	(μ)	10^{-6}
Nano	(n)	10^{-9}
Pico	(p)	10^{-12}

The rule of thumb is that prefixes greater than 10^3 are capitalized when abbreviating. Abbreviations do not need a period after them. A decimeter (dm) is a tenth of a meter, a deciliter (dL) is a tenth of a liter, and a decigram (dg) is a tenth of a gram. Pluralization is understood. For example, when referring to 5 mL of water, no "s" needs to be added to the abbreviation.

Basic SI Units of Measurement

SI uses **second(s)** to measure time. Fractions of seconds are usually measured in metric terms using prefixes such as millisecond ($\frac{1}{1,000}$ of a second) or nanosecond ($\frac{1}{1,000,000,000}$ of a second). Increments of time larger than a second are measured in **minutes** and **hours**, which are multiples of 60 and 24. An example of this is a swimmer's time in the 800-meter freestyle being described as 7:32.67, meaning 7 minutes, 32 seconds, and 67 one-hundredths of a second. One second is equal to $\frac{1}{60}$ of a minute, $\frac{1}{3,600}$ of an hour, and $\frac{1}{86,400}$ of a day. Other SI base units are the **ampere** (A) (used to measure electric current), the **kelvin** (K) (used to measure thermodynamic temperature), the **candela** (cd) (used to measure luminous intensity), and the **mole** (mol) (used to measure the amount of a substance at a molecular level). **Meter** (m) is used to measure length and **kilogram** (kg) is used to measure mass.

Significant Figures

The mathematical concept of **significant figures** or **significant digits** is often used to determine the accuracy of measurements or the level of confidence one has in a specific measurement. The significant figures of a measurement include all the digits known with certainty plus one estimated or uncertain digit. There are a number of rules for determining which digits are considered "important" or "interesting." They are: all non-zero digits are *significant*, zeros between digits are *significant*, and leading and trailing zeros are *not significant* unless they appear to the right of the non-zero digits in a decimal. For example, in 0.01230 the significant digits are 1230, and this number would be said to be accurate to the hundred-thousandths place. The zero indicates that the amount has actually been measured as 0. Other zeros are considered place holders, and are not important. A decimal point may be placed after zeros to indicate their importance (in 100. for example). **Estimating**, on the other hand, involves approximating a value rather than calculating the exact number. This may be used to quickly determine a value that is close to the actual number when complete accuracy does not matter or is not possible. In science, estimation may be used when it is impossible to measure or calculate an exact amount, or to quickly approximate an answer when true calculations would be time consuming.

Graphs and Charts

Graphs and charts are effective ways to present scientific data such as observations, statistical analyses, and comparisons between dependent variables and independent variables. On a line chart, the **independent variable** (the one that is being manipulated for the experiment) is represented on the horizontal axis (the x-

axis). Any **dependent variables** (the ones that may change as the independent variable changes) are represented on the y-axis. An **XY** or **scatter plot** is often used to plot many points. A "best fit" line is drawn, which allows outliers to be identified more easily. Charts and their axes should have titles. The x and y interval units should be evenly spaced and labeled. Other types of charts are **bar charts** and **histograms**, which can be used to compare differences between the data collected for two variables. A **pie chart** can graphically show the relation of parts to a whole.

Review Video: Identifying Variables
Visit mometrix.com/academy and enter code: 627181

Review Video: Data Interpretation of Graphs
Visit mometrix.com/academy and enter code: 200439

Data Presentation

Data collected during a science lab can be organized and **presented** in any number of ways. While **straight narrative** is a suitable method for presenting some lab results, it is not a suitable way to present numbers and quantitative measurements. These types of observations can often be better presented with **tables** and **graphs**. Data that is presented in tables and organized in rows and columns may also be used to make graphs quite easily. Other methods of presenting data include illustrations, photographs, video, and even audio formats. In a **formal report**, tables and figures are labeled and referred to by their labels. For example, a picture of a bubbly solution might be labeled Figure 1, Bubbly Solution. It would be referred to in the text in the following way: "The reaction created bubbles 10 mm in size, as shown in Figure 1, Bubbly Solution." Graphs are also labeled as figures. Tables are labeled in a different way. Examples include: Table 1, Results of Statistical Analysis, or Table 2, Data from Lab 2.

Review Video: Understanding Charts and Tables
Visit mometrix.com/academy and enter code: 882112

Statistical Precision and Errors

Errors that occur during an experiment can be classified into two categories: random errors and systematic errors. **Random errors** can result in collected data that is wildly different from the rest of the data, or they may result in data that is indistinguishable from the rest. Random errors are not consistent across the data set. In large data sets, random errors may contribute to the variability of data, but they will not affect the average. Random errors are sometimes referred to as noise. They may be caused by a student's inability to take the same measurement in exactly the same way or by outside factors that are not considered variables, but influence the data. A **systematic error** will show up consistently across a sample or data set, and may be the result of a flaw in the experimental design. This type of error affects the average, and is also known as bias.

Scientific Notation

Scientific notation is used because values in science can be very large or very small, which makes them unwieldy. A number in **decimal notation** is 93,000,000. In **scientific notation**, it is 9.3×10^7. The first number, 9.3, is the **coefficient**. It is always greater than or equal to 1 and less than 10. This number is followed by a multiplication sign. The base is always 10 in scientific notation. If the number is greater than ten, the exponent is positive. If the number is between zero and one, the exponent is negative. The first digit of the number is followed by a decimal point and then the rest of the number. In this case, the number is 9.3, and the decimal point was moved seven places to the right from the end of the number to get 93,000,000. The number of places moved, seven, is the exponent.

Statistical Terminology

Mean - The average, found by taking the sum of a set of numbers and dividing by the number of numbers in the set.

Median - The middle number in a set of numbers sorted from least to greatest. If the set has an even number of entries, the median is the average of the two in the middle.

Mode - The value that appears most frequently in a data set. There may be more than one mode. If no value appears more than once, there is no mode.

Range - The difference between the highest and lowest numbers in a data set.

Standard deviation - Measures the dispersion of a data set or how far from the mean a single data point is likely to be.

Regression analysis - A method of analyzing sets of data and sets of variables that involves studying how the typical value of the dependent variable changes when any one of the independent variables is varied and the other independent variables remain fixed.

> **Review Video: Mean, Median, and Mode**
> Visit mometrix.com/academy and enter code: 286207
>
> **Review Video: Standard Deviation**
> Visit mometrix.com/academy and enter code: 419469

Biology

Differences Between Prokaryotic and Eukaryotic Cells

Prokaryotes and Eukaryotes

Sizes and Metabolism

Cells of the domains of Bacteria and Archaea are **prokaryotes**. Bacteria cells and Archaea cells are much smaller than cells of eukaryotes. Prokaryote cells are usually only 1 to 2 micrometers in diameter, but eukaryotic cells are usually at least 10 times and possibly 100 times larger than prokaryotic cells. Eukaryotic cells are usually 10 to 100 micrometers in diameter. Most prokaryotes are unicellular organisms, although some prokaryotes live in colonies. Because of their large surface-area-to-volume ratios, prokaryotes have a very high metabolic rate. **Eukaryotic cells** are much larger than prokaryotic cells. Due to their larger sizes, they have a much smaller surface-area-to-volume ratio and consequently have much lower metabolic rates.

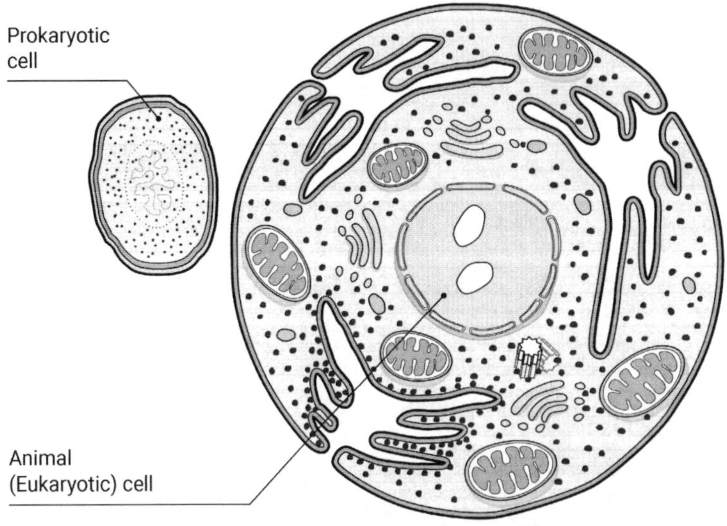

> **Review Video: Eukaryotic and Prokaryotic Cells**
> Visit mometrix.com/academy and enter code: 231438
>
> **Review Video: Cell Structure**
> Visit mometrix.com/academy and enter code: 591293

Membrane-Bound Organelles

Prokaryotic cells are much simpler than eukaryotic cells. Prokaryote cells do not have a nucleus due to their small size and their DNA is located in the center of the cell in a region referred to as a **nucleoid**. Eukaryote cells have a **nucleus** bound by a double membrane. Eukaryotic cells typically have hundreds or thousands of additional **membrane-bound organelles** that are independent of the cell membrane. Prokaryotic cells do not have any membrane-bound organelles that are independent of the cell membrane. Once again, this is probably due to the much larger size of the eukaryotic cells. The organelles of eukaryotes give them much higher levels of intracellular division than is possible in prokaryotic cells.

Cell Walls

Not all cells have cell walls, but most prokaryotes have cell walls. The cell walls of organisms from the domain Bacteria differ from the cell walls of the organisms from the domain Archaea. Some eukaryotes, such as some fungi, some algae, and plants, have cell walls that differ from the cell walls of the Bacteria and Archaea domains. The main difference between the cell walls of different domains or kingdoms is the composition of the cell walls. For example, most bacteria have cell walls outside of the plasma membrane that contains the molecule peptidoglycan. **Peptidoglycan** is a large polymer of amino acids and sugars. The peptidoglycan helps maintain the strength of the cell wall. Some of the Archaea cells have cell walls containing the molecule pseudopeptidoglycan, which differs in chemical structure from the peptidoglycan but basically provides the same strength to the cell wall. Some fungi cell walls contain **chitin**. The cell walls of diatoms, a type of yellow algae, contain silica. Plant cell walls contain cellulose, and woody plants are further strengthened by lignin. Some algae also contain lignin. Animal cells do not have cell walls.

Chromosome Structure

Prokaryote cells have DNA arranged in a **circular structure** that should not be referred to as a chromosome. Due to the small size of a prokaryote cell, the DNA material is simply located near the center of the cell in a region called the nucleoid. A prokaryotic cell may also contain tiny rings of DNA called plasmids. Prokaryote cells lack histone proteins, and therefore the DNA is not actually packaged into chromosomes. Prokaryotes reproduce by binary fission, while eukaryotes reproduce by mitosis with the help of **linear chromosomes** and histone proteins. During mitosis, the chromatin is tightly wound on the histone proteins and packaged as a chromosome. The DNA in a eukaryotic cell is located in the membrane-bound nucleus.

Review Video: Chromosomes
Visit mometrix.com/academy and enter code: 132083

Structure and Function of Cells and Organelles

Cells and Organelles of Plant Cells and Animal Cells

Plant cells and animal cells both have a nucleus, cytoplasm, cell membrane, ribosomes, mitochondria, endoplasmic reticulum, Golgi apparatus, and vacuoles. Plant cells have only one or two extremely large vacuoles. Animal cells typically have several small vacuoles. Plant cells have chloroplasts for photosynthesis and use this process to produce their own food, distinguishing plants as **autotrophs**. Animal cells do not have chloroplasts and therefore cannot use photosynthesis to produce their own food. Instead animal cells rely on other sources for food, which classifies them as **heterotrophs**. Animal cells have centrioles, which are used to help organize microtubules and in in cell division, but only some plant cells have centrioles. Additionally, plant cells have a rectangular and more rigid shape due to the cell wall, while animal cells have more of a circular shape because they lack a cell wall.

Review Video: Difference Between Plant and Animal Cells
Visit mometrix.com/academy and enter code: 115568

Review Video: An Introduction to Cellular Biology
Visit mometrix.com/academy and enter code: 629967

Review Video: Cell Functions
Visit mometrix.com/academy and enter code: 883787

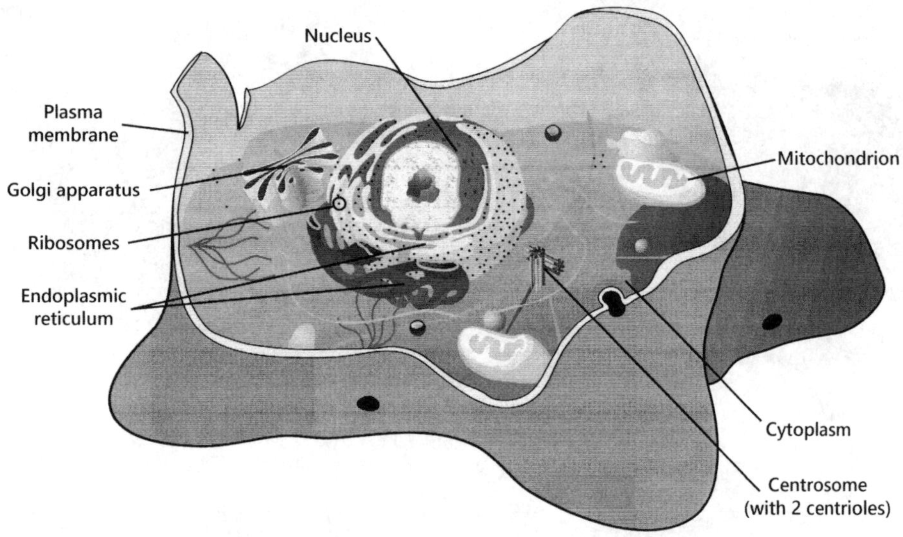

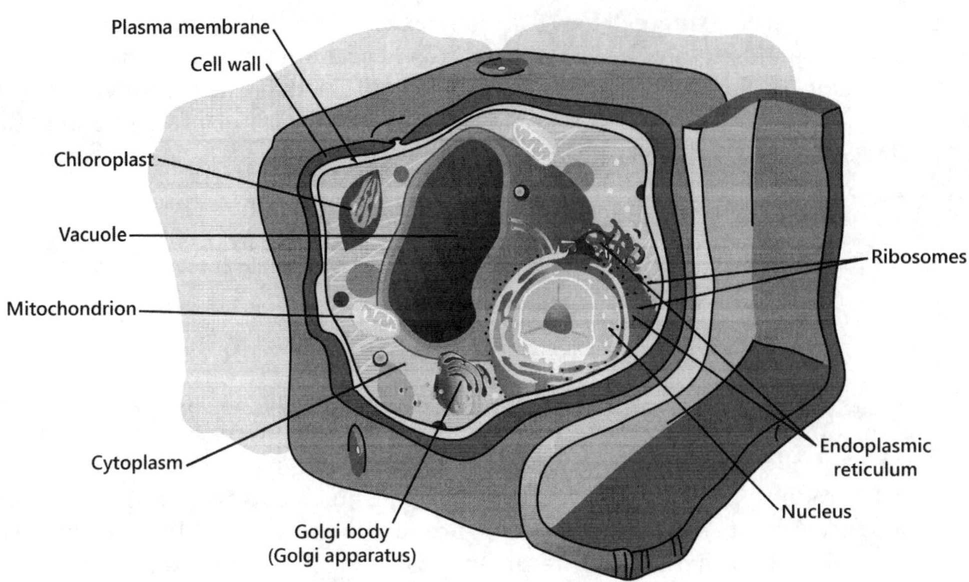

Cell Membranes

The **cell membrane**, also referred to as the plasma membrane, is a thin semipermeable membrane of lipids and proteins. The cell membrane isolates the cell from its external environment while still enabling the cell to communicate with that outside environment. It consists of a phospholipid bilayer, or double layer, with the hydrophilic ("water-loving") ends of the outer layer facing the external environment, the inner layer facing the inside of the cell, and the hydrophobic ("water-fearing") ends facing each other. Cholesterol in the cell membrane adds stiffness and flexibility. Glycolipids help the cell to recognize other cells of the organisms. The proteins in the cell membrane help give the cells shape. Special proteins help the cell communicate with its external environment, while other proteins transport molecules across the cell membrane.

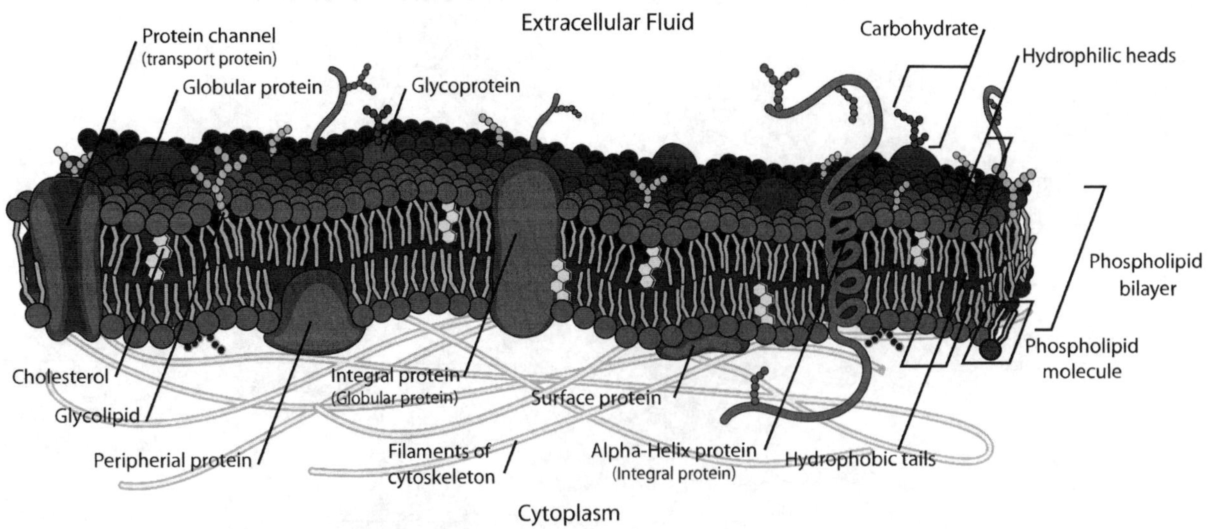

Review Video: Function of the Plasma Membrane
Visit mometrix.com/academy and enter code: 943095

Nucleus

Typically, a eukaryote has a single nucleus that takes up approximately 10% of the volume of the cell. Components of the nucleus include the nuclear envelope, nucleoplasm, chromatin, and nucleolus. The **nuclear**

envelope is a double-layered membrane with the outer layer connected to the endoplasmic reticulum. The nucleus can communicate with the rest of the cell through several nuclear pores. The chromatin consists of deoxyribonucleic acid (DNA) and histones that are packaged into chromosomes during mitosis. The **nucleolus**, which is the dense central portion of the nucleus, produced and assembles ribosomes with the help of ribosomal RNA and proteins. Functions of the nucleus include the storage of genetic material, production of ribosomes, and transcription of ribonucleic acid (RNA).

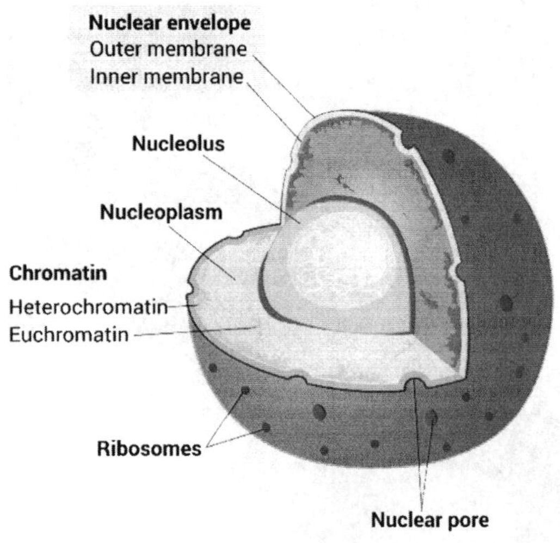

Review Video: Nucleic Acids
Visit mometrix.com/academy and enter code: 503931

CHLOROPLASTS

Chloroplasts are large organelles that are enclosed in a double membrane. Discs called **thylakoids** are arranged in stacks called **grana** (singular, *granum*). The thylakoids have chlorophyll molecules on their surfaces. **Stromal lamellae** separate the thylakoid stacks. Sugars are formed in the stroma, which is the inner portion of the chloroplast. Chloroplasts perform photosynthesis and make food in the form of sugars for the plant. The light reaction stage of photosynthesis occurs in the grana, and the dark reaction stage of photosynthesis occurs in the stroma. Chloroplasts have their own DNA and can reproduce by fission independently.

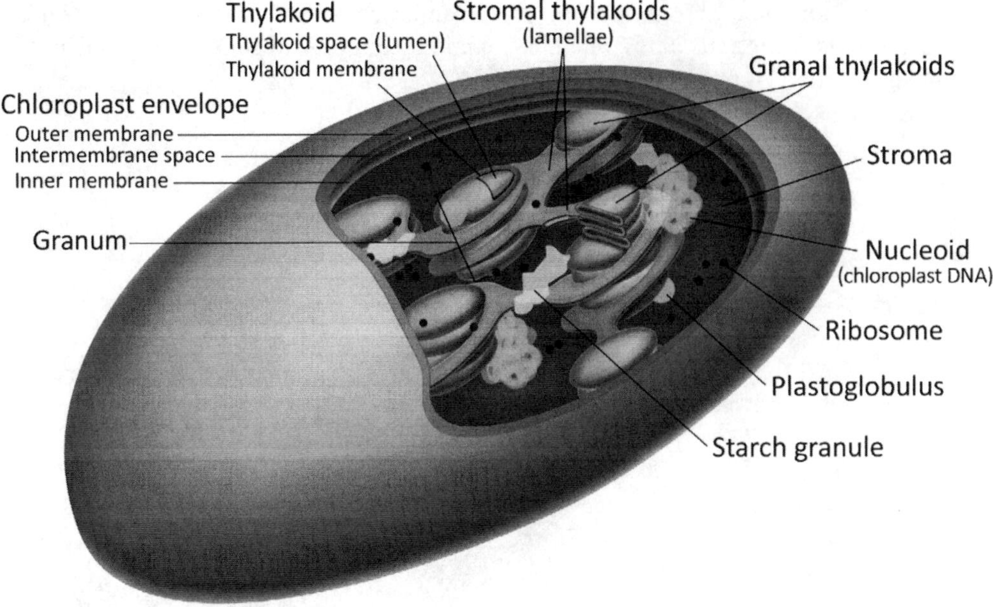

Plastids

Plastids are major organelles found in plants and algae that are used to synthesize and store food. Because plastids can differentiate, there are many forms of plastids. Specialized plastids can store pigments, starches, fats, or proteins. Two examples of plastids are amyloplasts and chloroplasts. **Amyloplasts** are the plastids that store the starch formed from long chains of glucose produced during photosynthesis. Amyloplasts synthesize and store the starch granules through the polymerization of glucose. When needed, amyloplasts also convert these starch granules back into sugar. Fruits and potato tubers have large numbers of amyloplasts. **Chloroplasts** can synthesize and store starch. Interestingly, amyloplasts can redifferentiate and transform into chloroplasts.

Mitochondria

Mitochondria break down sugar molecules and produce energy in the form of molecules of adenosine triphosphate (ATP). Both plant and animal cells contain mitochondria. Mitochondria are enclosed in a bilayer semi-membrane of phospholipids and proteins. The intermembrane space is the space between the two layers. The outer membrane has proteins called porins, which allow small molecules through. The inner membrane contains proteins that aid in the synthesis of ATP. The matrix consists of enzymes that help synthesize ATP. Mitochondria have their own DNA and can reproduce by fission independently. Mitochondria also help to maintain calcium concentrations, form blood components and hormones, and are involved in activating cell death pathways.

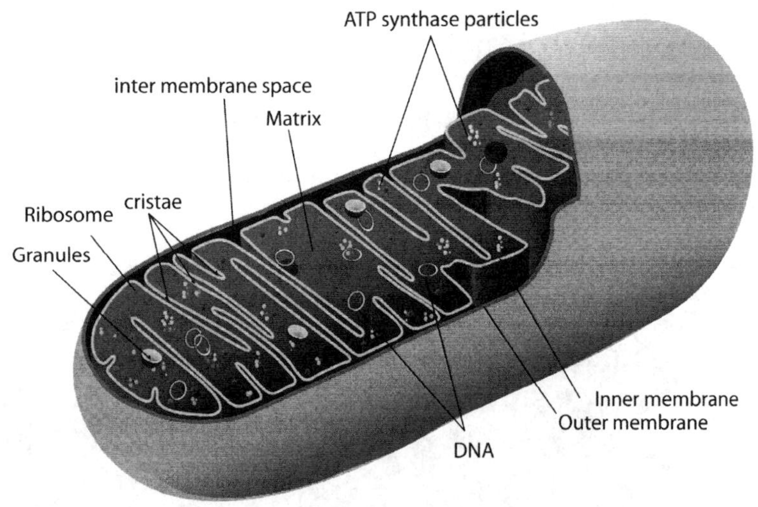

Review Video: Mitochondria
Visit mometrix.com/academy and enter code: 444287

Ribosomes

A **ribosome** consists of RNA and proteins. The RNA component of the ribosome is known as ribosomal RNA (rRNA). Ribosomes consist of two subunits, a large subunit and a small subunit. Few ribosomes are free in the cell. Most of the ribosomes in the cell are embedded in the rough endoplasmic reticulum located near the nucleus. Ribosomes are protein factories and translate the code of DNA into proteins by assembling long chains of amino acids. **Messenger RNA** (mRNA) is used by the ribosome to generate a specific protein sequence, while **transfer RNA** (tRNA) collects the needed amino acids and delivers them to the ribosome.

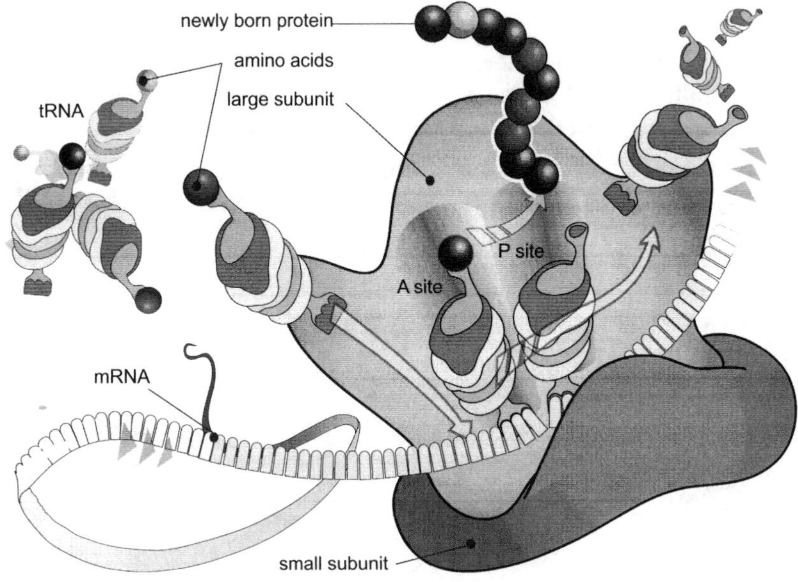

Golgi Apparatus

The **Golgi apparatus**, also called the Golgi body or Golgi complex, is a stack of flattened membranes called **cisternae** that package, ship, and distribute macromolecules such as carbohydrates, proteins, and lipids in shipping containers called **vesicles**. It also helps modify proteins and lipids before they are shipped. Most Golgi apparatuses have six to eight cisternae. Each Golgi apparatus has four regions: the cis region, the endo region, the medial region, and the trans region. Transfer vesicles from the rough endoplasmic reticulum (ER) enter at the cis region, and secretory vesicles leave the Golgi apparatus from the trans region.

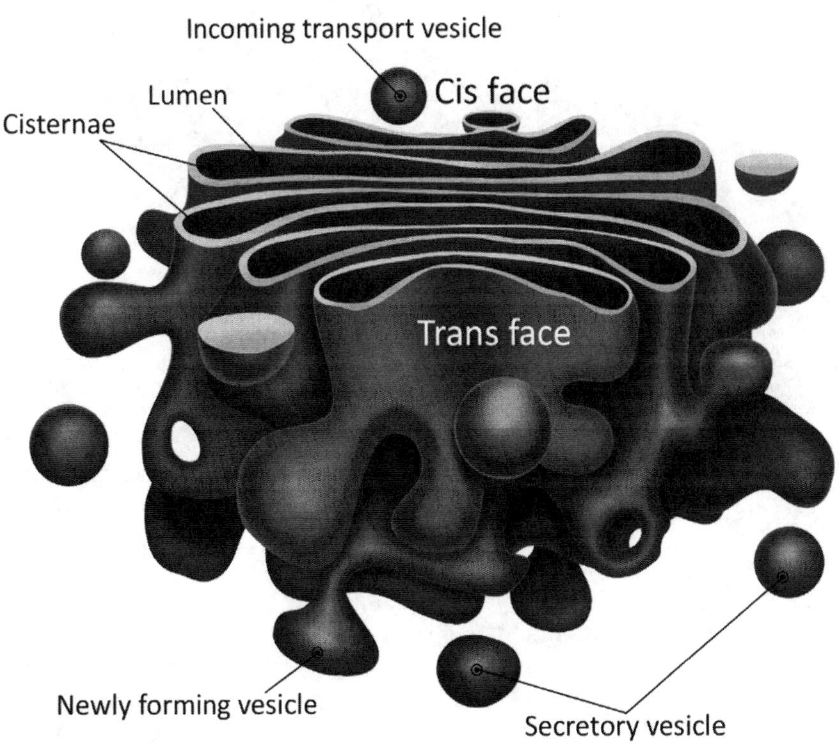

Cytoskeleton

The **cytoskeleton** is a scaffolding system located in the cytoplasm. The cytoskeleton consists of elongated organelles made of proteins called microtubules, microfilaments, and intermediate filaments. These organelles provide shape, support, and the ability to move. These structures also assist in moving the chromosomes during mitosis. Microtubules and microfilaments help transport materials throughout the cell and are the major components in cilia and flagella.

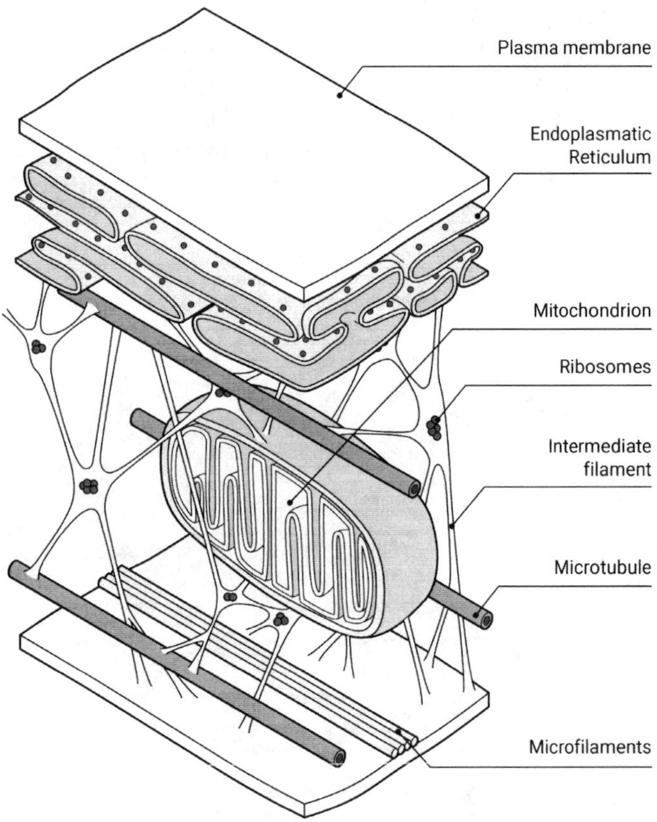

Cell Cycle and Cellular Division

Cell Cycle Stages

The cell cycle consists of three stages: interphase, mitosis, and cytokinesis. **Interphase** is the longest stage of the cell cycle and involves the cell growing and making a copy of its DNA. Cells typically spend more than 90% of the cell cycle in interphase. Interphase includes two growth phases called G_1 and G_2. The order of interphase is the first growth cycle, **GAP 1** (G_1 phase), followed by the **synthesis phase** (S), and ending with the second growth phase, **GAP 2** (G_2 phase). During the G_1 phase of interphase, the cell increases the number of organelles by forming diploid cells. During the S phase of interphase, the DNA is replicated, and the chromosomes are doubled. During the G_2 phase of interphase, the cell synthesizes needed proteins and organelles, continues to increase in size, and prepares for mitosis. Once the G_2 phase ends, mitosis can begin.

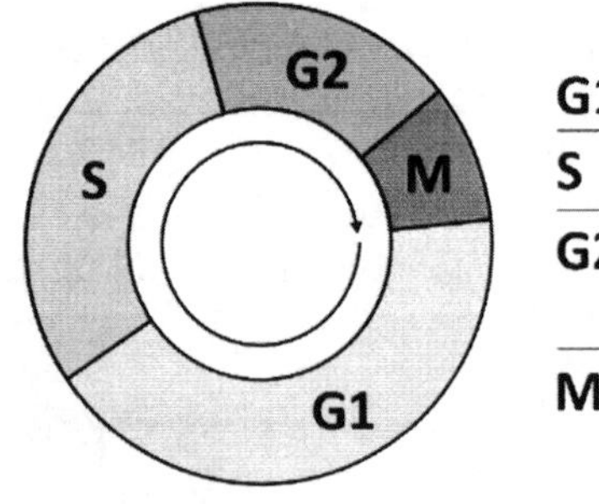

G1 - Growth

S - DNA synthesis

G2 - Growth and preparation for mitosis

M - Mitosis (cell division)

MITOSIS

Mitosis is the asexual process of cell division. During mitosis, one parent cell divides into two identical daughter cells. Mitosis is used for growth, repair, and replacement of cells. Some unicellular organisms reproduce asexually by mitosis. Some multicellular organisms can reproduce by fragmentation or budding, which involves mitosis. Mitosis consists of four phases: prophase, metaphase, anaphase, and telophase. During **prophase**, the spindle fibers appear and the DNA is condensed and packaged as chromosomes that become visible. The nuclear membrane also breaks down, and the nucleolus disappears. During **metaphase**, the spindle apparatus is formed and the centromeres of the chromosomes line up on the equatorial plane. During **anaphase**, the centromeres divide and the two chromatids separate and are pulled toward the opposite poles of the cell. During **telophase**, the spindle fibers disappear, the nuclear membrane reforms, and the DNA in the chromatids is decondensed.

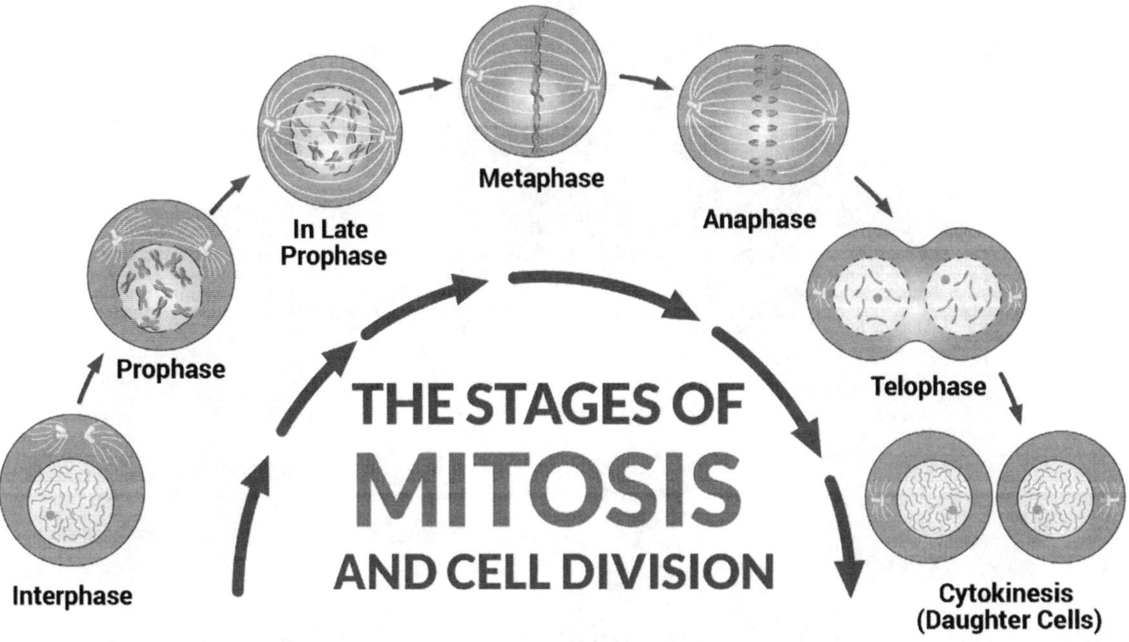

Review Video: Mitosis
Visit mometrix.com/academy and enter code: 849894

Review Video: Cellular Division: Mitosis and Meiosis
Visit mometrix.com/academy and enter code: 109813

CYTOKINESIS

Cytokinesis is the dividing of the cytoplasm and cell membrane by the pinching of a cell into two new daughter cells at the end of mitosis. This occurs at the end of telophase when the actin filaments in the cytoskeleton form a contractile ring that narrows and divides the cell. In plant cells, a cell plate forms across the phragmoplast, which is the center of the spindle apparatus. In animal cells, as the contractile ring narrows, the cleavage furrow forms. Eventually, the contractile ring narrows down to the spindle apparatus joining the two cells and the cells eventually divide. Diagrams of the cleavage furrow of an animal cell and cell plate of a plant are shown below.

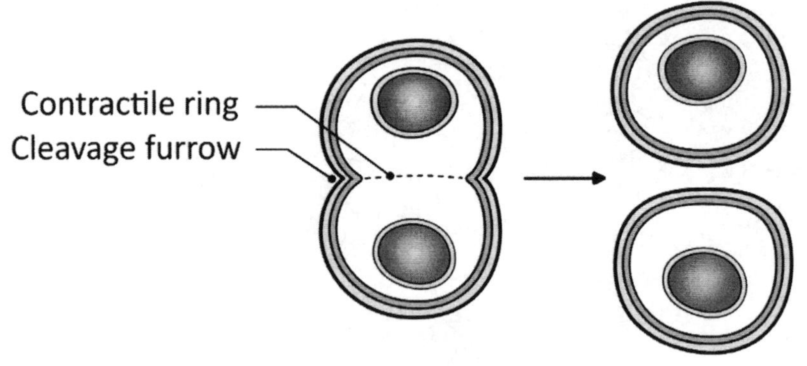

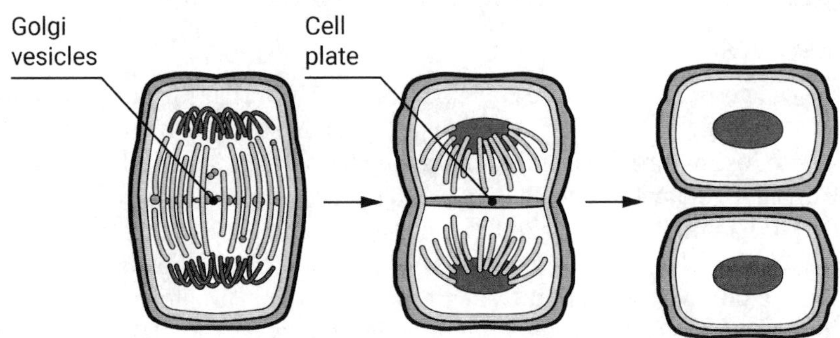

Meiosis

Meiosis is a type of cell division in which the number of chromosomes is reduced by half. Meiosis produces gametes, or egg and sperm cells. Meiosis occurs in two successive stages, which consist of a first mitotic division followed by a second mitotic division. During **meiosis I**, or the first meiotic division, the cell replicates its DNA in interphase and then continues through prophase I, metaphase I, anaphase I, and telophase I. At the end of meiosis I, there are two daughter cells that have the same number of chromosomes as the parent cell. During **meiosis II**, the cell enters a brief interphase but does not replicate its DNA. Then, the cell continues through prophase II, metaphase II, anaphase II, and telophase II. During prophase II, the unduplicated chromosomes split. At the end of telophase II, there are four daughter cells that have half the number of chromosomes as the parent cell.

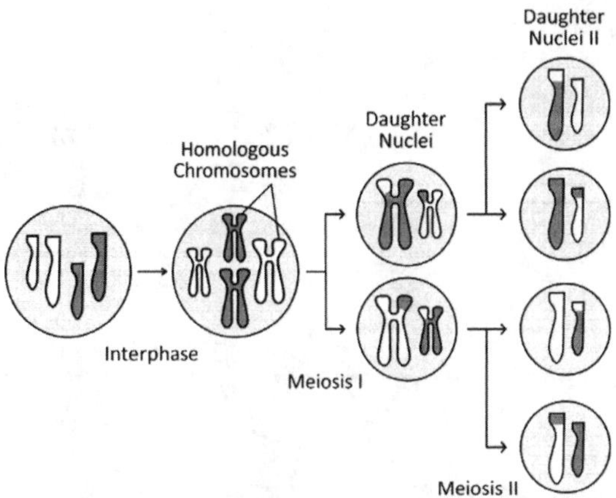

Review Video: Meiosis
Visit mometrix.com/academy and enter code: 247334

Cell Cycle Checkpoints

During the cell cycle, the cell goes through three checkpoints to ensure that the cell is dividing properly at each phase, that it is the appropriate time for division, and that the cell has not been damaged. The **first checkpoint** is at the end of the G_1 phase just before the cell undergoes the S phase, or synthesis. At this checkpoint, a cell may continue with cell division, delay the division, or rest. This **resting phase** is called G_0. In animal cells, the G_1 checkpoint is called **restriction.** Proteins called cyclin D and cyclin E, which are dependent on enzymes cyclin-dependent kinase 4 and cyclin-dependent kinase 2 (CDK4 and CDK2), respectively, largely control this first checkpoint. The **second checkpoint** is at the end of the G_2 phase just before the cell begins prophase during mitosis. The protein cyclin A, which is dependent on the enzyme CDK2, largely controls this checkpoint. During mitosis, the **third checkpoint** occurs at metaphase to check that the chromosomes are lined up along the equatorial plane. This checkpoint is largely controlled by cyclin B, which is dependent upon the enzyme CDK1.

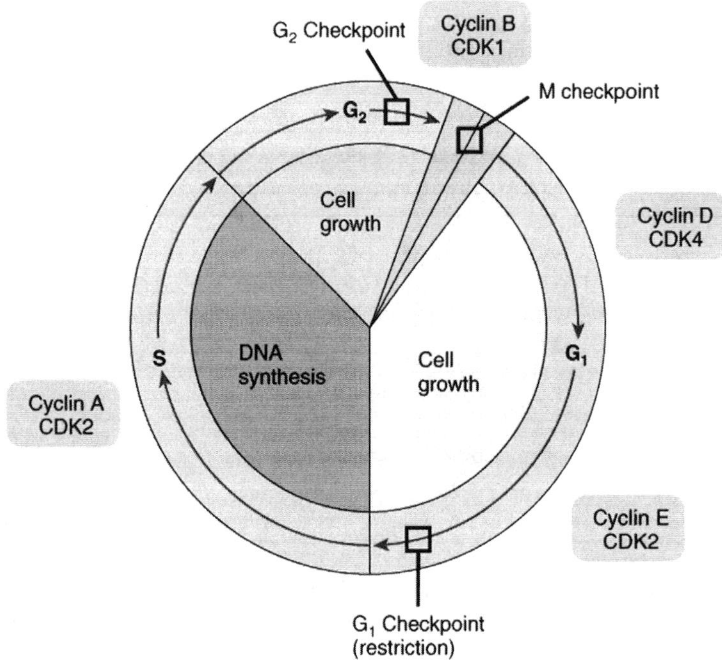

MUTATIONS

MUTATIONS

MISSENSE MUTATIONS, SILENT MUTATIONS, AND NONSENSE MUTATIONS

Mutations are changes in DNA sequences. **Point mutations** are changes in a single nucleotide in a DNA sequence. Three types of point mutations are missense, silent, and nonsense.

- **Missense mutations** result in a codon for a different amino acid. An example is mutating TGT (Cysteine codon) to TGG (Tryptophan codon).
- **Silent mutations** result in a codon for the same amino acid as the original sequence. An example is mutating TGT (Cysteine codon) to TGC (a different Cysteine codon).
- **Nonsense mutations** insert a premature stop codon, typically resulting in a non-functional protein. An example is mutating TGT (Cysteine codon) to TGA (STOP codon).

Review Video: Codons
Visit mometrix.com/academy and enter code: 978172

FRAMESHIFT MUTATIONS AND INVERSION MUTATIONS

Deletions and insertions can result in the addition of amino acids, the removal of amino acids, or cause a frameshift mutation. A **frameshift mutation** changes the reading frame of the mRNA (a new group of codons will be read), resulting in the formation of a new protein product. Mutations can also occur on the chromosomal level. For example, an **inversion** is when a piece of the chromosome inverts or flips its orientation.

GERMLINE MUTATIONS AND SOMATIC MUTATIONS

Mutations can occur in somatic (body) cells and germ cells (egg and sperm). **Somatic mutations** develop after conception and occur in an organism's body cells such as bone cells, liver cells, or brain cells. Somatic mutations cannot be passed on from parent to offspring. The mutation is limited to the specific descendent of the cell in which the mutation occurred. The mutation is not in the other body cells unless they are descendants of the originally mutated cell. Somatic mutations may cause cancer or diseases. Some somatic mutations are silent. **Germline mutations** are present at conception and occur in an organism's germ cells, which are only egg and sperms cells. Germline mutations may be passed on from parent to offspring. Germline mutations will be present in every cell of an offspring that inherits a germline mutation. Germline mutations may cause diseases. Some germline mutations are silent.

Mutagens

Mutagens are physical and chemical agents that cause changes or errors in DNA replication. Mutagens are external factors to an organism. Examples include ionizing radiation such as ultraviolet radiation, x-rays, and gamma radiation. Viruses and microorganisms that integrate their DNA into host chromosomes are also mutagens. Mutagens include environmental poisons such as asbestos, coal tars, tobacco, and benzene. Alcohol and diets high in fat have been shown to be mutagenic. Not all mutations are caused by mutagens. **Spontaneous mutations** can occur in DNA due to molecular decay.

Mendel's Laws

Law of Segregation

The **law of segregation** states that the alleles for a trait separate when gametes are formed, which means that only one of the pair of alleles for a given trait is passed to the gamete. This can be shown in monohybrid crosses, which can be used to show which allele is **dominant** for a single trait. A **monohybrid cross** is a genetic cross between two organisms with a different variation for a single trait. The first monohybrid cross typically occurs between two **homozygous** parents. Each parent is homozygous for a separate allele (gg or GG) for a particular trait. For example, in pea plants, green seeds (G) are dominant over yellow seeds (g). Therefore, in a genetic cross of two pea plants that are homozygous for seed color, the F_1 generation will be 100% **heterozygous** green seeds.

	g	**g**
G	Gg	Gg
G	Gg	Gg

Review Video: Gene & Alleles
Visit mometrix.com/academy and enter code: 363997

Review Video: Punnett Square
Visit mometrix.com/academy and enter code: 853855

Monohybrid Cross for a Cross Between Two Gg Parents

If the plants with the heterozygous green seeds are crossed, the F_2 generation should be 50% heterozygous green (Gg), 25% homozygous green (GG), and 25% homozygous yellow (gg).

	G	**g**
G	GG	Gg
g	Gg	gg

Law of Independent Assortment

Mendel's law of independent assortment states that alleles of one characteristic or trait separate independently of the alleles of another characteristic. Therefore, the allele a gamete receives for one gene does not influence the allele received for another gene due to the allele pairs separating independently during gamete formation. This means that traits are transmitted independently of each other. This can be shown in dihybrid crosses.

GENE, GENOTYPE, PHENOTYPE, AND ALLELE

A **gene** is a portion of DNA that identifies how traits are expressed and passed on in an organism. A gene is part of the genetic code. Collectively, all genes form the **genotype** of an individual. The genotype includes genes that may not be expressed, such as recessive genes. The **phenotype** is the physical, visual manifestation of genes. It is determined by the basic genetic information and how genes have been affected by their environment.

An **allele** is a variation of a gene. Also known as a trait, it determines the manifestation of a gene. This manifestation results in a specific physical appearance of some facet of an organism, such as eye color or height. The genetic information for eye color is a gene. The gene variations responsible for blue, green, brown, or black eyes are called alleles. **Locus** (plural, *loci*) refers to the location of a gene or alleles.

Review Video: Genotype vs Phenotype
Visit mometrix.com/academy and enter code: 922853

DOMINANT AND RECESSIVE GENES

Gene traits are represented in pairs with an uppercase letter for the **dominant trait** (A) and a lowercase letter for the **recessive trait** (a). Genes occur in pairs (AA, Aa, or aa). There is one gene on each chromosome half supplied by each parent organism. Since half the genetic material is from each parent, the offspring's traits are represented as a combination of these. A dominant trait only requires one gene of a gene pair for it to be expressed in a phenotype, whereas a recessive requires both genes in order to be manifested. For example, if the mother's genotype is Dd and the father's is dd, the possible combinations are Dd and dd. The dominant trait will be manifested if the genotype is DD or Dd. The recessive trait will be manifested if the genotype is dd. Both DD and dd are **homozygous** pairs. Dd is **heterozygous**.

DIHYBRID CROSS FOR THE F_2 GENERATION OF A CROSS BETWEEN *GGRR* AND *ggrr* PARENTS

A **dihybrid cross** is a genetic cross for two traits that each have two alleles. For example, in pea plants, green seeds (G) are dominant over yellow seeds (g), and round seeds (R) are dominant over wrinkled seeds (r). In a genetic cross of two pea plants that are homozygous for seed color and seed shape (GGRR or ggRR), the F_1 generation will be 100% heterozygous green and round seeds (GgRr). If these F_1 plants (GgRr) are crossed, the resulting F_2 generation is shown below. Out of the 16 total genotypes for the cross of green, round seeds, there are only four possible phenotypes, or physical traits of the seed: green and round seed (GGRR, GGRr, GgRR, or GgRr), green and wrinkled seed (GGrr or Ggrr), yellow and round seed (ggRR or ggRr) , or yellow and wrinkled seed (ggrr). There are nine green and round seed plants, three green and wrinkled seed plants, three yellow and round seed plants, and only one yellow and wrinkled seed plant. This cross has a **9:3:3:1 ratio**.

	GR	**gR**	**Gr**	**gr**
GR	GGRR	GgRR	GGRr	GgRr
gR	GgRR	ggRR	GgRr	ggRr
Gr	GGRr	GgRr	GGrr	Ggrr
gr	GgRr	ggRr	Ggrr	ggrr

PEDIGREE

Pedigree analysis is a type of genetic analysis in which an inherited trait is studied and traced through several generations of a family to determine how that trait is inherited. A **pedigree** is a chart arranged as a type of family tree using symbols for people and lines to represent the relationships between those people. Squares usually represent males, and circles represent females. Horizontal lines represent a male and female mating, and the vertical lines beneath them represent their children. Usually, family members who possess the trait are fully shaded and those who only carry the trait are half-shaded. Genotypes and phenotypes are determined for each individual if possible. The pedigree below shows the family tree of a family in which the first male who was red-green color blind mated with the first female who was unaffected. They had five children. The three sons were unaffected, and the two daughters were carriers.

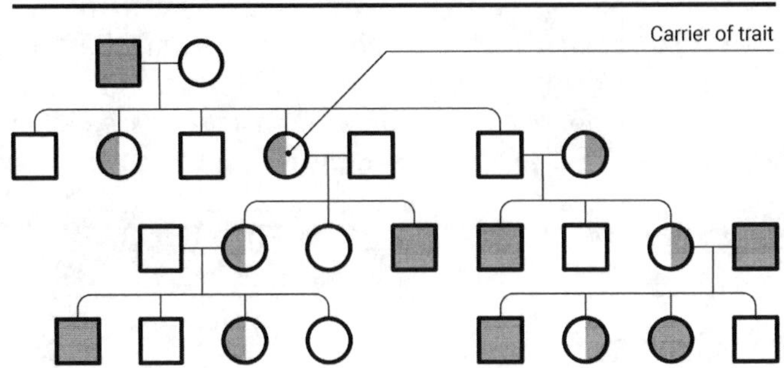

Processes Affecting the Gene Pool

Genetic Drift

Genetic drift is a microevolutionary process that causes random changes in allele frequencies that are not the result of natural selection. Genetic drift can result in a loss of genetic diversity. Genetic drift greatly impacts small populations. Two special forms of genetic drift are the genetic bottleneck and the founder effect. A **genetic bottleneck** occurs when there is a drastic reduction in population due to some change such as overhunting, disease, or habitat loss. When a population is greatly reduced in size, many alleles can be lost. Even if the population size greatly increases again, the lost alleles represent lost genetic diversity. The **founder effect** occurs when one individual or a few individuals populate a new area such as an island. This new population is limited to the alleles of the founder(s) unless mutations occur or new individuals immigrate to the region.

Gene Flow

Gene flow is a microevolutionary process in which alleles enter a population by immigration and leave a population by emigration. Gene flow helps counter genetic drift. When individuals from one genetically distinct population immigrate to a different genetically distinct population, alleles and their genetic information are added to the new population. The added alleles will change the gene frequencies within the population. This increases genetic diversity. If individuals with rare alleles emigrate from a population, the genetic diversity is decreased. Gene flow reduces the genetic differences between populations.

Mechanics of Evolution

Mechanisms of Evolution

Natural and Artificial Selection

Natural selection and artificial selection are both mechanisms of evolution. **Natural selection** is a process of nature in which a population can change over generations. Every population has variations in individual heritable traits and organisms best suited for survival typically reproduce and pass on those genetic traits to offspring to increase the likelihood of them surviving. Typically, the more advantageous a trait is, the more common that trait becomes in a population. Natural selection brings about evolutionary **adaptations** and is responsible for biological diversity. Artificial selection is another mechanism of evolution. **Artificial selection** is a process brought about by humans. Artificial selection is the selective breeding of domesticated animals and plants such as when farmers choose animals or plants with desirable traits to reproduce. Artificial selection has led to the evolution of farm stock and crops. For example, cauliflower, broccoli, and cabbage all evolved due to artificial selection of the wild mustard plant.

Sexual Selection

Sexual selection is a special case of natural selection in animal populations. **Sexual selection** occurs because some animals are more likely to find mates than other animals. The two main contributors to sexual selection are **competition** of males and **mate selection** by females. An example of male competition is in the mating practices of the redwing blackbird. Some males have huge territories and numerous mates that they defend. Other males have small territories, and some even have no mates. An example of mate selection by females is the mating practices of peacocks. Male peacocks display large, colorful tail feathers to attract females. Females are more likely to choose males with the larger, more colorful displays.

Coevolution

Coevolution describes a rare phenomenon in which two populations with a close ecological relationship undergo reciprocal adaptations simultaneously and evolve together, affecting each other's evolution. General examples of coevolution include predator and prey, or plant and pollinator, and parasites and their hosts. A specific example of coevolution is the yucca moths and the yucca plants. Yucca plants can only be pollinated by the yucca moths. The yucca moths lay their eggs in the yucca flowers, and their larvae grow inside the ovary.

Adaptive Radiation

Adaptive radiation is an evolutionary process in which a species branches out and adapts and fills numerous unoccupied ecological niches. The adaptations occur relatively quickly, driven by natural selection and resulting in new phenotypes and possibly new species eventually. An example of adaptive radiation is the finches that Darwin studied on the Galápagos Islands. Darwin recorded 13 different varieties of finches, which differed in the size and shape of their beaks. Through the process of natural selection, each type of finch adapted to the specific environment and specifically the food sources of the island to which it belonged. On newly formed islands with many unoccupied ecological niches, the adaptive radiation process occurred quickly due to the lack of competing species and predators.

Evidence Supporting Evolution

Evidence Supporting Evolution

Molecular Evidence

Because all organisms are made up of cells, all organisms are alike on a fundamental level. Cells share similar components, which are made up of molecules. Specifically, all cells contain DNA and RNA. This should indicate that all species descended from a **common ancestor**. Humans and chimpanzees share approximately 98% of their genes in common, while humans and bacteria share approximately 7% of their genes in common suggesting that bacteria and humans are not closely related. Biologists have been able to use DNA sequence comparisons of modern organisms to reconstruct the "root" of the tree of life. The fact that RNA can store information, replicate itself, and code for proteins suggests that RNA could have could have evolved first, followed by DNA.

Homology

Homology is the similarity of structures of different species based on a similar anatomy in a common evolutionary ancestor. For instance, the forelimbs of humans, dogs, birds, and whales all have the same basic pattern of the bones. Specifically, all of these organisms have a humerus, radius, and ulna. They are all modifications of the same basic evolutionary structure from a common ancestor. Tetrapods resemble the fossils of extinct transitional animal called the *Eusthenopteron*. This would seem to indicate that evolution primarily modifies preexisting structures.

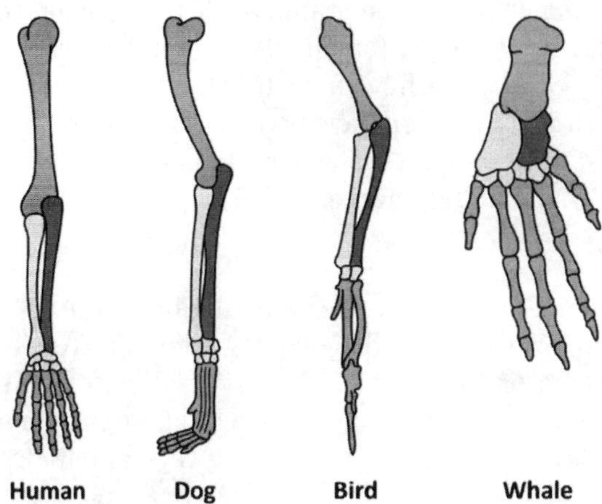

Review Video: Homologous vs Analogous Structures
Visit mometrix.com/academy and enter code: 355157

Embryology

The stages of **embryonic development** reveal homologies between species. These homologies are evidence of a **common ancestor**. For example, in chicken embryos and mammalian embryos, both include a stage in which slits and arches appear in the embryo's neck region that are strikingly similar to gill slits and gill arches in fish embryos. Adult chickens and adult mammals do not have gills, but this embryonic homology indicates that birds and mammals share a common ancestor with fish. As another example, some species of toothless whales have embryos that initially develop teeth that are later absorbed, which indicates that these whales have an ancestor with teeth in the adult form. Finally, most tetrapods have five-digit limbs, but birds have three-digit limbs in their wings. However, embryonic birds initially have five-digit limbs in their wings, which develop into a three-digit wing. Tetrapods such as reptiles, mammals, and birds all share a common ancestor with five-digit limbs.

Endosymbiosis Theory

The endosymbiosis theory is foundational to evolution. Endosymbiosis provides the path for prokaryotes to give rise to eukaryotes. Specifically, **endosymbiosis** explains the development of the organelles of mitochondria in animals and chloroplasts in plants. This theory states that some eukaryotic organelles such as mitochondria and chloroplasts originated as free living cells. According to this theory, primitive, heterotrophic eukaryotes engulfed smaller, autotrophic bacteria prokaryotes, but the bacteria were not digested. Instead, the eukaryotes and the bacteria formed a symbiotic relationship. Eventually, the bacteria transformed into mitochondrion or chloroplasts.

Supporting Evidence

Several facts support the endosymbiosis theory. Mitochondria and chloroplasts contain their own DNA and can both only arise from other preexisting mitochondria and chloroplasts. The genomes of mitochondria and chloroplasts consist of single, circular DNA molecules with no histones. This is similar to bacteria genomes, not eukaryote genomes. Also, the RNA, ribosomes, and protein synthesis of mitochondria and chloroplasts are remarkably similar to those of bacteria, and both use oxygen to produce ATP. These organelles have a double phospholipid layer that is typical of engulfed bacteria. This theory also involves a secondary endosymbiosis in which the original eukaryotic cells that have engulfed the bacteria are then engulfed themselves by another free-living eukaryote.

Convergent Evolution

Convergent evolution is the evolutionary process in which two or more unrelated species become increasingly similar in appearance. In convergent evolution, similar adaptations in these unrelated species occur due to these species inhabiting the same kind of environment. For example, the mammals shown below, although found in different parts of the world, developed similar appearances due to their similar environments.

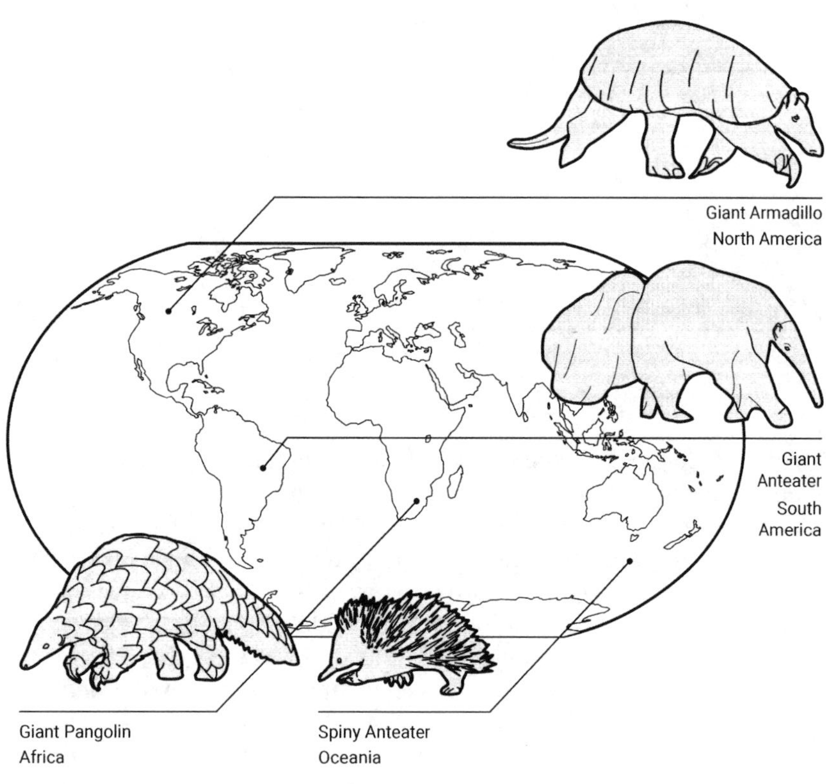

Divergent Evolution

Divergent evolution is the evolutionary process in which organisms of one species become increasingly dissimilar in appearance. As several small adaptations occur due to natural selection, the organisms will finally reach a point at which two new species are formed, also known as **speciation.** Then, these two species will further diverge from each other as they continue to evolve. Adaptive radiation is an example of divergent evolution. Another example is the divergent evolution of the wooly mammoth and the modern elephant from a common ancestor.

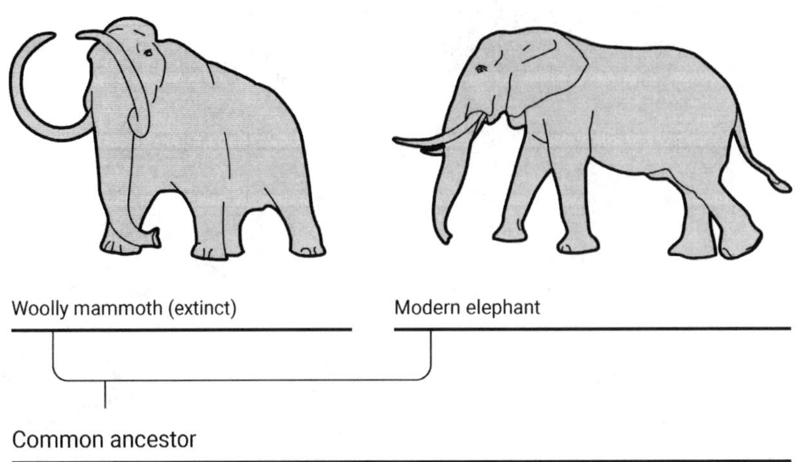

Fossil Record

The **fossil record** provides many types of support for evolution including comparisons from rock layers, transition fossils, and homologies with modern organisms. First, fossils from rock layers from all over the world have been compared, enabling scientists to develop a sequence of life from simple to complex. Based on the fossil record, the **geologic timeline** chronicles the history of all living things. For example, the fossil record clearly indicates that invertebrates developed before vertebrates and that fish developed before amphibians. Second, numerous transitional fossils have been found. **Transitional fossils** show an intermediate state between an ancestral form of an organism and the form of its descendants. These fossils show the path of evolutionary change. For example, many transition fossils documenting the evolutionary change from fish to amphibians have been discovered. In 2004, scientists discovered *Tiktaalik roseae*, or the "fishapod," which is a 375-million-year-old fossil that exhibits both fish and amphibian characteristics. Another example would be *Pakicetus,* an extinct land mammal, that scientists determined is an early ancestor of modern whales and dolphins based on the specialized structures of the inner ear. Most fossils exhibit homologies with modern organisms. For example, extinct horses are similar to modern horses, indicating a common ancestor.

Cephalization and Multicellularity

Cephalization is the evolutionary trend that can be summarized as "the evolution of the head." In most animals, nerve tissue has been concentrated into a brain at one end of an organism over many generations. Eventually, a head enclosing a brain and housing sensory organs was produced at one end of the organism. Many invertebrates, such as arthropods and annelids and all vertebrates, have undergone cephalization. However, some invertebrates, such as echinoderms and sponges, have not undergone cephalization, and these organisms literally do not have a head.

Another evolutionary trend is **multicellularity**. Life has evolved from simple, single-celled organisms to complex, multicellular organisms. Over millions of years, single-celled organisms gave rise to biofilms, which gave rise to multicellular organisms, which gave rise to all of the major phyla of multicellular organisms present today.

Scientific Explanations for the Origin of Life on Earth

Explanations for the Origin of Life on Earth

Panspermia

The word *panspermia* is a Greek work that means "seeds everywhere." **Panspermia** is one possible explanation for the origin of life on Earth that states that "seeds" of life exist throughout the universe and can be transferred from one location to another. Three types of panspermia based on the seed-dispersal method have been proposed. **Lithopanspermia** is described as rocks or dust transferring microorganisms between solar systems. **Ballistic panspermia** is described as rocks or dust transferring microorganisms between planets within the same solar system. **Directed panspermia** is described as intelligent extraterrestrials purposely spreading the seeds to other planets and solar systems. The panspermia hypothesis only proposes the origin of life on Earth. It does not offer an explanation for the origin of life in the universe or explain the origin of the seeds themselves.

Abiotic Synthesis of Organic Compounds

Scientists have performed sophisticated experiments to determine how the first organic compounds appeared on Earth. First, scientists performed controlled experiments that closely resembled the conditions similar to an early Earth. In the classic **Miller–Urey experiment** (1953), the Earth's early atmosphere was simulated with water, methane, ammonia, and hydrogen that were stimulated by an electric discharge. The Miller–Urey experiment produced complex organic compounds including several amino acids, sugars, and hydrocarbons. Later experiments by other scientists produced nucleic acids. Recently, Jeffrey Bada, a former student of Miller, was able to produce amino acids in a simulation using the Earth's current atmospheric conditions with the addition of iron and carbonate to the simulation. This is significant because in previous studies using Earth's current atmosphere, the amino acids were destroyed by the nitrites produced by the nitrogen.

Atmospheric Composition

The early atmosphere of Earth had little or possibly no oxygen. Early rocks had high levels of iron at their surfaces. Without oxygen, the iron just entered into the early oceans as ions. In the same time frame, early photosynthetic algae were beginning to grow abundantly in the early ocean. During photosynthesis, the algae would produce oxygen gas, which oxidized the iron at the rocks' surfaces, forming an iron oxide. This process basically kept the algae in an oxygen-free environment. As the algae population grew much larger, it eventually produced such a large amount of oxygen that it could not be removed by the iron in the rocks. Because the algae at this time were intolerant to oxygen, the algae became extinct. Over time, a new iron-rich layer of sediments formed, and algae populations reformed, and the cycle began again. This cycle repeated itself for millions of years. Iron-rich layers of sediment alternated with iron-poor layers. Gradually, algae and other life forms evolved that were tolerant to oxygen, stabilizing the oxygen concentration in the atmosphere at levels similar to those of today.

Development of Self-Replication

Several hypotheses for the origin of life involve the self-replication of molecules. In order for life to have originated on Earth, proteins and RNA must have been replicated. Hypotheses that combine the replication of proteins and RNA seem promising. One such hypothesis is called **RNA world**. RNA world explains how the pathway of DNA to RNA to protein may have originated by proposing the reverse process. RNA world proposes that self-replicating RNA was the precursor to DNA. Scientists have shown that RNA can actually function both as a gene and as an enzyme and could therefore have carried genetic information in earlier life stages. Also, RNA can be transcribed into DNA using reverse transcription. In RNA world, RNA molecules self-replicated and evolved through recombination and mutations. RNA molecules developed the ability to act as enzymes.

Eventually, RNA began to synthesize proteins. Finally, DNA molecules were copied from the RNA in a process of reverse transcription.

Historical and Current Biological Classification Systems of Organisms

Historical and Current Kingdom Systems

In 1735 Carolus Linnaeus devised a two-kingdom classification system. He placed all living things into either the *Animalia* kingdom or the *Plantae* kingdom. Fungi and algae were classified as plants. Also, Linnaeus developed the binomial nomenclature system that is still used today. In 1866, Ernst Haeckel introduced a three-kingdom classification system, adding the *Protista* kingdom to Linnaeus's animal and plant kingdoms. Bacteria were classified as protists and cyanobacteria were still classified as plants. In 1938, Herbert Copeland introduced a four-kingdom classification system in which bacteria and cyanobacteria were moved to the *Monera* kingdom. In 1969, Robert Whittaker introduced a five-kingdom system that moved fungi from the plant kingdom to the *Fungi* kingdom. Some algae were still classified as plants. In 1977, Carl Woese introduced a six-kingdom system in which in the *Monera* kingdom was replaced with the *Eubacteria* kingdom and the *Archaebacteria* kingdom.

Domain Classification System

In 1990, Carl Woese introduced his domain classification system. **Domains** are broader groupings above the kingdom level. This system consists of three domains—*Archaea*, *Bacteria*, and *Eukarya*. All eukaryotes such as plants, animals, fungi, and protists are classified in the *Eukarya* domain. The *Bacteria* and *Archaea* domains consist of prokaryotes. Organisms previously classified in the *Monera* kingdom are now classified into either the *Bacteria* or *Archaea* domain based on their ribosomal RNA structure. Members of the *Archaea* domain often live in extremely harsh environments.

Review Video: Biological Classification Systems
Visit mometrix.com/academy and enter code: 736052

Viruses, Bacteria, Protists, Fungi, Plants, and Animals

Viruses

Viruses are nonliving, infectious particles that act as parasites in living organisms. Viruses are acellular, which means that they lack cell structure. Viruses cannot reproduce outside of living cells. The structure of a virus is a nucleic acid genome, which may be either DNA or RNA, surrounded by a protective protein coat or **capsid**. In some viruses, the capsid may be surrounded by a lipid membrane or envelope. Viruses can contain up to 500 genes and have various shapes. They usually are too small to be seen without the aid of an electron microscope. Viruses can infect plants, animals, fungi, protists, and bacteria. Viruses can attack only specific types of cells that have specific receptors on their surfaces. Viruses do not divide or reproduce like living cells. Instead, they use the host cell they infect by "reprogramming" it, using the nucleic acid genome, to make more copies of the virus. The host cell usually bursts to release these copies.

Review Video: Viruses and Antiviral Drugs
Visit mometrix.com/academy and enter code: 984455

Bacteria

Bacteria are small, prokaryotic, single-celled organisms. Bacteria have a circular loop of DNA (plasmid) that is not contained within a nuclear membrane. Bacterial ribosomes are not bound to the endoplasmic reticulum, as in eukaryotes. A cell wall containing peptidoglycan surrounds the bacterial plasma membrane. Some bacteria such as pathogens are further encased in a gel-like, sticky layer called the **capsule**, which enhances their ability to cause disease. Bacteria can be autotrophs or heterotrophs. Some bacterial heterotrophs are saprophytes that function as decomposers in ecosystems. Many types of bacteria share commensal or mutualistic relationships with other organisms. Most bacteria reproduce asexually by binary fission. Two identical daughter cells are produced from one parent cell. Some bacteria can transfer genetic material to other bacteria through a process called conjugation, while some bacteria can incorporate DNA from the environment in a process called transformation.

Protists

Protists are small, eukaryotic, single-celled organisms. Although protists are small, they are much larger than prokaryotic bacteria. Protists have three general forms, which include plantlike protists, animal-like protists, and fungus-like protists. **Plantlike protists** are algae that contain chlorophyll and perform photosynthesis. Animal-like protists are **protozoa** with no cell walls that typically lack chlorophyll and are grouped by their method of locomotion, which may use flagella, cilia, or a different structure. **Fungus-like protists**, which do not have chitin in their cell walls, are generally grouped as either slime molds or water molds. Protists may be autotrophic or heterotrophic. Autotrophic protists include many species of algae, while heterotrophic protists include parasitic, commensal, and mutualistic protozoa. Slime molds are heterotrophic fungus-like protists, which consume microorganisms. Some protists reproduce sexually, but most reproduce asexually by binary fission. Some reproduce asexually by spores while others reproduce by alternation of generations and require two hosts in their life cycle.

Fungi

Fungi are nonmotile organisms with eukaryotic cells and contain chitin in their cell walls. Most fungi are multicellular, but a few including yeast are unicellular. Fungi have multicellular filaments called **hyphae** that are grouped together into the mycelium. Fungi do not perform photosynthesis and are considered heterotrophs. Fungi can be parasitic, mutualistic or free living. Free-living fungi include mushrooms and toadstools. Parasitic fungi include fungi responsible for ringworm and athlete's foot. Mycorrhizae are mutualistic fungi that live in or near plant roots increasing the roots' surface area of absorption. Almost all fungi reproduce asexually by spores, but most fungi also have a sexual phase in the production of spores. Some fungi reproduce by budding or fragmentation.

Review Video: Feeding Among Heterotrophs
Visit mometrix.com/academy and enter code: 836017

Review Video: Kingdom Fungi
Visit mometrix.com/academy and enter code: 315081

Plants

Plants are multicellular organisms with eukaryotic cells containing cellulose in their cell walls. Plant cells have chlorophyll and perform photosynthesis. Plants can be vascular or nonvascular. **Vascular plants** have true leaves, stems, and roots that contain xylem and phloem. **Nonvascular plants** lack true leaves, stems and roots and do not have any true vascular tissue but instead rely on diffusion and osmosis to transport most of materials or resources needed to survive. Almost all plants are autotrophic, relying on photosynthesis for food. A small number do not have chlorophyll and are parasitic, but these are extremely rare. Plants can reproduce sexually or asexually. Many plants reproduce by seeds produced in the fruits of the plants, while some plants reproduce by seeds on cones. One type of plant, ferns, reproduce by a different system that utilizes spores. Some plants can even reproduce asexually by vegetative reproduction.

Review Video: Kingdom Plantae
Visit mometrix.com/academy and enter code: 710084

Structure, Organization, Modes of Nutrition, and Reproduction of Animals

Animals are multicellular organism with eukaryotic cells that do not have cell walls surrounding their plasma membranes. Animals have several possible structural body forms. Animals can be relatively simple in structure such as sponges, which do not have a nervous system. Other animals are more complex with cells organized into tissues, and tissues organized into organs, and organs even further organized into systems. Invertebrates such as arthropods, nematodes, and annelids have complex body systems. Vertebrates including fish, amphibians, reptiles, birds, and mammals are the most complex with detailed systems such as those with gills, air sacs, or lungs designed to exchange respiratory gases. All animals are heterotrophs and obtain their nutrition by consuming autotrophs or other heterotrophs. Most animals are motile, but some animals move their environment to bring food to them. All animals reproduce sexually at some point in their life cycle. Typically, this involves the union of a sperm and egg to produce a zygote.

Review Video: Kingdom Animalia
Visit mometrix.com/academy and enter code: 558413

Characteristics of the Major Animal Phyla

Characteristics of the Major Animal Phyla

Body Planes

Animals can exhibit bilateral symmetry, radial symmetry, or asymmetry. With **bilateral symmetry**, the organism can be cut in half along only one plane to produce two identical halves. Most animals, including all vertebrates such as mammals, birds, reptiles, amphibians, and fish, exhibit bilateral symmetry. Many invertebrates including arthropods and crustaceans also exhibit bilateral symmetry. With **radial symmetry**, the organism can be cut in half along several planes to produce two identical halves. Starfish, sea urchins, and jellyfish exhibit radial symmetry. With **asymmetry**, the organism exhibits no symmetry. Very few organisms in the animal phyla exhibit asymmetry, but a few species of sponges are asymmetrical.

Body Cavities

Animals can be grouped based on their types of body cavities. A **coelom** is a fluid-filled body cavity between the alimentary canal and the body wall. The three body plans based on the formation of the coelom are coelomates, pseudocoelomates, and acoelomates. **Coelomates** have a true coelom located within the mesoderm. Most animals including arthropods, mollusks, annelids, echinoderms, and chordates are coelomates. **Pseudocoelomates** have a body cavity called a pseudocoelom. **Pseudocoeloms** are not considered true coeloms. Pseudocoeloms are located between mesoderm and endoderm instead of actually in the mesoderm as in a true coelom. Pseudocoelomates include roundworms and rotifers. **Acoelomates** do not have body cavities. Simple or primitive animals such as sponges, jellyfish, sea anemones, hydras, flatworms, and ribbon worms are acoelomates.

Modes of Reproduction

Animals can reproduce sexually or asexually. Most animals reproduce sexually. In **sexual reproduction**, males and females have different reproductive organs that produce **gametes**. Males have testes that produce sperm, and females have ovaries that produce eggs. During fertilization, a sperm cell unites with an egg cell, forming a **zygote**. Fertilization can occur internally such as in most mammals and birds or externally such as aquatic animals such as fish and frogs. The zygote undergoes cell division, which develops into an embryo and eventually develops into an adult organism. Some embryos develop in eggs such as in fish, amphibians, reptiles, and birds. Some mammals are **oviparous** meaning that they lay eggs, but most are **viviparous** meaning they have a uterus in which the embryo develops. One particular type of mammal called **marsupials** give birth to an immature fetus that finishes development in a pouch. However, there are some animals reproduce **asexually**. For example, hydras reproduce by budding, and starfish and planarians can reproduce by fragmentation and regeneration. Some fish, frogs, and insects can even reproduce by parthenogenesis, which is a type of self-reproduction without fertilization.

Modes of Temperature Regulation

Animals can be classified as either homeotherms or poikilotherms. **Homeotherms**, also called warm-blooded animals or **endotherms**, maintain a constant body temperature regardless of the temperature of the environment. Homeotherms such as mammals and birds have a high metabolic rate because a lot of energy is needed to maintain the constant temperature. **Poikilotherms**, also called cold-blooded animals or **ectotherms**, do not maintain a constant body temperature. Their body temperature fluctuates with the temperature of the environment. Poikilotherms such as arthropods, fish, amphibians, and reptiles have metabolic rates that fluctuate with their body temperature.

Hierarchy of Multicellular Organisms

Organizational Hierarchy within Multicellular Organisms

Cells are the smallest living units of organisms. Tissues are groups of cells that work together to perform a specific function. Organs are groups of tissues that work together to perform a specific function. Organ systems are groups of organs that work together to perform a specific function. An organism is an individual that contains several body systems.

Cells

Cells are the basic structural units of all living things. Cells are composed of various molecules including proteins, carbohydrates, lipids, and nucleic acids. All animal cells are eukaryotic and have a nucleus, cytoplasm, and a cell membrane. Organelles include mitochondria, ribosomes, endoplasmic reticulum, Golgi apparatuses, and vacuoles. Specialized cells are numerous, including but not limited to, muscle cells, nerve cells, epithelial cells, bone cells, blood cells, and cartilage cells. Cells can be grouped together in tissues to perform specific functions.

Tissues

Tissues are groups of cells that work together to perform a specific function. Tissues can be grouped into four broad categories: muscle tissue, connective tissue, nerve tissue, and epithelial tissue. Muscle tissue is involved in body movement. **Muscle tissues** can be composed of skeletal muscle cells, cardiac muscle cells, or smooth muscle cells. Skeletal muscles include the muscles commonly called biceps, triceps, hamstrings, and quadriceps. Cardiac muscle tissue is found only in the heart. Smooth muscle tissue provides tension in the blood vessels, controls pupil dilation, and aids in peristalsis. **Connective tissues** include bone tissue, cartilage, tendons, ligaments, fat, blood, and lymph. **Nerve tissue** is located in the brain, spinal cord, and nerves. **Epithelial tissue** makes up the layers of the skin and various membranes. Tissues are grouped together as organs to perform specific functions.

Organs and Organ Systems

Organs are groups of tissues that work together to perform specific functions. **Organ systems** are groups of organs that work together to perform specific functions. Complex animals have several organs that are grouped together in multiple systems. In mammals, there are 11 major organ systems: integumentary system, respiratory system, cardiovascular system, endocrine system, nervous system, immune system, digestive system, excretory system, muscular system, skeletal system, and reproductive system.

Homeostasis

Maintenance of Homeostasis in Organisms

Role of Feedback Mechanisms

Homeostasis is the regulation of internal chemistry to maintain a constant internal environment. This state is controlled through various feedback mechanisms that consist of receptors, an integrator, and effectors. **Receptors** such as mechanoreceptors or thermoreceptors in the skin detect the stimuli. Then, an **integrator**, such as the brain or spinal cord, receives the information concerning the stimuli and sends out signals to other parts of the body. Finally, **effectors**, such as muscles or glands, respond to the stimulus. Basically, the receptors receive the stimuli and notify an integrator, which signals the effectors to respond.

Feedback mechanisms can be negative or positive. **Negative-feedback** mechanisms are mechanisms that provide a decrease in response with an increase in stimulus that inhibits the stimulus, which in turn decreases the response. **Positive-feedback** mechanisms are mechanisms that provide an increase in response with an increase in stimulus, which actually increases the stimulus, which in turn increases the response.

Role of Hypothalamus

The hypothalamus plays a major role in the homoeostasis of vertebrates. The **hypothalamus** is the central portion of the brain just above the brainstem and is linked to the endocrine system through the pituitary gland. The hypothalamus releases special hormones that influence the secretion of pituitary hormones. The hypothalamus regulates the fundamental physiological state by controlling body temperature, hunger, thirst, sleep, behaviors related to attachment, sexual development, fight-or-flight stress response, and circadian rhythms.

Role of Endocrine System and Hormones

All vertebrates have an **endocrine system** that consists of numerous ductless glands that produce hormones to help coordinate many functions of the body. **Hormones** are signaling molecules that are received by receptors. Many hormones are secreted in response to signals from the pituitary gland and hypothalamus gland. Other hormones are secreted in response to signals from inside the body. Hormones can consist of amino acids, proteins, or lipid molecules such as steroid hormones. Hormones can affect target cells, which have the correct receptor that is able to bind to that particular hormone. Most cells have receptors for more than one type of hormone. Hormones are distributed to the target cells in the blood by the cardiovascular system. Hormones incorporate feedback mechanisms to help the body maintain homeostasis.

Role of Antidiuretic Hormone

Antidiuretic hormone (ADH) helps maintain homeostasis in vertebrates. ADH is produced by the posterior pituitary gland, and it regulates the reabsorption of water in the kidneys and concentrates the urine. The stimulus in this feedback mechanism is a drop in blood volume due to water loss. This signal is picked up by the hypothalamus, which signals the pituitary gland to secrete ADH. ADH is carried by the cardiovascular system to the nephrons in the kidneys signaling them to reabsorb more water and send less out as waste. As more water is reabsorbed, the blood volume increases, which is monitored by the hypothalamus. As the blood volume reaches the set point, the hypothalamus signals for a decrease in the secretion of ADH, and the cycle continues.

Role of Insulin and Glucagon

Insulin and glucagon are hormones that help maintain the glucose concentration in the blood. Insulin and glucagon are secreted by the clumps of endocrine cells called the **pancreatic islets** that are located in the pancreas. Insulin and glucagon work together to maintain the blood glucose level. **Insulin** stimulates cells to remove glucose from the blood. **Glucagon** stimulates the liver to convert glycogen to glucose. After eating, glucose levels increase in the blood. This stimulus signals the pancreas to stop the secretion of glucagon and to start secreting insulin. Cells respond to the insulin and remove glucose from the blood, lowering the level of glucose in the blood. Later, after eating, the level of glucose in the blood decreases further. This stimulus signals the pancreas to secrete glucagon and decrease the secretion of insulin. In response to the stimulus, the liver converts glycogen to glucose, and the level of glucose in the blood rises. When the individual eats, the cycle begins again.

Thermoregulation

Animals exhibit many adaptations that help them achieve homeostasis, or a stable internal environment. Some of these adaptions are behavioral. Most organisms exhibit some type of behavioral thermoregulation. **Thermoregulation** is the ability to keep the body temperature within certain boundaries. The type of behavioral thermoregulation depends on whether the animal is an ectotherm or an endotherm. **Ectotherms** are "cold-blooded," and their body temperature changes with their external environment. **Endotherms** are "warm-blooded" and maintain a stable body temperature by internal means.

To regulate their temperature, ectotherms often move to an appropriate location. For example, fish move to warmer waters while animals will climb to higher grounds. **Diurnal ectotherms** such as reptiles often bask in the sun to increase their body temperatures. Butterflies are special ectotherms classified as **heliotherms** since they get nearly all of their heat from basking in the sun.

While they have internal systems that regulate temperature, many endotherms that live in hot environments have adapted to the nocturnal lifestyle. Desert animals are often nocturnal to escape high daytime temperatures. Other nocturnal animals sleep during the day in underground burrows or dens.

REPRODUCTION, DEVELOPMENT, AND GROWTH IN ANIMALS

GAMETE FORMATION

Gametogenesis is the formation of gametes, or reproductive cells. Gametes are produced by meiosis. **Meiosis** is a special type of cell division that consists of two consecutive mitotic divisions referred to as meiosis I and meiosis II. **Meiosis I** is a reduction division in which a diploid cell is reduced to two haploid daughter cells that contain only one of each pair of homologous chromosomes. During **meiosis II**, those haploid cells are further divided to form four haploid cells. **Spermatogenesis** in males produces four viable sperm cells from each complete cycle of meiosis. **Oogenesis** produces four daughter cells, but only one is a viable egg and the other three are polar bodies.

FERTILIZATION

Fertilization is the union of a sperm cell and an egg cell to produce a zygote. Many sperm may bind to an egg, but only one joins with the egg and injects its nuclei into the egg. Fertilization can be external or internal. **External fertilization** takes place outside of the female's body. For example, many fish, amphibians, crustaceans, mollusks, and corals reproduce externally by **spawning** or releasing gametes into the water simultaneously or right after each other. Reptiles and birds reproduce by **internal fertilization**. All mammals except monotremes (e.g. platypus) reproduce by internal fertilization.

EMBRYONIC DEVELOPMENT

Embryonic development in animals is typically divided into four stages: cleavage, patterning, differentiation, and growth. **Cleavage** occurs immediately after fertilization when the large single-celled zygote immediately begins to divide into smaller and smaller cells without an increase in mass. A hollow ball of cells forms a blastula. Next, during patterning, gastrulation occurs. During gastrulation, the cells are organized into three primary germ layers: ectoderm, mesoderm, and endoderm. Then, the cells in these layers differentiate into special tissues and organs. For example, the nervous system develops from the ectoderm. The muscular system develops from the mesoderm. Much of the digestive system develops from the endoderm. The final stage of embryonic development is growth and further tissue specialization. The embryo continues to grow until ready for hatching or birth.

POSTNATAL GROWTH

Postnatal growth occurs from hatching or birth until death. The length of the postnatal growth depends on the species. Elephants can live 70 years, but mice only about 4 years. Right after animals are hatched or born, they go through a period of rapid growth and development. In vertebrates, bones lengthen, muscles grow in bulk, and fat is deposited. At maturity, bones stop growing in length, but bones can grow in width and repair themselves throughout the animal's lifetime, and muscle deposition slows down. Fat cells continue to increase and decrease in size throughout the animal's life. Growth is controlled by genetics but is also influenced by nutrition and disease. Most animals are sexually mature in less than two years and can produce offspring.

CHARACTERISTICS OF MAJOR PLANT DIVISIONS

VASCULAR AND NONVASCULAR PLANTS

Vascular plants, also referred to as **tracheophytes**, have dermal tissue, meristematic tissue, ground tissues, and vascular tissues. Nonvascular plants, also referred to as **bryophytes**, do not have the vascular tissue xylem and phloem. Vascular plants can grow very tall, whereas nonvascular plants are short and close to the ground. Vascular plants can be found in dry regions, but nonvascular plants typically grow near or in moist areas. Vascular plants have leaves, roots, and stems, but nonvascular plants have leaf-like, root-like, and stem-like structures that do not have true vascular tissue. Nonvascular plants have hair-like **rhizoids**, that act like roots by anchoring them to the ground and absorbing water. Vascular plants include angiosperms, gymnosperms, and ferns. Nonvascular plants include mosses and liverworts.

Flowering Versus Nonflowering Plants

Angiosperms and gymnosperms are both vascular plants. **Angiosperms** are flowering plants, and **gymnosperms** are non-flowering plants. Angiosperms reproduce by seeds that are enclosed in an ovary, usually in a fruit, while gymnosperms reproduce by unenclosed or "naked" seeds on scales, leaves, or cones. Angiosperms can be further classified as either monocots or dicots, depending on if they have one or two cotyledons, respectively. Angiosperms include grasses, garden flowers, vegetables, and broadleaf trees such as maples, birches, elms, and oaks. Gymnosperms include conifers such as pines, spruces, cedars, and redwoods.

Review Video: Fruits in Flowering Plants
Visit mometrix.com/academy and enter code: 867090

Review Video: Kingdom Plantae Characteristics
Visit mometrix.com/academy and enter code: 710084

Monocots and Dicots

Angiosperms can be classified as either monocots or dicots. The seeds of **monocots** have one cotyledon, and the seeds of **dicots** have two cotyledons. The flowers of monocots have petals in multiples of three, and the flowers of dicots have petals in multiples of four or five. The leaves of monocots are slender with parallel veins, while the leaves of dicots are broad and flat with branching veins. The vascular bundles in monocots are distributed throughout the stem, whereas the vascular bundles in dicots are arranged in rings. Monocots have a **fibrous root system**, and dicots have a **taproot system**.

Major Plant Tissues and Organs

Plant Dermal Tissue

Plant dermal tissue is called the epidermis, and is usually a single layer of closely-packed cells that covers leaves and young stems. The epidermis protects the plant by secreting the cuticle, which is a waxy substance that helps prevent water loss and infections. The epidermis in leaves has tiny pores called **stomata**. Guard cells in the epidermis control the opening and closing of the stomata. The epidermis usually does not have chloroplasts. The epidermis may be replaced by periderm in older plants. The **periderm** is also referred to as bark. The layers of the periderm are cork cells or phellem, phelloderm, and cork cambium or phellogen. Cork is the outer layer of the periderm and consists of nonliving cells. The periderm protects the plant and provides insulation.

Plant Vascular Tissue

The two major types of plant vascular tissue are xylem and phloem. Xylem and phloem are bound together in vascular bundles. A meristem called vascular cambium is located between the xylem and phloem and produces new xylem and phloem. **Xylem** is made up of tracheids and vessel elements. All vascular plants contain tracheids, but only angiosperms contain vessel elements. Xylem provides support and transports water and dissolved minerals unidirectionally from the roots upward using processes like transpiration pull and root pressure. Phloem is made up of companion cells and sieve-tube cells. **Phloem** transports dissolved sugars produced during photosynthesis and other nutrients bidirectionally to non-photosynthetic areas of the plant. By active transport, the companion vessels move glucose in and out of the sieve-tube cells.

Plant Ground Tissue

The three major types of ground tissue are parenchyma tissue, collenchyma tissue, and sclerenchyma tissue. Most ground tissue is made up of parenchyma. **Parenchyma** is formed by parenchyma cells, and it function in photosynthesis, food storage, and tissue repair. The inner tissue of a leaf, mesophyll, is an example of parenchyma tissue. **Collenchyma** is made of collenchyma cells and provides support in roots, stems, and petioles. **Sclerenchyma** tissue is made of sclereid cells, which are more rigid than the collenchyma cells, and provides rigid support and protection. Plant sclerenchyma tissue may contain cellulose or lignin. Fabrics such as jute, hemp, and flax are made of sclerenchyma tissue.

Plant Meristematic Tissue

Meristems or meristematic tissues are regions of plant growth. The cells in meristems are undifferentiated and always remain **totipotent**, which means they can always develop into any type of special tissue. Meristem cells can divide and produce new cells, which can aid in the process of regenerating damaged parts. Cells of meristems reproduce asexually through mitosis or cell division that is regulated by hormones. The two types of meristems are lateral meristems and apical meristems. **Primary growth** occurs at **apical meristems**, located at the tip of roots and shoots, and increases the length of the plant. Primary meristems include the protoderm, which produces epidermis; the procambium, which produces cambium, or lateral meristems; xylem and phloem; and the ground meristem, which produces ground tissue including parenchyma. **Secondary growth** occurs at the lateral or secondary meristems and causes an increase in diameter or thickness.

Flowers

The primary function of flowers is to produce seeds for reproduction of the plant. Flowers have a **pedicel**, a stalk with a receptacle or enlarged upper portion, which holds the developing seeds. Flowers also can have sepals and petals. **Sepals** are leaflike structures that protect the bud. **Petals**, which are collectively called the corolla, help to attract pollinators. Plants can have stamens, pistils, or both depending on the type of plant. The **stamen** consists of the anther and filament. The end of the stamen is called the **anther** and is where pollen is produced. Pollen also contains sperm, which is needed in order for a proper plant zygot to form. The **pistil** consists of the stigma, style, and ovary. The ovary contains the ovules, which house the egg cells.

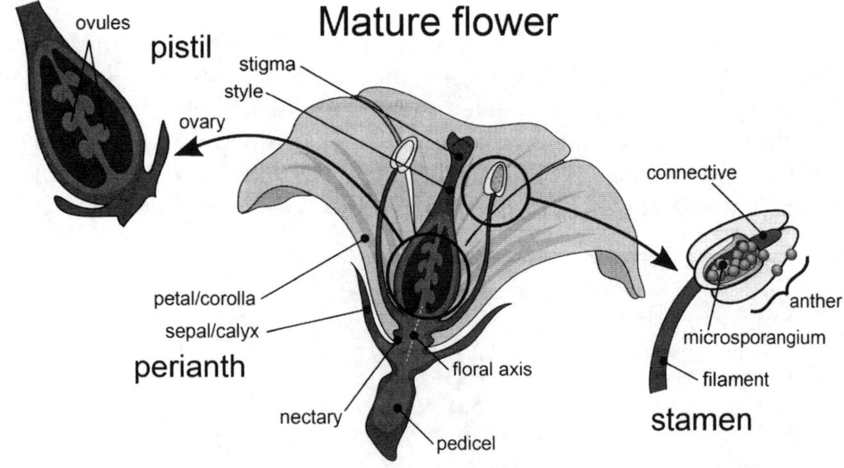

Stems

Plants can have either woody or nonwoody (herbaceous) stems. **Woody** stems consist of wood, or bark, as a structural tissue, while **herbaceous** stems are very flexible. The stem is divided into nodes and internodes. Buds are located at the nodes and may develop into leaves, roots, flowers, cones, or more stems. Stems consist of dermal tissue, ground tissue, and vascular tissue. **Monocot stems have vascular bundles distributed through the stem. Dicots have rings of vascular bundles**. Stems have four main functions: (1) they provide support to leaves, flowers, and fruits; (2) they transport materials in the xylem and phloem; (3) they store food; and (4) they have meristems, which provide all of the new cells for the plant.

MONOCOT	DICOT
Single Cotyledon	Two Cotyledon
Long Narrow Leaf Parallel Veins	Broad Leaf Network of Veins
Vascular Bundles Scattered	Vascular Bundles in a Ring
Floral Parts in Multiples of 3	Floral Parts in Multiples of 4 or 5

LEAVES

The primary function of a **leaf** is to manufacture food through photosynthesis. The leaf consists of a flat portion called the **blade** and a stalk called the **petiole**. The edge of the leaf is called the margin and can be entire, toothed, or lobed. Veins transport food and water and make up the skeleton of the leaf. The large central vein is called the **midrib**. The blade has an upper and lower epidermis. The epidermis is covered by a protective cuticle. The lower epidermis contains many stomata, which are pores that allow air to enter and leave the leaf. Stomata also regulate transpiration. The middle portion of the leaf is called the **mesophyll**. The mesophyll consists of the palisade mesophyll and the spongy mesophyll. Most photosynthesis occurs in chloroplasts located in the palisade mesophyll.

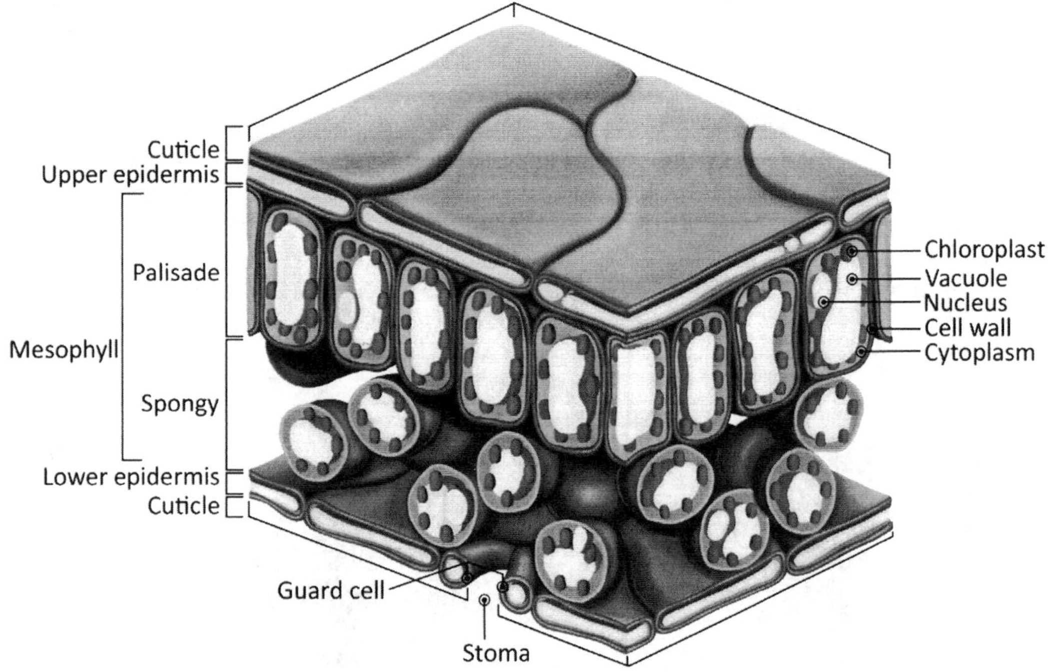

Roots

The primary functions of roots are to anchor the plant, absorb materials, and store food. The two basic types of root systems are taproot systems and fibrous root systems. **Taproot systems** have a primary root with many smaller secondary roots. **Fibrous root systems**, which lack a primary root, consist of a mass of many small secondary roots. The root has three main regions: the area of maturation, the area of elongation, and the area of cell division or the meristematic region. The root is covered by an epidermal cell, some of which develops into root hairs. **Root hairs** absorb water and minerals by osmosis, and capillary action helps move the water upward through the roots to the rest of the plant. The center of the root is the **vascular cylinder**, which contains the xylem and phloem. The vascular cylinder is surrounded by the cortex where the food is stored. Primary growth occurs at the root tip. Secondary growth occurs at the vascular cambium located between the xylem and phloem.

Plant Life Cycles and Reproductive Strategies

Pollination Strategies

Pollination is the transfer of pollen from the anther of the stamen to the stigma of the pistil on the same plant or on a different plant. Pollinators can be either **abiotic** (not derived from a living organism) or **biotic** (derived from a living organism). Abiotic pollinators include wind and water. Approximately 20% of pollination occurs by abiotic pollinators. For example, grasses are typically pollinated by wind, and aquatic plants are typically pollinated by water. Biotic pollinators include insects, birds, mammals, and occasionally reptiles. Most biotic pollinators are insects. Many plants have colored petals and strong scents, which attract insects. Pollen rubs off on the insects and is transferred as they move from plant to plant.

Seed Dispersal Methods

Methods of **seed dispersal** can be abiotic or biotic. Methods of seed dispersal include gravity, wind, water, and animals. Some plants produce seeds in fruits that get eaten by animals and then are distributed to new locations in the animals' waste. Some seeds (e.g. dandelions) have structures to aid in dispersal by wind. Some seeds have barbs that get caught in animal hair or bird feathers and are then carried to new locations by the animals. Interestingly, some animals bury seeds for food storage but do not return for the seeds. The seeds of aquatic plants can be dispersed by water, while the seeds of plants near rivers, streams, lakes, and beaches (e.g. coconuts) are also often dispersed by water. Some plants, in a method called **mechanical dispersal**, can propel or shoot their seeds away from them even up to several feet. For example, touch-me-nots and violets utilize mechanical dispersal.

Alternation of Generations

Alternation of generations, also referred to as **metagenesis**, contains both a sexual phase and an asexual phase in the life cycle of the plant. Mosses and ferns reproduce by alternation of generations: the sexual phase is called the **gametophyte**, and the asexual phase is called the **sporophyte**. During the sexual phase, a sperm fertilizes an egg to form a zygote. By mitosis, the zygote develops into the sporophyte. The sporangia in the sori of the sporophyte produce the spores through meiosis. The spores germinate and by mitosis produce the gametophyte.

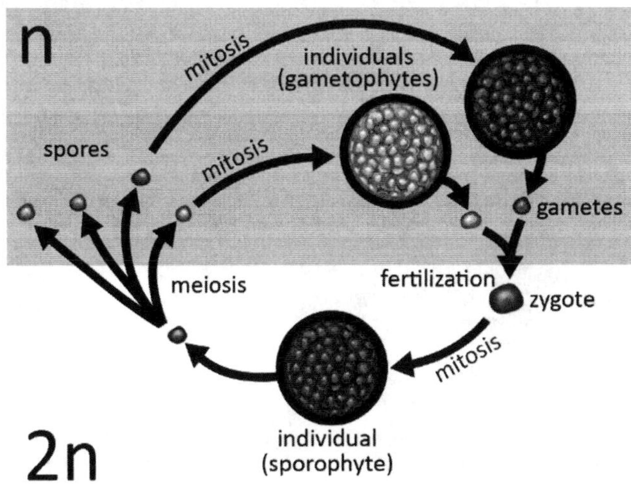

Plant Transportation of Water and Nutrients

Obtaining and Transporting Water and Inorganic Nutrients

Inorganic nutrients and water enter plants through the root hair and travel to the xylem. Once the water, minerals, and salts have crossed the endodermis, they must be moved upward through the xylem by water uptake. Most of a plant's water is lost through the stomata by transpiration. This loss is necessary to provide the tension needed to pull the water and nutrients up through the xylem. In order to maintain the remaining water that is necessary for the functioning of the plant, guard cells control the stomata. Whether an individual stoma is closed or open is controlled by two guard cells. When the guard cells lose water and become flaccid, they collapse together, closing the stoma. When the guard cells swell with water and become turgid, they move apart, opening the stoma.

Use of Roots

Plant roots have numerous root hairs that absorb water and inorganic nutrients such as minerals and salts. Root hairs are thin, hair-like outgrowths of the root's epidermal cells that exponentially increase the root's surface area. Water molecules cross the cell membranes of the root hairs by **osmosis** and then travel on to the vascular cylinder. Inorganic nutrients are transported across the cell membranes of the root endodermis by **active transport**. The endodermis is a single layer of cells that the water and nutrients must pass through by osmosis or active transport. To control mineral uptake by the roots, Casparian strips act as an extracellular diffusion barrier, and forces nutrients to be pulled into the plant. While water passes through by osmosis, mineral uptake is controlled by transport proteins.

Use of Xylem

The xylem contains dead, water-conducting cells called tracheids and vessels. The movement of water upward through the tracheids and vessels is explained by the **cohesion-tension theory**. First, water is lost through evaporation of the plant's surface through transpiration. This can occur at any surface exposed to air but is mainly through the stomata in the epidermis. This transpiration puts the water inside the xylem in a state of tension. Because water is cohesive due to the strong hydrogen bonds between molecules, the water is pulled up the xylem as long as the water is transpiring.

Products of Photosynthesis

Glucose Produced During Photosynthesis

Plants produce glucose, a simple carbohydrate or monosaccharide, during photosynthesis. Plants do not transport glucose molecules directly, but instead glucose undergoes reactions to form sucrose, starch, and cellulose which are then used in different ways. Glucose is joined to a fructose molecule to form **sucrose**, a disaccharide, which is transported in sap. Like glucose, sucrose is also considered a simple carbohydrate. Starches and cellulose are complex carbohydrates consisting of long chains of glucose molecules called polysaccharides. Plants use **starch** to store glucose, and **cellulose** for rigidity in cell walls.

Use of Phloem to Transport Products of Photosynthesis

The movement of sugars and other materials from the leaves to other tissues throughout the plants is called **translocation**. Nutrients are translocated from **sources**, or areas with excess sugars such as mature leaves, to **sinks**, areas where sugars are needed (i.e. roots or developing seeds). Phloem vessels are found in the vascular bundles along with the xylem. Phloem contains conducting cells called sieve elements, which are connected end to end in sieve tubes. **Sieve tubes** carry sap from sugar sources to sugar sinks. Phloem sap contains mostly sucrose dissolved in water. The sap can also contain proteins, amino acids, and hormones. Some plants transport sugar alcohols. Loading the sugar into the sieve tubes causes water to enter the tubes by osmosis, creating a higher hydrostatic pressure at the source end of the tube. This pressure is what causes nutrients to move upward towards the sink areas. Sugar is removed from the sieve tube at the sink end and the solute potential is increased, thus causing water to leave the phloem. This process is referred to as the **pressure-flow mechanism**.

Hierarchical Structure of the Biosphere

Biosphere

Components

The **biosphere** is the region of the earth inhabited by living things. The components of the biosphere from smallest to largest are organisms, populations, communities, ecosystems, and biomes. Organisms of the same species make up a **population**. All of the populations in an area make up the **community**. The community combined with the physical environment for a region forms an **ecosystem**. Several ecosystems are grouped together to form large geographic regions called **biomes**.

Population

A **population** is a group of all the individuals of one species in a specific area or region at a certain time. A **species** is a group of organisms that can breed and produce fertile offspring. There may be many populations of a specific species in a large geographic region. **Ecologists** study the size, density, and growth rate of populations to determine their stability. Population size continuously changes with births, deaths, and migrations. The population density is the number of individuals per unit of area. Growth rates for a population may be exponential or logistic. Ecologists also study how the individuals are dispersed within a population. Some species form clusters, while others are evenly or randomly spaced. However, every population has limiting factors. Changes in the environment or geography can reduce or limit population size. The individuals of a population interact with each other and with other organisms in the community in various ways, including competition and predation, which have direct impacts population size.

Community Interactions

A **community** is all of the populations of different species that live in an area and interact with each other. Community interaction can be intraspecific or interspecific. **Intraspecific interactions** occur between members of the same species. **Interspecific interactions** occur between members of different species. Different types of interactions include competition, predation, and symbiosis. Communities with high diversity are more complex and more stable than communities with low diversity. The level of diversity can be seen in a food web of the community, which shows all the feeding relationships within the community.

Ecosystems

An **ecosystem** is the basic unit of ecology. An ecosystem is the sum of all the biotic and abiotic factors in an area. **Biotic factors** are all living things such as plants, animals, fungi, and microorganisms. **Abiotic factors** include the light, water, air, temperature, and soil in an area. Ecosystems obtain the energy they need from sunlight. Ecosystems also contain biogeochemical cycles such as the hydrologic cycle and the nitrogen cycle. Ecosystems are generally classified as either terrestrial or aquatic. All of the living things within an ecosystem are called its community. The number and variety of living things within a community describes the ecosystem's **biodiversity**. However, each ecosystem can only support a limited number of organisms known as the **carrying capacity**.

Relationships between Species

Symbiosis

Many species share a special nutritional relationship with another species, called **symbiosis**. The term symbiosis means "living together." In symbiosis, two organisms share a close physical relationship that can be helpful, harmful, or neutral for each organism. Three forms of symbiotic relationships are parasitism, commensalism, and mutualism. **Parasitism** is a relationship between two organisms in which one organism is the parasite, and the other organism is the host. The parasite benefits from the relationship because the parasite obtains its nutrition from the host. The host is harmed from the relationship because the parasite is using the host's energy and giving nothing in return. For example, a tick and a dog share a parasitic relationship in which the tick is the parasite, and the dog is the host. **Commensalism** is a relationship between two organisms in which one benefits, and the other is not affected. For example, a small fish called a remora can attach to the belly of a shark and ride along. The remora is safe under the shark, and the shark is not affected. **Mutualism** is a relationship between two organisms in which both organisms benefit. For example, a rhinoceros usually can be seen with a few tick birds perched on its back. The tick birds are helped by the easy food source of ticks, and the rhino benefits from the tick removal.

Predation

Predation is a special nutritional relationship in which one organism is the predator, and the other organism is the prey. The predator benefits from the relationship, but the prey is harmed. The predator hunts and kills the prey for food. The predator is specially adapted to hunt its prey, and the prey is specially adapted to escape its predator. While predators harm (kill) their individual prey, predation usually helps the prey species. Predation keeps the population of the prey species under control and prevents them from overshooting the carrying capacity, which often leads to starvation. Also, predation usually helps to remove weak or slow members of the prey species leaving the healthier, stronger, and better adapted individuals to reproduce. Examples of predator-prey relationships include lions and zebras, snakes and rats, and hawks and rabbits.

Competition and Territoriality

Competition is a relationship between two organisms in which the organisms compete for the same vital resource that is in short supply. Typically, both organisms are harmed, but one is usually harmed more than the other, which provides an avenue for natural selection. Organisms compete for resources such as food, water, mates, and space. **Interspecific competition** is between members of different species, while

intraspecific competition is between members of the same species. **Territoriality** can be considered to be a type of interspecific competition for space. Many animals including mammals, birds, reptiles, fish, spiders, and insects have exhibited territorial behavior. Once territories are established, there are fewer conflicts between organisms. For example, a male redwing blackbird can establish a large territory. By singing and flashing his red patches, he is able to warn other males to avoid his territory, and they can avoid fighting.

Altruistic Behaviors Between Animals

Altruism is a self-sacrificing behavior in which an individual animal may serve or protect another animal. For example, in a honey bee colony there is one queen with many workers (females). There are also drones (males), but only during the mating seasons. Adult workers do all the work of the hive and will die defending it. Another example of altruism is seen in a naked mole rat colony. Each colony has one queen that mates with a few males, and the rest of the colony is nonbreeding and lives to service the queen, her mates, and her offspring.

Review Video: Mutualism, Commensalism, and Parasitism
Visit mometrix.com/academy and enter code: 757249

Energy Flow in the Environment

Energy Flow in the Environment

Using Trophic Levels with an Energy Pyramid

Energy flow through an ecosystem can be tracked through an energy pyramid. An **energy pyramid** shows how energy is transferred from one trophic level to another. **Producers** always form the base of an energy pyramid, and the consumers form successive levels above the producers. Producers only store about 1% of the solar energy they receive. Then, each successive level only uses about 10% of the energy of the previous level. That means that **primary consumers** use about 10% of the energy used by primary producers, such as grasses and trees. Next, **secondary consumers** use 10% of primary consumers' 10%, or 1% overall. This continues up for as many trophic levels as exist in a particular ecosystem.

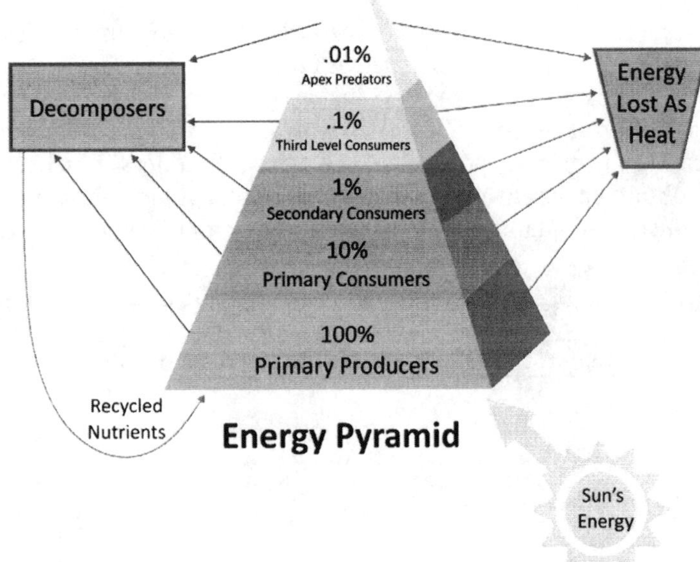

FOOD WEB

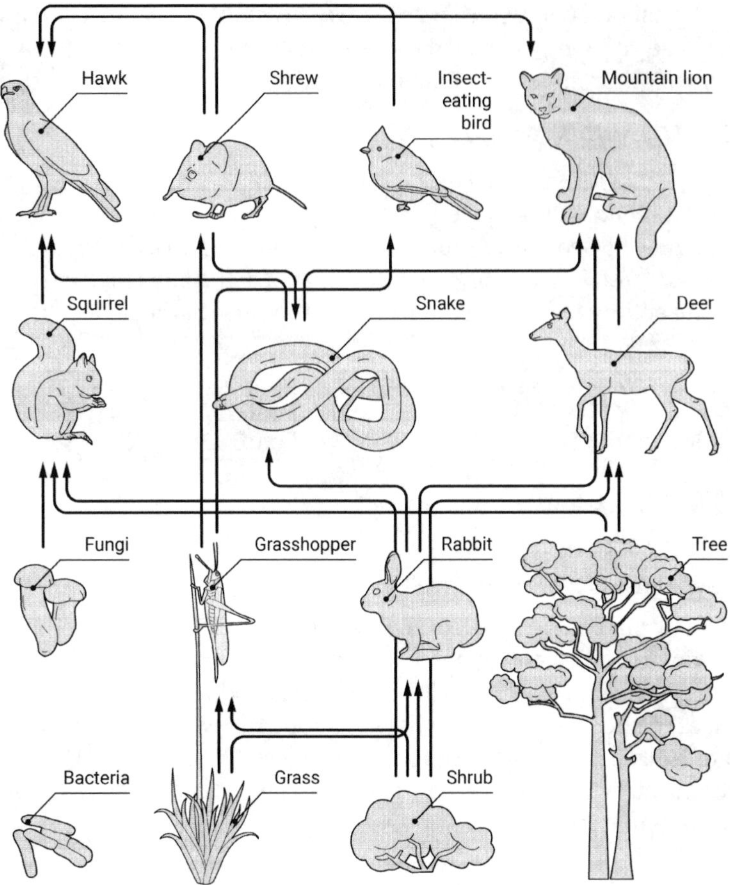

Energy flow through an ecosystem can be illustrated by a **food web**. Energy moves through the food web in the direction of the arrows. In the food web, producers such as grass, trees, and shrubs use energy from the sun to produce food through photosynthesis. Herbivores or primary consumers such as squirrels, grasshoppers, and rabbits obtain energy by eating the producers. Secondary consumers, which are carnivores such as snakes and shrews, obtain energy by eating the primary consumers. Tertiary consumers, which are carnivores such as hawks and mountain lions, obtain energy by eating the secondary consumers. Note that the hawk and the mountain lion can also be considered quaternary consumers in this food web if a different food chain within the web is followed.

Review Video: Food Webs
Visit mometrix.com/academy and enter code: 853254

Anatomy and Physiology

Human Body Systems

The Three Primary Body Planes

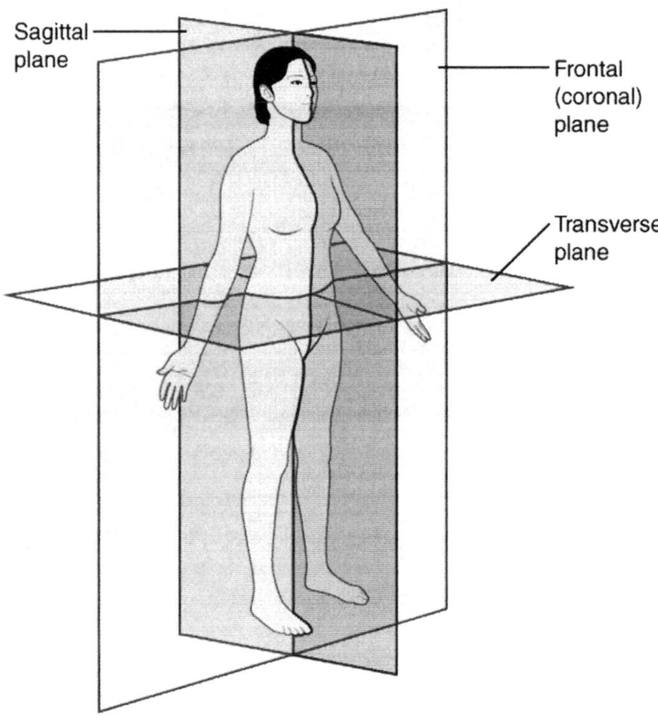

The **transverse (or horizontal) plane** divides the patient's body into imaginary upper (*superior*) and lower (*inferior or caudal*) halves.

The **sagittal plane** divides the body, or any body part, vertically into right and left sections. The sagittal plane runs parallel to the midline of the body.

The **coronal (or frontal) plane** divides the body, or any body structure, vertically into front and back (*anterior* and *posterior*) sections. The coronal plane runs vertically through the body at right angles to the midline.

Integumentary System

The **integumentary system** refers to the **skin**, **hair**, and **nails**. It is the largest organ system in the body, encompassing 15-20% of its total mass. This system serves as a barrier to physical, chemical, and biological agents, prevents the loss of body water, and regulates temperature. Many signs of illness and disease are first indicated by changes in the skin.

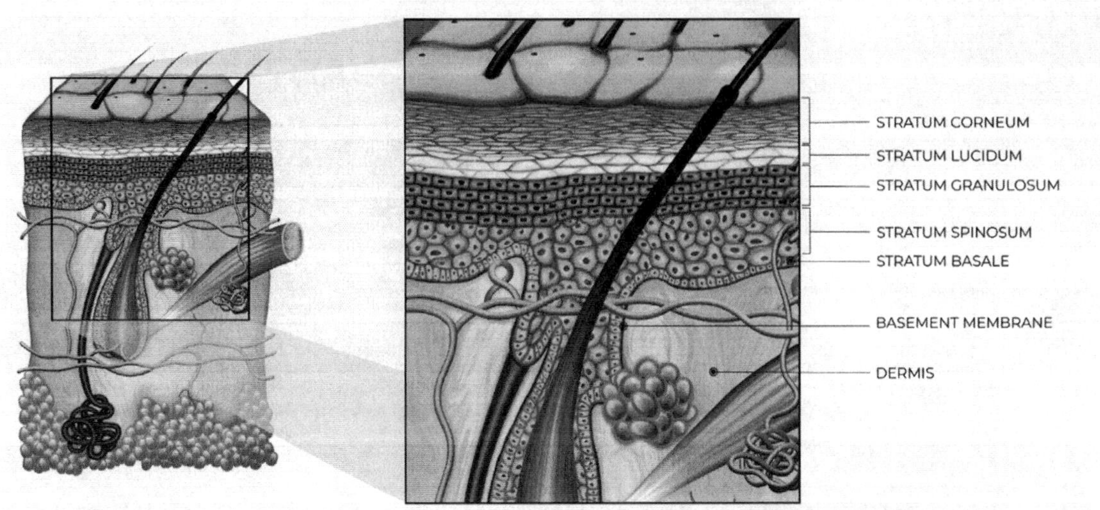

Review Video: Integumentary System
Visit mometrix.com/academy and enter code: 655980

Muscular System

The **muscular system** works in concert with the **skeletal system** to move the body and perform such core functions as cardiac activity. Key elements include:

- **Smooth muscles** - found in organs such as the heart and digestive tract.
- **Cardiac muscles** - found in the heart and responsible for circulatory activity.
- **Skeletal muscles** - surround the skeleton and function primarily to move the body as directed from the brain. Skeletal muscles also produce heat and are responsible for posture

Review Video: Muscular System
Visit mometrix.com/academy and enter code: 967216

Lymphatic System

The **lymphatic system** consists of the **thymus**, **lymph nodes**, **bone marrow**, and **spleen**. They primarily serve to distribute filtered fluids throughout the body and to remove excess fluid and debris. **White blood cells** are a key element of the lymphatic system which serve to prevent disease and repair the body after infection to prevent further illness.

Skeletal System

The **skeletal system** serves as the "framework" for the body by supporting and protecting internal organs and allowing the body to move. Its key elements are **bones**, which store key body chemicals, such as calcium, and produce blood cells in soft bone tissue. The **skull** is one of the most important bones in the skeletal system, as it protects the brain, which controls all bodily functions.

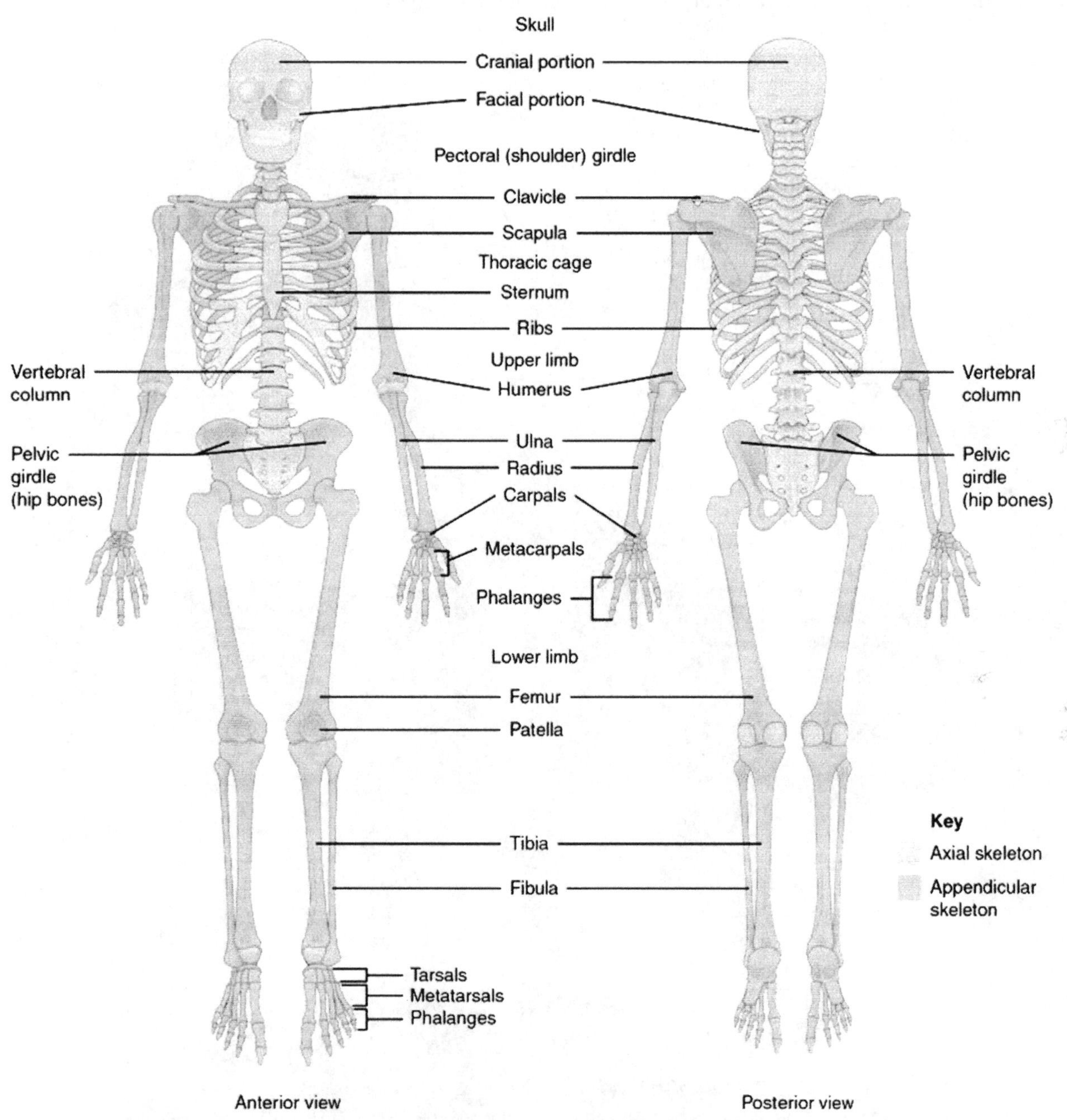

Review Video: Skeletal System
Visit mometrix.com/academy and enter code: 256447

Respiratory System

The main organs in the **respiratory system** are the nasal cavity, trachea, and lungs. They distribute oxygen throughout the body and remove waste particles of carbon dioxide. The respiratory system also functions to enhance speech and smell. The respiratory system works jointly with the **cardiovascular system** by taking **oxygenated blood** (red blood cells) and distributing them through arteries and capillaries. **Deoxygenated blood** (carbon dioxide) is transported via the venous system back to the lungs to exhaled.

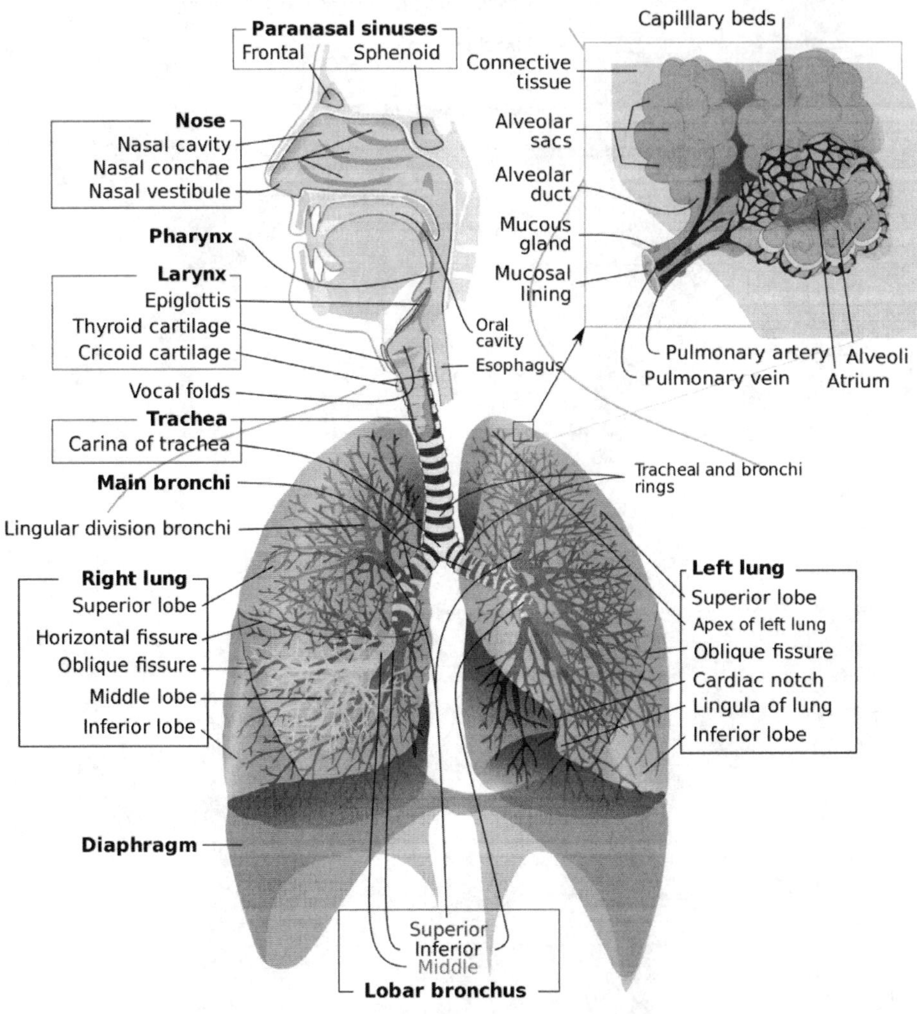

Review Video: Respiratory System
Visit mometrix.com/academy and enter code: 783075

Review Video: Pulmonary Circuit
Visit mometrix.com/academy and enter code: 955608

CARDIOVASCULAR SYSTEM

The **cardiovascular system** pumps blood throughout the body via the arterial and venous systems. The **blood** carries oxygen, carbon dioxide, nutrients, and other waste throughout the body. Working with the **respiratory system**, the cardiovascular system provides muscles and other organs with nourishment. A healthy heart can more efficiently distribute nutrients and remove waste than distressed or failing heart.

Review Video: Cardiovascular System
Visit mometrix.com/academy and enter code: 376581

DIGESTIVE AND URINARY SYSTEMS

The **digestive system** consists of the oral cavity, esophagus, stomach, liver, large and small intestines, rectum, and anus. The digestive system is responsible for breaking down food, absorbing nutrients, and working with the **cardiovascular system** to distribute nutrients throughout the body, while also removing waste products.

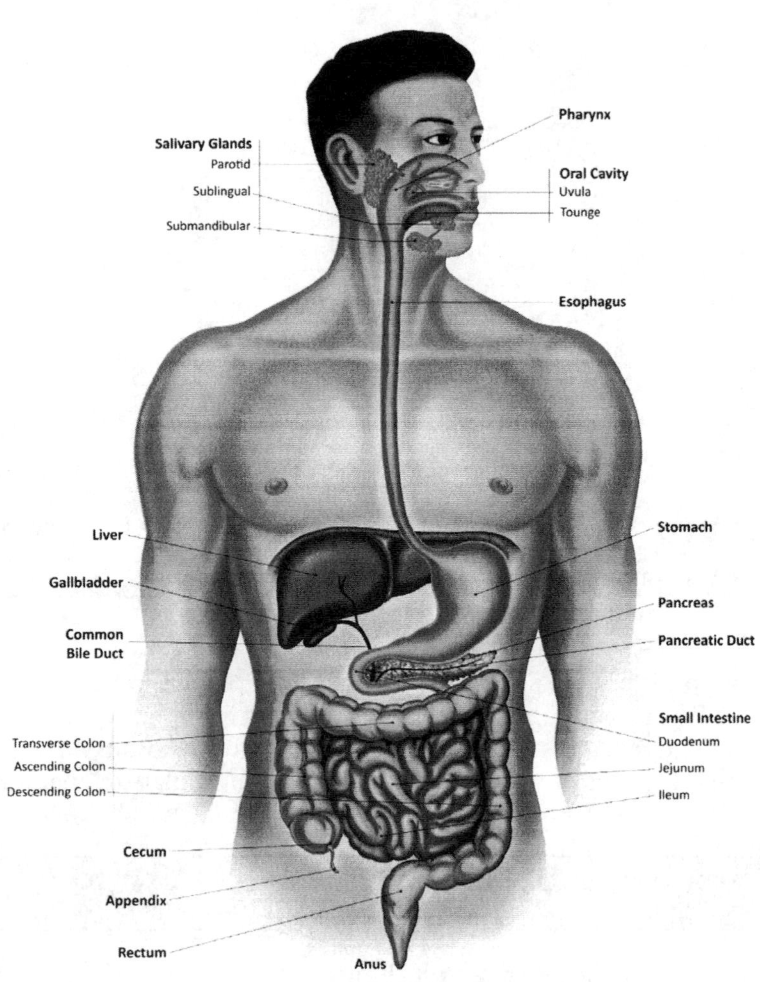

Review Video: Gastrointestinal System
Visit mometrix.com/academy and enter code: 378740

The **urinary system** consists of the bladder, kidneys, ureter, and urethra. Their main function is to eliminate waste products by expelling urine. This system also maintains homeostatic balance of water by excreting excess urine, maintaining electrolytes in the blood stream, and regulating blood Ph levels. This balance of water is crucial to body functioning as dehydration can lead to low blood pressure, which in turn can result in metabolic shock. **Metabolic shock** is characterized by low blood pressure that affects the kidneys, liver, and brain. **Dehydration** can also affect the muscular, system resulting in cramps from poor thermal regulation and altered fluid movement across tissue membranes.

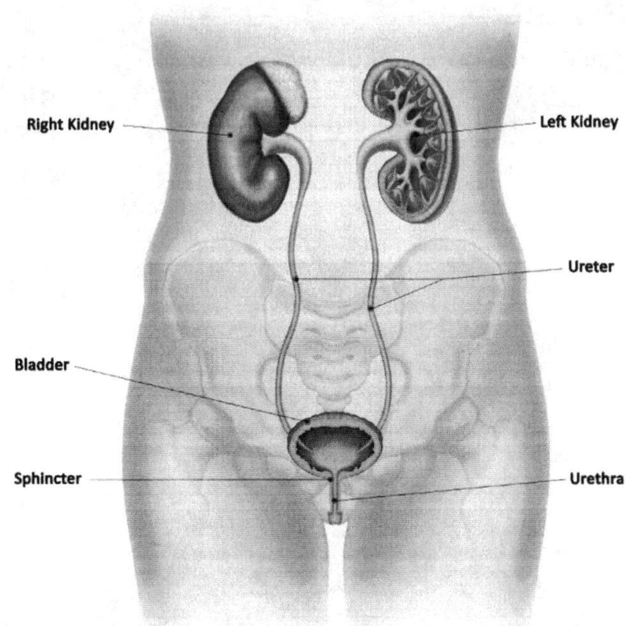

Review Video: Urinary System Visit mometrix.com/academy and enter code: 601053

Nervous and Reproductive Systems

The human **nervous system** consists of the **central nervous system** (i.e., brain and spinal cord) and the **peripheral nervous system** (i.e., nerves). They deliver voluntary and involuntary messages throughout the body. Core functions, such as digestion and respiration, are controlled by the brain via messages sent through the peripheral nervous system. The brain also receives external cues to regulate temperature and activate certain muscle groups.

Review Video: What is the Function of the Nervous System? Visit mometrix.com/academy and enter code: 708428

The **reproductive system** consists of the prostate, testicle, penis, and scrotum in males and ovaries, uterus, vagina, fallopian tubes, and mammary glands in females. The primary function is the creation of human life. **Sperm** is produced by the testes and is delivered to the ovary-produced **eggs** in the fallopian tubes for fertilization. The uterus then serves as the home for the developing fetus. **Mammary glands** secrete nutrients for the newborn child.

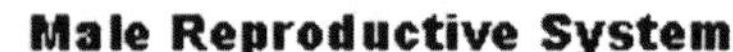

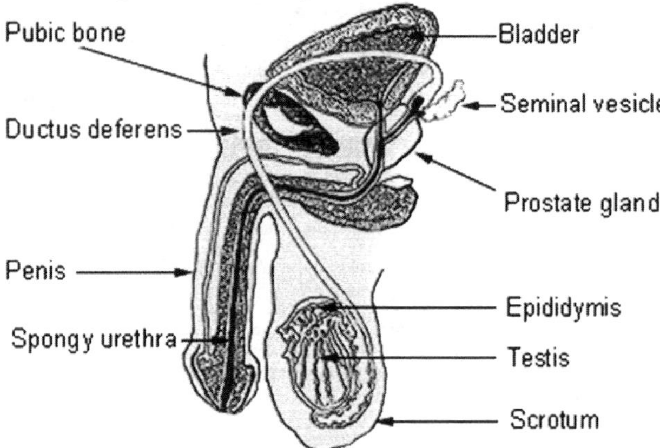

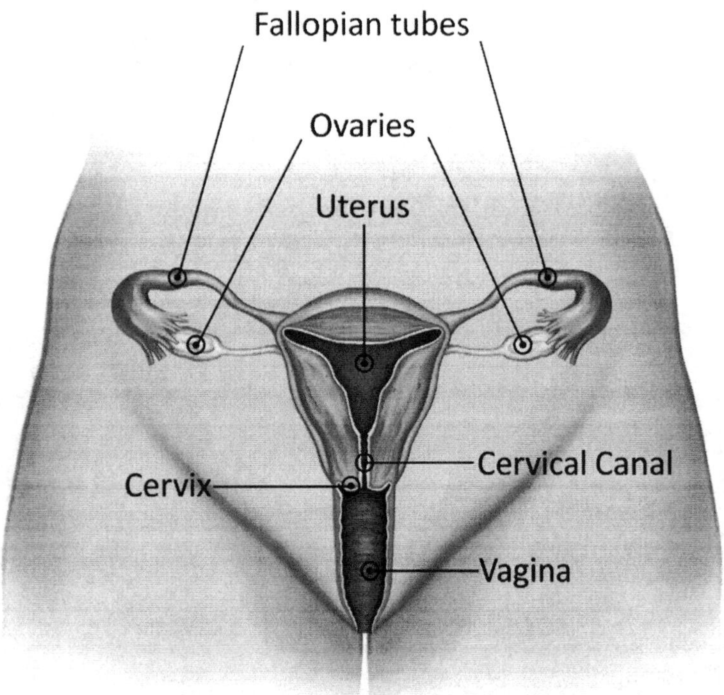

Review Video: Reproductive Systems
Visit mometrix.com/academy and enter code: 505450

Endocrine System

The **endocrine system** consists of the pituitary, adrenal, pancreas, and thyroid glands. They circulate **hormones** throughout the body that regulate growth, metabolism, and reproduction. The endocrine system controls heart rate, blood pressure, appetite, sleep patterns, body temperature, and the levels of **glucose** (blood sugars) in the bloodstream. **Diabetes** (both Types I and II) are diseases of the endocrine system.

Gland	Hormones	Disease
Adrenal Cortex	Aldosterone Cortisol Androgens	Addison's Disease Cushing's Disease
Adrenal Medulla	Epinephrine Norepinephrine	Anxiety Attacks Depression
Anterior Pituitary	Adrenocorticotropic hormone (ACTH) Follicle-stimulating hormone (FSH) Gonadotropic hormones Growth hormone (GH) Luteinizing hormone (LH) Prolactin Thyroid Stimulating Hormone (TSH)	Dwarfism Gigantism
Hypothalamus/ Posterior Pituitary	Inhibiting hormones (stop the release of other hormones) Antidiuretic hormone (ADH) Oxytocin Releasing hormones (trigger the release of other hormones)	Diabetes Insipidus
Kidneys	Calcitriol Erythropoietin	Hypertension
Ovaries	Estrogen Progesterone	Endometriosis Menometrorrhagia
Pancreas	Insulin Glucagon	Diabetes Mellitus
Parathyroid	Parathyroid hormone	Tetany Renal calculi
Pineal	Melatonin	Alzheimer's Disease
Testes	Testosterone	Gynecomastia Klinefelter Syndrome
Thymus	Thymic factor (TF) Thymosin Thymic humoral factor (THF) Thymopoietin	DiGeorge Syndrome
Thyroid	Calcitonin Thyroxine (T4) Triiodothyronine (T3)	Cretinism Hypo/Hyperthyroidism Goiter Myxedema
Digestive tract	Gastrin Cholecystokinin Secretin Ghrelin Motilin	Gastritis Gastroesophageal reflux

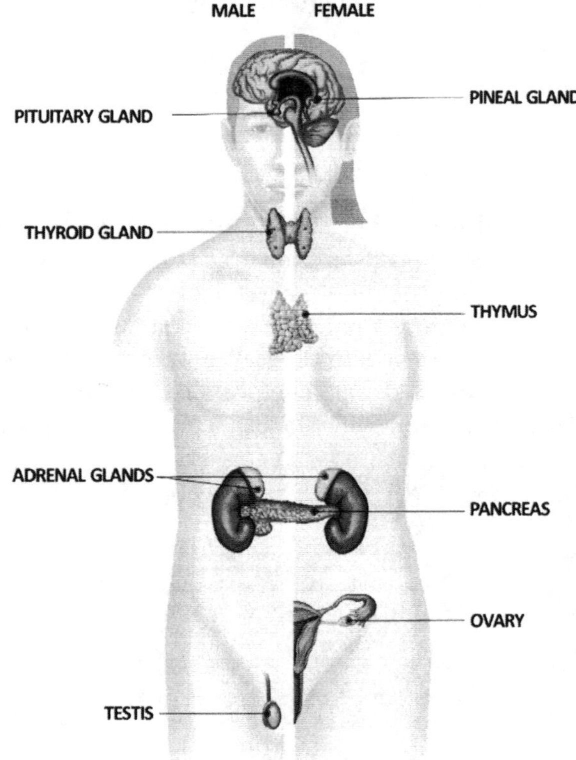

Review Video: Endocrine System
Visit mometrix.com/academy and enter code: 678939

RESPIRATORY AND CIRCULATORY SYSTEMS WORKING TOGETHER

Body systems work in concert with each other to respond to increasing and decreasing demands on the body and regulate **homeostasis**, the manner in which the human body regulates itself based on internal and external conditions in order to maintain a physiological balance. For example, the heart pumps blood through the **circulatory system** to distribute oxygenated blood throughout the body to meet physiological demands at any given time. Blood becomes oxygenated in the lungs (**respiratory system**) after excess **carbon dioxide** is released from the body through respiration. Inspiration of **oxygen** into the lungs allows the blood to become oxygen-rich so as to be distributed throughout the body. When physiological demands of the body increase (i.e., quickly climbing stairs), inspiration of oxygen increases and the heart pumps faster in order to more efficiently increase the delivery of oxygenated blood throughout the body. When the intense physical activity subsides, breathing slows and the heart returns to a normal resting heart rate.

IMPACT OF DIET AND EXERCISE ON THE CIRCULATORY SYSTEM

The delivery of **oxygenated blood** throughout the body can be accomplished more efficiently with a pattern of consistent exercise and good dietary habits. **Aerobic** activity strengthens the heart by increasing the oxygen carrying capacity of the red blood cells (**hemoglobin**) while also lowering resting blood pressure. In addition, aerobic exercise helps increase high density lipoproteins (HDL) (i.e., "good cholesterol") and decreasing low density lipoproteins (i.e., "bad cholesterol") which helps keep the arteries (**circulatory system**) clear. Consistent and adequate physical activity also helps regulate blood sugars, which can reduce the likelihood of developing Type II diabetes. A high fiber, low fat diet also directly contributes to lower blood sugar levels, cholesterol management, and helps maintain healthy bowels (**digestive system**). Combining regular aerobic physical activity with a high fiber, low fat diet is one of the most effective methods to improve one's cardiovascular health, maintain a healthy weight, and increase personal longevity.

Chemistry

Phase Transitions

States of Matter

The four states of matter are solid, liquid, gas, and plasma. **Solids** have a definite shape and a definite volume. Because solid particles are held in fairly rigid positions, solids are the least compressible of the four states of matter. **Liquids** have definite volumes but no definite shapes. Because their particles are free to slip and slide over each other, liquids take the shape of their containers, but they still remain fairly incompressible by natural means. **Gases** have no definite shape or volume. Because gas particles are free to move, they move away from each other to fill their containers. Gases are compressible. **Plasmas** are high-temperature, ionized gases that exist only under very high temperatures at which electrons are stripped away from their atoms.

Review Video: States of Matter
Visit mometrix.com/academy and enter code: 742449

Review Video: Properties of Liquids
Visit mometrix.com/academy and enter code: 802024

Review Video: States of Matter [Advanced]
Visit mometrix.com/academy and enter code: 298130

The following table shows similarities and differences between solids, liquids, and gases:

	Solid	**Liquid**	**Gas**
Shape	Fixed shape	No fixed shape (assumes shape of container)	No fixed shape (assumes shape of container)
Volume	Fixed	Fixed	Changes to assume shape of container
Fluidity	Does not flow easily	Flows easily	Flows easily
Compressibility	Hard to compress	Hard to compress	Compresses

Six Different Types of Phase Change

A substance that is undergoing a change from a solid to a liquid is said to be melting. If this change occurs in the opposite direction, from liquid to solid, this change is called freezing. A liquid which is being converted to a gas is undergoing vaporization. The reverse of this process is known as condensation. Direct transitions from gas to solid and solid to gas are much less common in everyday life, but they can occur given the proper conditions. Solid to gas conversion is known as sublimation, while the reverse is called deposition.

Review Video: Chemical and Physical Properties of Matter
Visit mometrix.com/academy and enter code: 717349

Phase Diagram and Critical Point

A **phase diagram** is a graph or chart of pressure versus temperature that represents the solid, liquid, and gaseous phases of a substance and the transitions between these phases. Typically, **pressure** is located on the vertical axis, and temperature is located along the horizontal axis. The curves drawn on the graph represent points at which different phases are in an equilibrium state. These curves indicate at which pressure and temperature the phase changes of sublimation, melting, and boiling occur. Specifically, the curve between the liquid and gas phases indicates the pressures and temperatures at which the liquid and gas phases are in equilibrium. The curve between the solid and liquid phases indicates the temperatures and pressures at which the solid and liquid phases are in equilibrium. The open spaces on the graph represent the distinct phases solid, liquid, and gas. The point on the curve at which the graph splits is referred to as the **critical point.** At the critical point, the solid, liquid, and gas phases all exist in a state of equilibrium.

Lettered Regions of a Phase Diagram

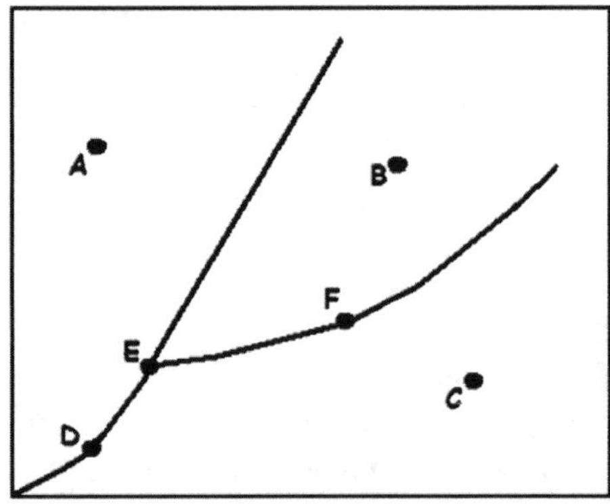

A—**Solid phase**: This is a region of high pressure and low temperature where the substance always exists as a solid.

B—**Liquid phase**: This is a region of pressure and temperature where the substance is in the liquid phase.

C—**Gas phase**: This is a region of pressure and temperature where the substance is in the gaseous phase.

D—**Sublimation point**: The portion of the curve that contains point D shows all the combinations of pressure and temperature at which the solid phase is in equilibrium with the gaseous phase.

E—**Critical point**: The point at which the solid, liquid, and gaseous phases are all in equilibrium.

F—**Boiling point**: The line that contains point F indicates all the combinations of pressure and temperature at which the liquid phase and gas phase are in equilibrium.

Historical Models of the Atom

Atomic Models and Theories

There have been many theories regarding the **structure** of atoms and their particles. Part of the challenge in developing an understanding of matter is that atoms and their particles are too small to be seen. It is believed that the first conceptualization of the atom was developed by **Democritus** in 400 B.C. Some of the more notable models are the solid sphere or billiard ball model postulated by **John Dalton**, the plum pudding or raisin bun model by **J.J. Thomson**, the planetary or nuclear model by **Ernest Rutherford**, the Bohr or orbit model by **Niels Bohr**, and the electron cloud or quantum mechanical model by **Louis de Broglie** and **Erwin Schrodinger**. Rutherford directed the alpha scattering experiment that discounted the plum pudding model. The shortcoming of the Bohr model was the belief that electrons orbited in fixed rather than changing ecliptic orbits.

Review Video: Atomic Models
Visit mometrix.com/academy and enter code: 434851

Review Video: John Dalton
Visit mometrix.com/academy and enter code: 565627

THOMSON "PLUM PUDDING" MODEL

J.J. Thomson, the discoverer of the electron, suggested that the arrangement of protons and electrons within an atom could be approximated by dried fruit in a **plum pudding**. Thomson, whose discovery of the electron preceded that of the proton or neutron, hypothesized that an atom's electrons, the dried plums, were **positioned uniformly** inside the atom within a cloud of positive charge, the pudding. This model was later disproved.

RUTHERFORD SCATTERING

Ernest Rutherford concluded from the work of Geiger and Marsden that the majority of the mass was concentrated in a minute, positively charged region, the **nucleus**, which was surrounded by **electrons**. When a positive alpha particle approached close enough to the nucleus, it was strongly repelled, enough so that it had the ability to rebound at high angles. The small nucleus size explained the small number of alpha particles that were repelled in this fashion. The scattering led to development of the **planetary model of the atom**, which was further developed by Niels Bohr into what is now known as the Bohr model.

BOHR MODEL

Niels Bohr postulated that the electrons orbiting the nucleus must occupy **discrete orbits**. These discrete orbits also corresponded to discrete levels of energy and angular momentum. Consequently, the only way that electrons could move between orbits was by making nearly instantaneous jumps between them. These jumps, known as **quantum leaps**, are associated with the absorption or emission of a quantum of energy, known as a **photon**. If the electron is jumping to a higher energy state, a photon must be absorbed. Similarly, if the electron is dropping to a lower energy state, a photon must be emitted.

Review Video: Structure of Atoms
Visit mometrix.com/academy and enter code: 905932

ATOMIC AND SUBATOMIC STRUCTURE

BASIC ORGANIZATION OF MATTER

An **element** is the most basic type of matter. It has unique properties and cannot be broken down into other elements. The smallest unit of an element is the **atom**. Most elements are found somewhere in nature in single-atom form, but a few elements only exist naturally in pairs. These are called diatomic elements, and some of the most common of these are hydrogen, nitrogen, and oxygen. A chemical combination of two or more types of elements is called a compound. **Compounds** often have properties that are very different from those of their constituent elements. The smallest independent unit of an element or compound of two or more atoms is known as a **molecule**. Elements and compounds are represented by chemical symbols, one or two letters, most often the first in the element name. More than one atom of the same element in a compound is represented with a subscript number designating how many atoms of that element are present. Water, for instance, contains two hydrogens and one oxygen. Thus, the chemical formula is H_2O. Methane contains one carbon and four hydrogens, so its formula is CH_4.

Review Video: Molecules
Visit mometrix.com/academy and enter code: 349910

PROTONS, NEUTRONS, AND ELECTRONS

The three major subatomic particles are the proton, neutron, and electron. The **proton**, which is located in the nucleus, has a relative charge of +1. The **neutron**, which is located in the nucleus, has a relative charge of 0. The **electron**, which is located outside the nucleus, has a relative charge of –1. The proton and neutron, which are essentially the same mass, are much more massive than the electron and make up the mass of the atom. The electron's mass is insignificant compared to the mass of the proton and neutron.

Review Video: Nuclear Charge
Visit mometrix.com/academy and enter code: 412575

Orbits and Orbitals

An orbit is a definite path, but an orbital is a region in space. The Bohr model described electrons as orbiting or following a definite path in space around the nucleus of an atom. But, according to **Heisenberg's uncertainty principle**, it is impossible to determine the location and the momentum of an electron simultaneously. Therefore, it is impossible to draw a definite path or orbit of an electron. An **orbital**, as described by the quantum-mechanical model or the electron-cloud model, is a region in space that is drawn in such a way as to indicate the probability of finding an electron at a specific location. The distance an orbital is located from the nucleus corresponds to the principal quantum number. The orbital shape corresponds to the subshell or azimuthal quantum number. The orbital orientation corresponds to the magnetic quantum number.

Quantum Numbers

The **principal quantum number** (n) describes an electron's shell or energy level and actually describes the size of the orbital. Electrons farther from the nucleus are at higher energy levels. The **subshell** or azimuthal quantum number (l) describes the electron's sublevel or subshell (s, p, d, or f) and specifies the shape of the orbital. Typical shapes include spherical, dumbbell, and clover leaf. The **magnetic quantum number** (m_l) describes the orientation of the orbital in space. The spin or magnetic moment quantum number (m_s) describes the direction of the spin of the electron in the orbital.

Atomic Number and Mass Number

The **atomic number** of an element is the number of protons in the nucleus of an atom of that element. This is the number that identifies the type of an atom. For example, all oxygen atoms have eight protons, and all carbon atoms have six protons. Each element is identified by its specific atomic number.

The **mass number** is the number of protons and neutrons in the nucleus of an atom. Although the atomic number is the same for all atoms of a specific element, the mass number can vary due to the varying numbers of neutrons in various isotopes of the atom.

Isotopes

Isotopes are atoms of the same element that vary in their number of neutrons. Isotopes of the same element have the same number of protons and thus the same atomic number. Because isotopes vary in the number of neutrons, they are identified by their mass numbers. For example, two naturally occurring carbon isotopes are carbon-12 and carbon-13, which have mass numbers 12 and 13, respectively. The symbols ${}^{12}_{6}C$ and ${}^{13}_{6}C$ also represent the carbon isotopes. The general form of the symbol is ${}^{M}_{A}X$, where X is the element symbol, M is the mass number, and A is the atomic number.

Average Atomic Mass

The **average atomic mass** is the weighted average of the masses of all the naturally occurring isotopes of an atom in comparison to the carbon-12 isotope. The unit for average atomic mass is the atomic mass unit (u). Atomic masses of isotopes are measured using a mass spectrometer by bombarding a gaseous sample of the isotope and measuring its relative deflections. Atomic masses can be calculated if the percent abundances and the atomic masses of the naturally occurring isotopes are known.

Cathode Ray Tube (CRT)

Electrons were discovered by Joseph John Thomson through scientific work with cathode ray tubes (CRTs). **Cathode rays** had been studied for many years, but it was Thomson who showed that cathode rays were **negatively charged particles**. Although Thomson could not determine an electron's charge or mass, he was able to determine the ratio of the charge to the mass. Thomson discovered that this ratio was constant regardless of the gas in the CRT. He was able to show that the cathode rays were actually streams of negatively charged particles by deflecting them with a positively charged plate.

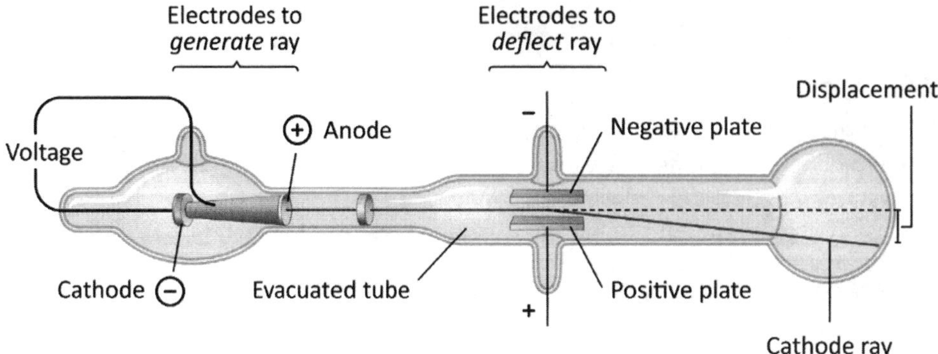

Gold Foil Experiment

After Thomson determined the ratio of the charge to the mass of an electron from studying cathode rays, he proposed the plum pudding model, in which he compared electrons to the raisins embedded in plum pudding. This model of the atom was disproved by the gold foil experiment. The gold foil experiment led to the discovery of the nucleus of an atom. Scientists at Rutherford's laboratory bombarded a thin gold foil with high-speed helium ions. Much to their surprise, some of the ions were reflected by the foil. The scientists concluded that the atom has a **hard central core**, which we now know to be the **nucleus**.

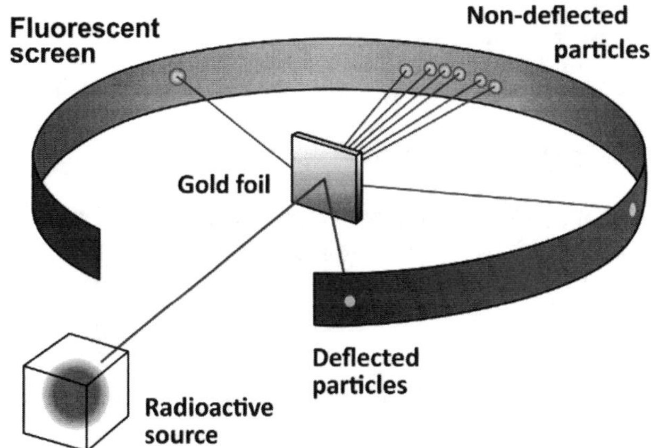

Problems that Rutherford's Model Had with Spectral Lines

Rutherford's model allowed for the electrons of an atom to be in an **infinite number of orbits** based on Newton's laws of motion. Rutherford believed that electrons could orbit the nucleus at any distance from the nucleus and that electrons could change velocity and direction at any moment. But, according to Rutherford's model, the electrons would lose energy and spiral into the nucleus. Unfortunately, if this was in fact true, then every atom would be **unstable**. Rutherford's model also does not correspond to the spectral lines emitted from gases at low pressure. The **spectral lines** are discrete bands of light at specific energy levels. These spectral lines indicate that electrons must be at specific distances from the nucleus. If electrons could be located at any distance from the nucleus, then these gases should emit continuous spectra instead of spectral lines.

Pure Substances and Mixtures

Pure Substances

Pure substances are substances that cannot be further broken down into simpler components or pieces and still retain their characteristics. Pure substances are categorized as either **elements** or **compounds**. Elements consist of only one type of atom may be monatomic, diatomic, or polyatomic. For example, helium (He) and copper (Cu) are monatomic elements, and hydrogen (H_2) and oxygen (O_2) are diatomic elements. Phosphorus (P_4) and sulfur (S_8) are polyatomic elements. Compounds consist of molecules of more than one type of atom. For example, pure water (H_2O) is made up of molecules consisting of two atoms of hydrogen bonded to one atom of oxygen, and glucose ($C_6H_{12}O_6$) is made up of molecules of six carbon atoms and twelve hydrogen atoms bonded together with six oxygen atoms.

Mixtures

Mixtures can be classified as either homogeneous or heterogeneous. The molecules of a **homogeneous mixture** are distributed uniformly throughout the mixture, whereas the molecules of a **heterogeneous mixture** are not. Air is an example of a homogeneous mixture, and a pile of sand and rock is an example of a heterogeneous mixture. Solutions are homogeneous mixtures consisting of a **solute** (the substance that is dissolved) and a **solvent** (the substance doing the dissolving).

Suspensions

Suspensions are heterogeneous mixtures in which the particle size of the substance **suspended** is too large to be kept in suspension by Brownian motion. Once left undisturbed, suspensions will settle out to form layers. An example of a suspension is sand stirred into water. Left undisturbed, the sand will fall out of suspension and the water will form a layer on top of the sand.

Mixtures with Compounds

Mixtures are similar to compounds in that they are produced when two or more substances are combined. However, there are some key differences as well. Compounds require a chemical combination of the constituent particles, while mixtures are simply the interspersion of particles. Unlike compounds, mixtures may be **separated** without a chemical change. A mixture retains the chemical properties of its constitutent particles, while a compound acquires a new set of properties. Given compounds can exist only in specific ratios, while mixtures may be any ratio of the involved substances.

Chemical and Physical Properties and Changes

Chemical and Physical Properties

Matter has both physical and chemical properties. **Physical properties** can be seen or observed without changing the identity or composition of matter. For example, the mass, volume, and density of a substance can be determined without permanently changing the sample. Other physical properties include color, boiling point, freezing point, solubility, odor, hardness, electrical conductivity, thermal conductivity, ductility, and malleability.

Chemical properties cannot be measured without changing the identity or composition of matter. Chemical properties describe how a substance reacts or changes to form a new substance. Examples of chemical properties include flammability, corrosivity, oxidation states, enthalpy of formation, and reactivity with other chemicals.

Intensive and Extensive Properties

Physical properties are categorized as either intensive or extensive. **Intensive properties** *do not* depend on the amount of matter or quantity of the sample. This means that intensive properties will not change if the sample size is increased or decreased. Intensive properties include color, hardness, melting point, boiling point, density, ductility, malleability, specific heat, temperature, concentration, and magnetization.

Extensive properties *do* depend on the amount of matter or quantity of the sample. Therefore, extensive properties do change if the sample size is increased or decreased. If the sample size is increased, the property increases. If the sample size is decreased, the property decreases. Extensive properties include volume, mass, weight, energy, entropy, number of moles, and electrical charge.

Atomic Properties of Neutral Atoms, Anions, and Cations

Neutral atoms have the same number of protons as electrons. **Cations** are positively-charged ions that are formed when atoms lose electrons. For example, the alkali metals sodium and potassium form the cations Na^+ and K^+, and the alkaline earth metals magnesium and calcium form the cations Mg^{2+} and Ca^{2+}. These elements easily lose electrons because the resulting ion is left with a full valence shell.

Anions are negatively-charged ions that are formed when atoms gain electrons. For example, the halogens fluorine and chlorine form the anions F^- and Cl^-. These elements easily gain electrons because the resulting ion has a full valence shell.

Chemical and Physical Changes

Physical changes do not produce new substances. The atoms or molecules may be rearranged, but no new substances are formed. **Phase changes** or changes of state such as melting, freezing, and sublimation are physical changes. For example, physical changes include the melting of ice, the boiling of water, sugar dissolving into water, and the crushing of a piece of chalk into a fine powder.

Chemical changes involve a **chemical reaction** and do produce new substances. When iron rusts, iron oxide is formed, indicating a chemical change. Other examples of chemical changes include baking a cake, burning wood, digesting food, and mixing an acid and a base.

Conservation of Energy and Matter

Law of Conservation of Energy

The **law of conservation of energy** states that in a closed system, energy cannot be created or destroyed but only changed from one form to another. This is also known as the first law of thermodynamics. Another way to state this is that the **total energy in an isolated system is constant**. Energy comes in many forms that may be transformed from one kind to another, but in a closed system, the total amount of energy is conserved or remains constant. For example, potential energy can be converted to kinetic energy, thermal energy, radiant energy, or mechanical energy. In an isolated chemical reaction, there can be no energy created or destroyed. The energy simply changes forms.

Law of Conservation of Mass

The **law of conservation of mass** is also known as the **law of conservation of matter**. This law states that for a chemical reaction in a closed system, the total mass of the products must equal the total mass of the reactants. This could also be stated that in a closed system, mass never changes. A consequence of this law is that matter is never created or destroyed during a typical chemical reaction. The atoms of the reactants are only rearranged to form the products. The number and type of each specific atom involved in the reactants is identical to the number and type of atoms in the products. This is the key principle used when balancing chemical equations. In a balanced chemical equation, the number of moles of each element on the reactant side equals the number of moles of each element on the product side.

Review Video: How Do You Balance Chemical Equations?
Visit mometrix.com/academy and enter code: 341228

Conversion of Energy Within Chemical Systems

Chemical energy is the energy stored in molecules in the bonds between the atoms of those molecules and the energy associated with the intermolecular forces. This stored **potential energy** may be converted into **kinetic energy** and then into heat. During a chemical reaction, atoms may be rearranged and chemical bonds may be formed or broken accompanied by a corresponding absorption or release of energy, usually in the form of heat. According to the first law of thermodynamics, during these energy conversions, the **total amount of energy must be conserved**.

Properties of Bonds

Relative Bond Length and Bond Strength of Single, Double, and Triple Covalent Bonds

The **bond length of a covalent bond** is the distance between the nuclei of two covalently bonded atoms. The higher the bond order, the shorter the bond length. **Single bonds** are between one pair of electrons, and they are the weakest. Because single bonds (bond order 1) are the weakest, they are the longest of the three types of covalent bonds. **Double bonds** are between two pairs of electrons. Because double bonds (bond order 2) are stronger than single bonds, double bonds are shorter than single bonds. **Triple bonds** are between three pairs of electrons. Because triple bonds (bond order 3) are stronger than double bonds and single bonds, triple bonds have the shortest bond length.

Bond Types

Bonds

Chemical bonds are the attractive forces that bind atoms together into molecules. Atoms form chemical bonds in an attempt to satisfy the octet rule. These bond types include covalent bonds, ionic bonds, and metallic bonds. **Covalent bonds** are formed from the sharing of electron pairs between two atoms in a molecule. **Ionic bonds** are formed from the transferring of electrons between one atom and another, which results in the formations of cations and anions. **Metallic bonding** results from the sharing of delocalized electrons among all of the atoms in a molecule.

Ionic Bonding

Ionic bonding results from the transfer of electrons between atoms. A **cation** or positive ion is formed when an atom loses one or more electrons. An **anion** or negative ion is formed when an atom gains one or more electrons. An ionic bond results from the electrostatic attraction between a cation and an anion. One example of a compound formed by ionic bonds is sodium chloride or NaCl. Sodium (Na) is an alkali metal and tends to form Na^+ ions. Chlorine (Cl) is a halogen and tends to form Cl^- ions. The Na^+ ion and the Cl^- ion are attracted to each other. This electrostatic attraction between these oppositely charged ions is what results in the ionic bond between them.

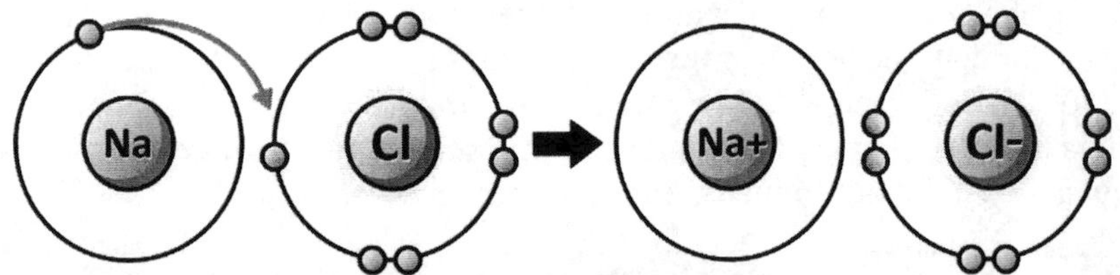

Review Video: Ionic Bonds
Visit mometrix.com/academy and enter code: 116546

Covalent Bonding

Covalent bonding results from the sharing of electrons between atoms. Atoms seek to fill their valence shell and will share electrons with another atom in order to have a full octet (except hydrogen and helium, which only hold two electrons in their valence shells). **Molecular compounds** have covalent bonds. **Organic compounds** such as proteins, carbohydrates, lipids, and nucleic acids are molecular compounds formed by covalent bonds. Methane (CH_4) is a molecular compound in which one carbon atom is covalently bonded to four hydrogen atoms as shown below.

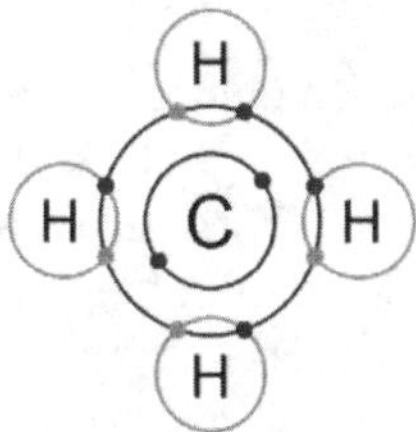

Polar Covalent Bonds, Nonpolar Covalent Bonds, and Hybridization

Polar covalent bonds result when electrons are shared unequally between atoms. **Nonpolar covalent bonds** result when electrons are shared equally between atoms. The unequal sharing of electrons is due to the differences in the electronegativities of the two atoms sharing the electrons. Partial charges develop due to this unequal sharing of electrons. The greater the difference in electronegativities between the two atoms, the stronger the dipole is. For example, the covalent bonds formed between the carbon atom and the two oxygen atoms in carbon dioxide are polar covalent bonds because the electronegativities of carbon and oxygen differ slightly. If the electronegativities are equal, then the covalent bonds are nonpolar. For example, the covalent double bond between two oxygen atoms is nonpolar because the oxygen atoms have the same electronegativities.

Review Video: Nonpolar Covalent Bonds
Visit mometrix.com/academy and enter code: 986465

Review Video: Covalent Bonds
Visit mometrix.com/academy and enter code: 482899

Metallic Bonding

Metallic bonding is a type of bonding between metals. Metallic bonds are similar to covalent bonds in that they are a type of sharing of electrons between atoms. However, in covalent bonding, the electrons are shared with only one other atom. In metallic bonding, the electrons are shared with all the surrounding atoms. These electrons are referred to as delocalized electrons. Metallic bonding is responsible for many of the characteristics in metals including conductivity, malleability, and ductility. An example of metallic bonding is the metallic bond between the copper atoms in a piece of copper wire.

Review Video: Metallic Bonds
Visit mometrix.com/academy and enter code: 230855

Reaction Types

Types of Reactions

One way to organize chemical reactions is to sort them into two categories: **oxidation/reduction reactions** (also called redox reactions) and **metathesis reactions** (which include acid/base reactions). Oxidation/reduction reactions can involve the transfer of one or more electrons, or they can occur as a result of the transfer of oxygen, hydrogen, or halogen atoms. The species that loses electrons (or increases its oxidation state) is oxidized and is referred to as the reducing agent. The species that gains electrons (or decreases its oxidation state) is reduced and is referred to as the oxidizing agent. **Single substitution reactions** are types of oxidation/reduction reactions. In a single substitution reaction, electrons are transferred from one chemical species to another. The transfer of electrons results in changes in the nature and charge of the species.

Review Video: Understanding Chemical Reactions
Visit mometrix.com/academy and enter code: 579876

Review Video: What is the Process of a Reaction?
Visit mometrix.com/academy and enter code: 808039

SUBSTITUTION REACTIONS

Single substitution reactions, also called **single displacement** or **single replacement reactions**, are those where one reactant is displaced by another to form the final product ($A + BC \rightarrow AB + C$). Single substitution reactions can be cationic or anionic. When a piece of copper (Cu) is placed into a solution of silver nitrate ($AgNO_3$), the solution turns blue. The copper appears to be replaced with a silvery-white material. The equation is $2AgNO_3 + Cu \rightarrow Cu(NO_3)_2 + 2Ag$. When this reaction takes place, the copper dissolves and the silver in the silver nitrate solution precipitates (becomes a solid), resulting in copper nitrate and silver. Copper and silver have switched places in the nitrate.

Double substitution reactions, also called **double displacement**, **double replacement**, **metathesis**, or **ion exchange reactions**, are those where ions or bonds are exchanged by two compounds to form different compounds ($AC + BD \rightarrow AD + BC$). An example of this is that silver nitrate and sodium chloride form two different products (silver chloride and sodium nitrate) when they react. The formula for this reaction is $AgNO_3 + NaCl \rightarrow AgCl + NaNO_3$.

Review Video: Single-Replacement Reactions
Visit mometrix.com/academy and enter code: 442975

COMBINATION AND DECOMPOSITION REACTIONS

Combination, or **synthesis**, **reactions**: In a combination reaction, two or more reactants combine to form a single product ($A + B \rightarrow AB$). These reactions are also called synthesis or **addition reactions**. An example is burning hydrogen in air to produce water. The equation is $2H_2(g) + O_2(g) \rightarrow 2H_2O(l)$. Another example is when water and sulfur trioxide react to form sulfuric acid. The equation is $H_2O + SO_3 \rightarrow H_2SO_4$.

Decomposition (or desynthesis, decombination, or deconstruction) reactions: In a decomposition reaction, a reactant is broken down into two or more products ($AB \rightarrow A + B$). These reactions are also called analysis reactions. **Thermal decomposition** is caused by heat. **Electrolytic decomposition** is due to electricity. An example of this type of reaction is the decomposition of water into hydrogen and oxygen gas. The equation is $2H_2O \rightarrow 2H_2 + O_2$.

A + B → A-B

A-B → A + B

A-B + C → A-C + B

A-B + C-D → A-D + C-B

ACID/BASE REACTIONS

In **acid/base reactions**, an **acid** is a compound that can donate a proton, while a **base** is a compound that can accept a proton. In these types of reactions, the acid and base react to form a salt and water. When the proton is donated, the base becomes water and the remaining ions form a salt. One method of determining whether a reaction is an oxidation/reduction or a metathesis reaction is that the oxidation number of atoms does not change during a metathesis reaction.

Isomerization and Neutralization Reactions

Isomerization, or **rearrangement**, is the process changing a compound to an isomer. Within a compound, bonds are reformed. The reactant and product have the same molecular formula, but different structural formulas and different properties (A → A'). For example, butane (C_4H_{10}) is a hydrocarbon consisting of four carbon atoms in a straight chain. Heating it to 100 °C or higher in the presence of a catalyst forms isobutane (methylpropane), which has a branched-chain structure. Boiling and freezing points are greatly different for butane and isobutane.

A **neutralization, acid-base**, or **proton transfer reaction** occurs when one compound acquires H^+ from another. These types of reactions are also usually double displacement reactions. The acid has an H^+ that is transferred to the base and the acid and base are neutralized in the form of a salt that, depending on the salt's solubility, may precipitate from the solution.

Chemical Kinetics

Chemical Kinetics

Chemical kinetics is the study of the **rates** of **chemical reactions** and the various factors that affect these rates. The rate of a reaction is the change in concentration of the reactants or products per unit of time. Another way to state this is that chemical kinetics is the study of the rate of change of the concentrations of the reactants and products and the factors that affect that rate of change. The study of catalysts is part of chemical kinetics. Catalysts are substances that speed up the rate of reactions without being consumed. Examples of reactions that occur at different rates include the explosion of trinitrotoluene (TNT), which occurs at a very fast rate, compared to the burning of a log, which occurs at a much slower rate.

Give the Rate Law for this General Reaction: $aA + bB + cC \rightarrow$ Products. Define Each Letter.

The rate of a chemical reaction can be defined as the following:

$$\text{rate} = \frac{\text{change in concentration}}{\text{change in time}}$$

This is usually represented by a rate law. The rate law for the general reaction $aA + bB + cC \rightarrow$ Products is given by rate $= k[A]^x[B]^y[C]^z$, where k is the rate constant; [A], [B], and [C] represent the concentrations of the reactants; and x, y, and z represent the reaction orders. The exponents x, y, and z must be experimentally determined. They do not necessarily equal the coefficients from the balanced chemical equation.

Activation Energy

Activation energy is the minimum amount of energy that must be possessed by reactant atoms or molecules in order to react. This is due to the fact that it takes a certain amount of energy to break bonds or form bonds between atoms. Reactants lacking the activation energy required will not be able to perform the necessary breaking or forming of bonds regardless of how often they collide. Catalysts lower the activation energy of a reaction and therefore increase the rate of reaction.

Reaction Mechanism

Often, when studying specific reactions, only the net reactions are given. Realistically, reactions take place in a series of steps or elementary reactions as shown in the reaction mechanism. **Reaction mechanisms** show how a reaction proceeds in a **series of steps**. Some steps are slow, and some are fast. Each step has its own reaction mechanism. The slowest step in the reaction mechanism coincides with the step with the greatest activation energy. This step is known as the rate-determining step.

Catalyst

A **catalyst** is a chemical that **accelerates** or speeds up a chemical reaction without being consumed or used up in the reaction. Although catalysts are not consumed or permanently changed during the process of the reaction, catalysts do participate in the elementary reaction of the reaction mechanisms. Catalysts lower the **activation energy** meaning more of the reactant molecules will have sufficient energy to react.

Review Video: Catalysts
Visit mometrix.com/academy and enter code: 288189

Factors That Affect Reaction Rate

Factors that affect reaction rate include concentration, surface area, and temperature. Increasing the **concentration** of the reactants increases the number of collisions between those reactants and therefore increases the reaction rate. Increasing the **surface area of contact** between the reactants also increases the number of collisions and therefore increases the reaction rate. Finally, increasing the **temperature** of the reactants increases the number of collisions but more significantly also increases the kinetic energy of the reactants, which in turn increases the fraction of molecules meeting the activation energy requirement. With more molecules at the activation energy, more of the reactants are capable of completing the reaction.

Terminology for Solutions and Solubility

Dilute and Concentrated

The terms *dilute* and *concentrated* have opposite meanings. In a **solution**, the **solute** is dissolved in the **solvent**. The more solute that is dissolved, the more **concentrated** is the solution. The less solute that is dissolved, the less concentrated and the more **dilute** is the solution. The terms are often associated with the preparation of a stock solution for a laboratory experiment. Stock solutions are typically acquired in a higly concentrated form. Typically, diluted forms of the solutions are used which must be prepared from the concentrated stock solutions. The desired dilutions are achieved by combining a specific amount of a solvent with a specific amount of stock solution.

Saturated, Unsaturated, and Supersaturated

Solutions can be categorized based on their saturation. In a **saturated** solution, the solute is added to the solvent until no more solute is able to dissolve. The undissolved solute will settle down to the bottom of the beaker. A solution is considered **unsaturated** as long as more solute is able to go into solution under ordinary conditions. The solubility of solids in liquids typically increases as temperature increases. If the temperature of a solution is increased as the solute is being added, more solute than is normally possible may go into solution, forming a **supersaturated** solution.

Mixture, Solution, and Colloid

A **mixture** is made of two or more substances that are combined in various proportions. The exact proportion of the constituents is the defining characteristic of any mixture. There are two types of mixtures: homogeneous and heterogeneous. **Homogeneous** means that the mixture's composition and properties are uniform throughout. Conversely, **heterogeneous** means that the mixture's composition and properties are not uniform throughout.

A **solution** is a homogeneous mixture of substances that cannot be separated by filtration or centrifugation. Solutions are made by dissolving one or more solutes into a solvent. For example, in an aqueous glucose solution, glucose is the solute and water is the solvent. If there is more than one liquid present in the solution, then the most prevalent liquid is considered the solvent. The exact mechanism of dissolving varies depending on the mixture, but the result is always individual solute ions or molecules surrounded by solvent molecules. The proportion of solute to solvent for a particular solution is its **concentration**.

A **colloid** is a heterogeneous mixture in which small particles (<1 micrometer) are suspended, but not dissolved, in a liquid. As such, they can be separated by centrifugation. A commonplace example of a colloid is milk.

Review Video: Solutions
Visit mometrix.com/academy and enter code: 995937

Factors Affecting Solubility

Effects of Temperature, Surface Area, Agitation, and Pressure on the Dissolution Rate

Temperature, pressure, surface area, and agitation affect the **dissolution rate**. Increasing the **temperature** increases the kinetic energy of the molecules, which increases the number of collisions with the solute particles. Increasing the **surface area** of contact by stirring (agitation) or crushing a solid solute also increases the dissolution rate and helps prevent recrystallization. Increasing the **pressure** will increase the dissolution rate for gas solutes in liquid solvents because the added pressure will make it more difficult for the gas to escape. Increasing the pressure will have virtually no effect on the dissolution rate for solid solutes in liquid solvents under normal conditions.

Effect of Temperature and Pressure on Solubility

Temperature and pressure affect **solubility**. For gas solutes in liquid solvents, increasing the **temperature** increases the kinetic energy causing more gas particles to escape the surface of the liquid solvents and therefore decreasing the solubility of the solutes. For solid solutes in liquid solvents, increasing the temperature generally increases the solubility, but there are exceptions. For gas solutes in liquid solvents, increasing the **pressure** increases the solubility. Increasing the pressure of liquid or solid solutes in liquid solvents has virtually no effect under normal conditions.

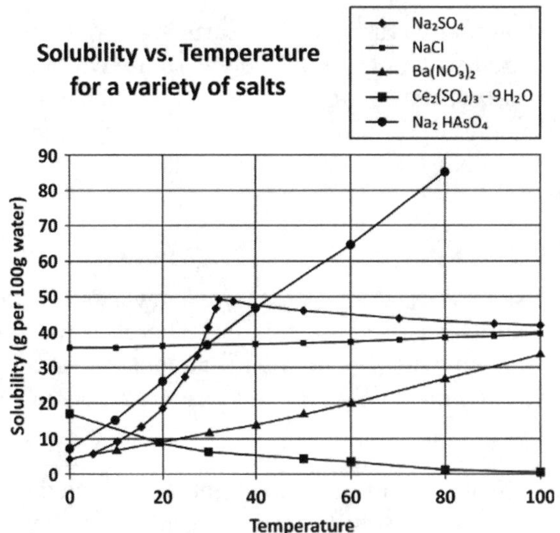

Equilibrium Relationships in Acid-Base Chemistry

Strong/Weak Acids and Bases

Acids or bases are categorized as strong or weak based on how completely they ionize in an aqueous solution. **Strong** acids and bases ionize essentially completely in an aqueous solution. **Weak** acids and bases ionize incompletely in an aqueous solution. Examples of strong acids include hydrochloric acid (HCl), sulfuric acid (H_2SO_4), and nitric acid (NO_3). Examples of weak acids are acetic acid ($HC_2H_3O_2$), hydrofluoric acid (HF), and carbonic acid (H_2CO_3). Examples of strong bases include sodium hydroxide (NaOH), potassium hydroxide (KOH), and calcium hydroxide ($Ca(OH)_2$). Ammonia (NH_3) is a common weak base.

Review Video: Strong and Weak Acids and Bases
Visit mometrix.com/academy and enter code: 268930

Monoprotic and Polyprotic Acids

Monoprotic acids are acids that have only one proton available to donate. **Polyprotic acids** have two or more protons available to donate. Typically, polyprotic acids donate their available protons in stages of one at a time. Specifically, diprotic acids can donate two protons, and triprotic acids can donate three protons. Common monoprotic acids include hydrochloric acid (HCl) and nitric acid (HNO_3). Common diprotic acids include sulfuric acid (H_2SO_4) and sulfurous acid (H_2SO_3). Phosphoric acid (H_3PO_4) is a common triprotic acid.

K_a of an Acid and the K_b of a Base

Given the general form $HA(aq) + H_2O(l) \leftrightarrow H_3O^+(aq) + A^-(aq)$ for the equilibrium of an acid in an aqueous solution, the equilibrium constant expression, called the **acid dissociation constant**, K_a, is:

$$K_a = \frac{[H_3O^+][A^-]}{[HA]}$$

Strong acids have high K_a values because strong acids ionize essentially completely in aqueous solution. Weak acids have low K_a values because weak acids do not ionize completely in aqueous solution.

Given the general form $B(aq) + H_2O(l) \leftrightarrow BH^+(aq) + OH^-(aq)$ for the equilibrium of a base in an aqueous solution, the equilibrium constant expression, called the **base dissociation constant**, K_b, is:

$$K_b = \frac{[BH^+][OH^-]}{[B]}$$

Strong bases have high K_b values because strong bases ionize essentially completely in aqueous solution. Weak bases have low K_b values because weak bases do not ionize completely in aqueous solution.

Hydrolysis

Hydrolysis is a chemical reaction between water and another reactant in which both compounds split apart. The water molecules split into hydrogen ions (H^+) and hydroxide ions (OH^-). The other compound splits into a cation and anion, too. Another way to state this is that hydrolysis is a decomposition reaction of a compound that is combined with water. The general form of a hydrolysis reaction is given by $X^-(aq) + H_2O(l) \leftrightarrow HX(aq) + OH^-(aq)$.

A hydrolysis reaction is the reverse process of a neutralization reaction. A neutralization reaction is given by the general form: acid + base → salt + water. In general, a hydrolysis reaction may be thought of as salt + water → acid + base.

Buffer Solution

A **buffer solution** is an aqueous solution that helps keep the pH constant. The addition of an acid or base to a buffer solution will not greatly affect the pH of that solution. A buffer consists of a weak acid and its conjugate base or a weak base and its conjugate acid. This combination of substances can remain in solution without the substances neutralizing each other. When acids or hydrogen ions (H^+) are added to a buffer solution, they are neutralized by the base in the buffer solution. When bases or hydroxide ions (OH^-) are added to a buffer solution, they are neutralized by the acid in the buffer solution.

Review Video: Buffer
Visit mometrix.com/academy and enter code: 389183

CHEMICAL STRUCTURES AND PROPERTIES OF BIOLOGICALLY IMPORTANT MOLECULES

CHEMICAL BONDING PROPERTIES OF CARBON

Carbon is considered to be the central atom of organic compounds. Carbon atoms each have four valence electrons and require four more electrons to have a stable outer shell. Due to the repulsion between the valence electrons, the bond sites are all equidistant from each other. This enables carbon to form longs chains and rings. Carbon atoms can form four single covalent bonds with other atoms. For example, methane (CH_4) consists of one carbon atom singly bonded to four separate hydrogen atoms. Carbon atoms can also form double or triple covalent bonds. For example, an oxygen atom can form a double bond with a carbon atom, and a nitrogen atom can form a triple bond with a carbon atom.

ORGANIC AND INORGANIC MOLECULES

Organic molecules contain carbon and hydrogen. Because carbon can form four covalent bonds, organic molecules can be very complex structures. Organic molecules can have carbon backbones that form long chains, branched chains, or even rings. Organic compounds tend to be less soluble in water than inorganic compounds. Organic compounds are often classified as either natural (found in plants and animals) or as synthetic (made via laboratory or industrial processes). **Inorganic molecules** generally do not contain carbon-carbon or carbon-hydrogen bonds, but there are some exceptions. Inorganic compounds include salts and metals. Specific examples of inorganic molecules include sodium chloride, oxygen, and carbon dioxide.

COVALENT BONDS

Chemical bonds are the attractive forces that bind atoms together to form molecules. Chemical bonds include covalent bonds, ionic bonds, and metallic bonds. **Covalent bonds** are formed from the sharing of electron pairs between two atoms in a molecule. In organic molecules, carbon atoms form single, double, or triple covalent bonds. Organic compounds including proteins, carbohydrates, lipids, and nucleic acids are molecular compounds formed by covalent bonds.

Review Video: What are Covalent Bonds?
Visit mometrix.com/academy and enter code: 482899

HYDROGEN BONDS

Intermolecular forces are the attractive forces between molecules. Intermolecular forces include hydrogen bonds, London or dispersion forces, and dipole-dipole forces. **Hydrogen bonds** are the attractive forces between molecules containing hydrogen atoms covalently bonded to oxygen, fluorine, or nitrogen. Hydrogen bonds bind the two strands of a DNA molecule to each other. Two hydrogen bonds join each adenosine and thymine, and three hydrogen bonds join each cytosine and guanine.

ATP

Adenosine triphosphate (ATP) is the energy source for most cellular functions. Each ATP molecule is a nucleotide consisting of a central ribose sugar flanked by a purine base and a chain of three phosphate groups. The purine base is adenine, and when adenine is joined to ribose, an adenosine is formed, explaining the name adenosine triphosphate. If one phosphate is removed from the end of the molecule, adenosine diphosphate (ADP) is formed.

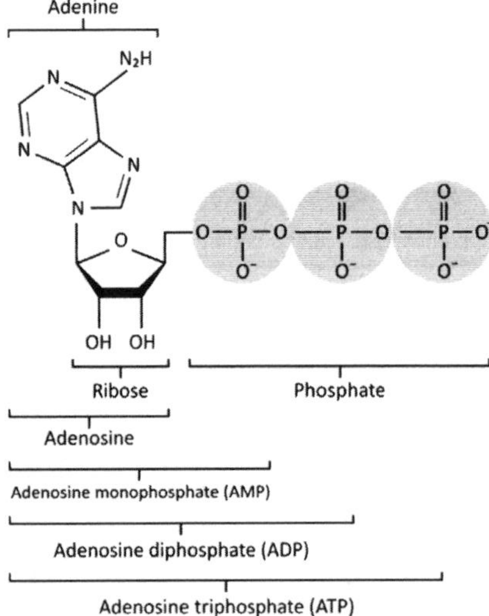

Properties of Water

Water exhibits numerous properties. Water has a high surface tension due to the cohesion between water molecules from the hydrogen bonds between the molecules. The capillary action of water is also due to this cohesion, and the adhesion of water is due to its polarity. Water is an excellent solvent due to its polarity and is considered the universal solvent. Water exists naturally as a solid, liquid, and gas. The density of water decreases as ice freezes and forms crystals in the solid phase. Water is most dense at 4 °C. Water can act as an acid or base in chemical reactions. Pure water is an insulator because it has virtually no ions. Water has a high specific heat capacity due to its low molecular mass and bent molecular shape.

> **Review Video: Properties of Water**
> Visit mometrix.com/academy and enter code: 279526

Biological Macromolecules

Macromolecules are large molecules made up of smaller organic molecules. Four classes of macromolecules include carbohydrates, nucleic acids, proteins, and lipids. Carbohydrates, proteins, and nucleic acids are polymers that are formed when the monomers are joined together in a dehydration process. In this dehydration process, the monomers are joined by a covalent bond and a water molecule is released. The monomers in carbohydrates are simple sugars such as glucose, while polysaccharides are polymers of carbohydrates. The monomers in proteins are amino acids. The amino acids form polypeptide chains, which are folded into proteins. The monomers in nucleic acids are nucleotides. Lipids are not actually considered to be polymers. Lipids typically are classified as fats, phospholipids, or steroids.

> **Review Video: Macromolecules**
> Visit mometrix.com/academy and enter code: 220156

Physics

Work, Energy, and Power

Basic Equation for Work

The equation for **work** (W) is $W = \boldsymbol{Fd}$, where $\boldsymbol{F}$ is the force exerted and $\boldsymbol{d}$ is the displacement of the object on which the force is exerted. For the simplest case, when the vectors of force and displacement have the same direction, the work done is equal to the product of the magnitudes of the force and displacement. If this is not the case, then the work may be calculated as $W = \boldsymbol{Fd}\cos\theta$, where θ is the angle between the force and displacement vectors. If force and displacement have the same direction, then work is positive; if they are in opposite directions, however, work is negative; and if they are perpendicular, the work done by the force is zero.

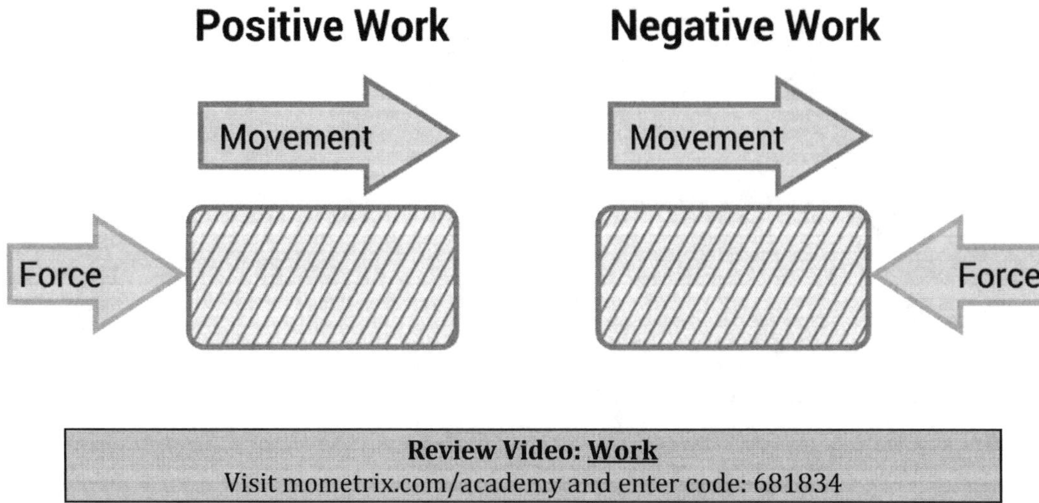

Review Video: Work
Visit mometrix.com/academy and enter code: 681834

For example, if a man pushes a block horizontally across a surface with a constant force of 10 N for a distance of 20 m, the work done by the man is 200 N-m or 200 J. If instead the block is sliding and the man tries to **slow its progress** by pushing against it, his work done is –200 J, since he is pushing in the direction opposite the motion. Also, if the man pushes vertically downward on the block while it slides, his work done is zero, since his force vector is perpendicular to the displacement vector of the block. It is important to note in each of these cases that neither the mass of the block nor the elapsed time is considered when calculating the amount of work done by the man.

Review Video: Push and Pull Forces
Visit mometrix.com/academy and enter code: 104731

POWER

Put simply, **power** is the **rate at which work is done**. Power, like work, is a scalar quantity. If we know the amount of work, W, that has been performed in a given amount of time, Δt, then we may find average power, $P_{avg} = \frac{W}{\Delta t}$. If we are instead looking for the instantaneous power, there are two possibilities. If the force on an object is constant, and the object is moving at a constant velocity, then the instantaneous power is the same as the average power. If either the force or the velocity is varying, the instantaneous power should be computed by the equation $P = \boldsymbol{Fv}$, where $\boldsymbol{F}$ and $\boldsymbol{v}$ are the instantaneous force and velocity, respectively. This equation may also be used to compute average power if the force and velocity are constant. Power is typically expressed in joules per second, or watts.

SIMPLE MACHINES

Simple machines include the pulley, lever, wheel and axle, wedge, inclined plane, and screw. These simple machines have no internal source of energy. More complex or compound machines can be formed from them. Simple machines provide a mechanical advantage and make it easier to accomplish a task. Single or double pulleys allow for easier direction of force. A lever enables a multiplication of force. The wheel and axle allows for movement with less resistance. The inclined plane enables a force less than an object's weight to be used to push it to a greater height. The wedge and screw are forms of the inclined plane. A wedge turns a smaller force working over a greater distance into a larger force. The screw is similar to an incline that is wrapped around a shaft.

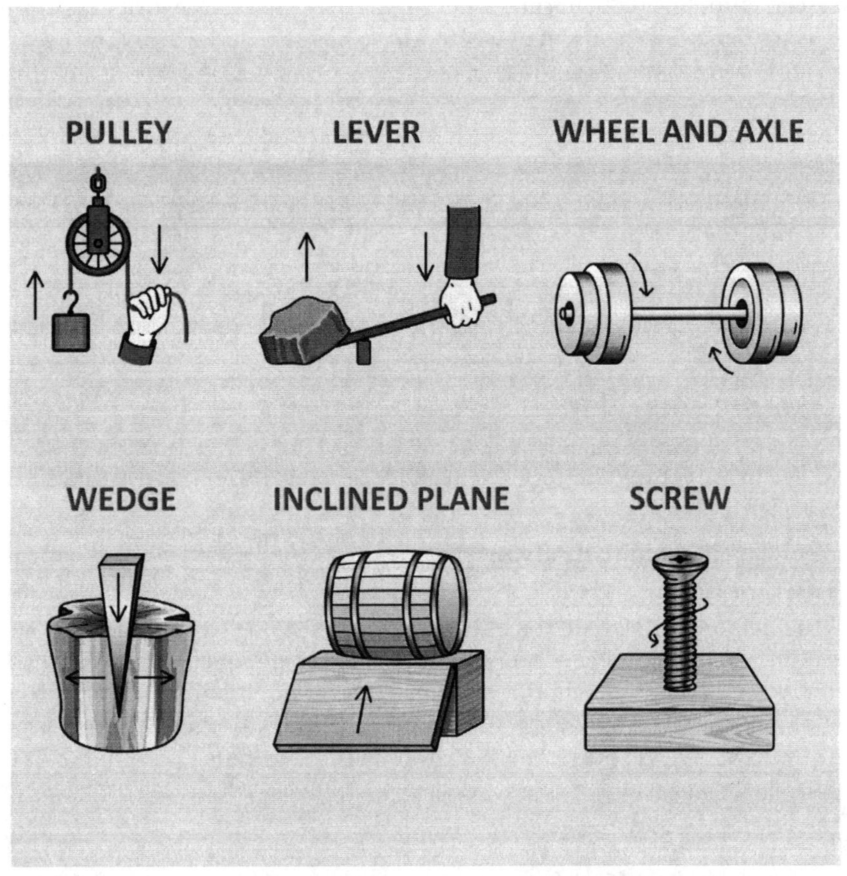

Review Video: Simple Machines
Visit mometrix.com/academy and enter code: 950789

Mechanical Advantage

There is a certain amount of **work** required to move an object that cannot be reduced. However, using one or more simple machines can increase either the distance or force needed. Since work is defined as a force multiplied by a distance, force and distance are inversely proportional.

$$\textbf{Work}_{\textbf{input}} = \textbf{Work}_{\textbf{output}}$$

$$\textbf{force}_{\textbf{input}} \times \textbf{distance}_{\textbf{input}} = \textbf{force}_{\textbf{output}} \times \textbf{distance}_{\textbf{output}}$$

Simple machines can either reduce the amount of input force needed by increasing the input distance or they can reduce the input distance needed by increasing the required input force. The ratio of the output force over the input force is a measure of the **mechanical advantage** of a machine. Due to the inverse relationship between force and distance for these machines, mechanical advantage can also be expressed as the ratio of input distance over the output distance.

$$\textbf{Mechanical Advantage} = \frac{\textbf{force}_{\textbf{output}}}{\textbf{force}_{\textbf{input}}} = \frac{\textbf{distance}_{\textbf{input}}}{\textbf{distance}_{\textbf{output}}}$$

LEVERS

The **lever** is the most common kind of simple machine. See-saws, shovels, and baseball bats are all examples of levers. There are three classes of levers which are differentiated by the relative orientations of the fulcrum, resistance, and effort. The **fulcrum** is the point at which the lever rotates, the **effort** is the point on the lever where force is applied, and the **resistance** is the part of the lever that acts in response to the effort.

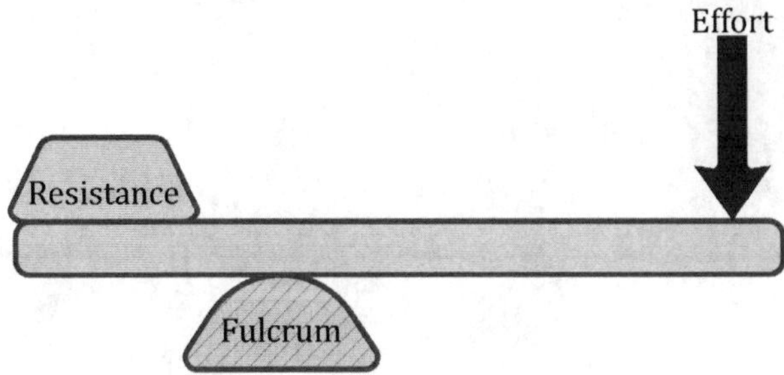

The mechanical advantage of a lever depends on the distances of the effort and resistance from the fulcrum.

$$\textbf{Mechanical Advantage} = \frac{\textbf{effort distance}}{\textbf{resistance distance}}$$

In a **first-class lever**, the fulcrum is between the effort and the resistance. A seesaw is a good example of a first-class lever when effort is applied to force one end up, the other end goes down, and vice versa. The shorter the distance between the fulcrum and the resistance, the easier it will be to move the resistance. As an example, consider whether it is easier to lift another person on a see-saw when they are sitting close to the middle or all the way at the end. A little practice will show you that it is much more difficult to lift a person the farther away he or she is on the see-saw.

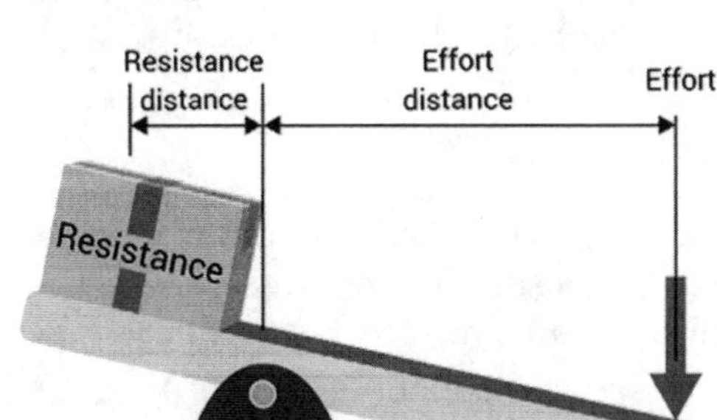

In a **second-class lever**, the resistance is in between the fulcrum and the effort. While a first-class lever is able to increase force and distance through mechanical advantage, a second-class lever is only able to increase force. A common example of a second-class lever is the wheelbarrow; the force exerted by your hand at one end of the wheelbarrow is magnified at the load. Basically, with a second-class lever, you are trading distance for force; by moving your end of the wheelbarrow a bit farther, you produce greater force at the load.

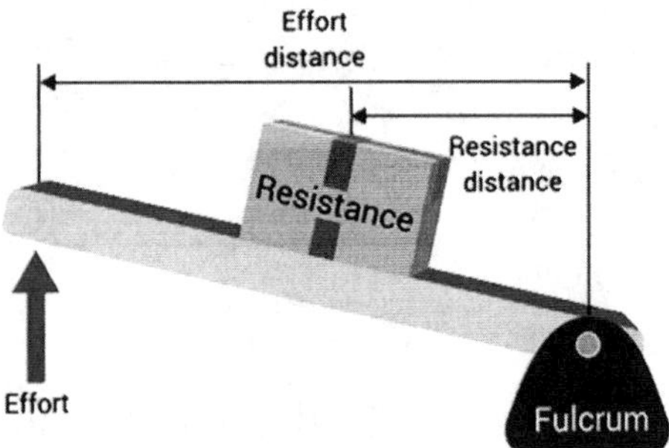

Third-class levers are used to produce greater distance. In a third-class lever, the force is applied in between the fulcrum and the resistance. A baseball bat is a classic example of a third-class lever; the bottom of the bat, below where you grip it, is considered the fulcrum. The end of the bat, where the ball is struck, is the resistance. By exerting effort at the base of the bat, close to the fulcrum, you are able to make the end of the bat fly quickly through the air. The closer your hands are to the base of the bat, the faster you will be able to make the other end of the bat travel.

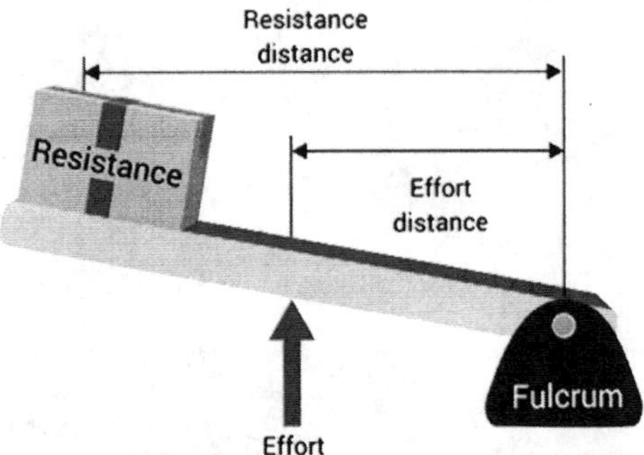

Review Video: Levers
Visit mometrix.com/academy and enter code: 103910

Wheel and Axle

Another basic arrangement that makes use of simple machines is called the wheel and axle. When most people think of a wheel and axle, they immediately envision an automobile tire. The steering wheel of the car, however, operates on the same mechanical principle, namely that the force required to move the center of a circle is much greater than the force required to move the outer rim of a circle. When you turn the steering wheel, you are essentially using a second-class lever by increasing the output force by increasing the input distance. The force required to turn the wheel from the outer rim is much less than would be required to turn the wheel from its center.

The equation for the mechanical advantage of a wheel and axle is:

$$\textbf{Mechanical Advantage} = \frac{\textbf{radius}_{\textbf{wheel}}}{\textbf{radius}_{\textbf{axle}}}$$

For instance, a steering wheel with a radius of 12 inches has a greater mechanical advantage than a steering wheel with a radius of 10 inches; the same amount of force exerted on the rim of each wheel will produce greater force on the axle of the larger wheel.

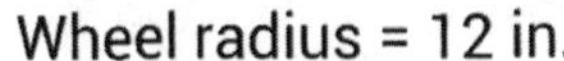

Wheel radius = 10 in.

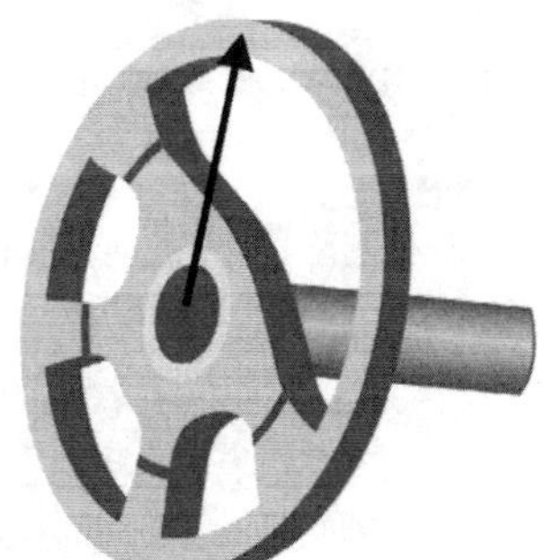

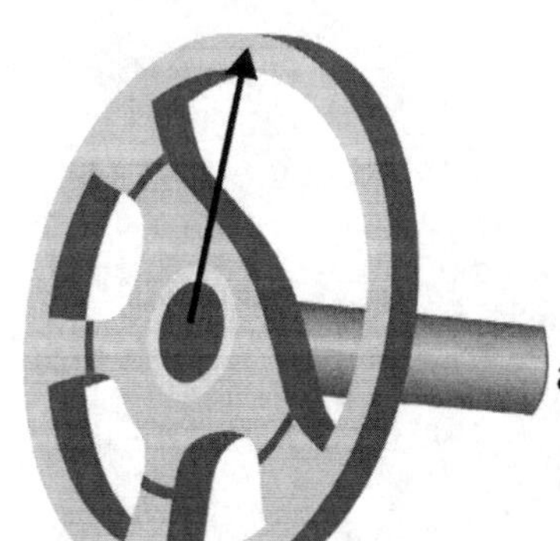

axle radius = 2 in.

Thus, the mechanical advantage for each is:

$$\frac{10 \text{ inches}}{2 \text{ inches}} = 5 \qquad \frac{12 \text{ inches}}{2 \text{ inches}} = 6$$

Review Video: Wheel and Axle
Visit mometrix.com/academy and enter code: 574045

Pulleys

The pulley is a simple machine in which a rope is carried by the rotation of a wheel. Another name for a pulley is a block. Pulleys are typically used to allow the force to be directed from a convenient location. For instance, imagine you are given the task of lifting a heavy and tall bookcase. Rather than tying a rope to the bookcase and trying to lift it, it would make sense to tie a pulley system to a rafter above the bookcase and run the rope through it, so that you could pull down on the rope and lift the bookcase. Pulling down allows you to incorporate your weight (normal force) into the act of lifting, thereby making it easier.

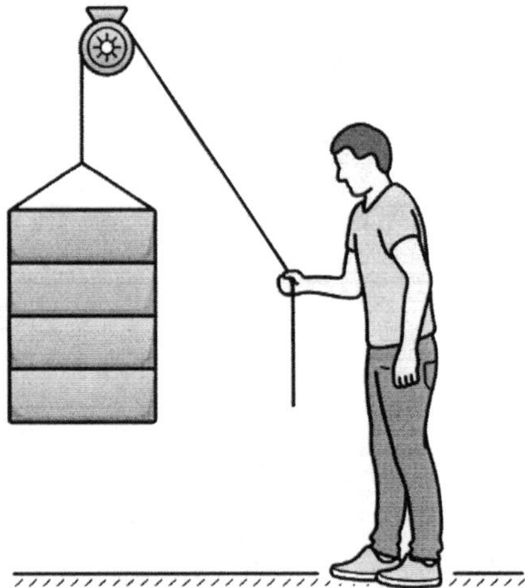

If there is just one pulley above the bookcase, you have created a first-class lever that will not diminish the amount of force that needs to be applied to lift the bookcase. There is another way to use a pulley, however, that can make the job of lifting a heavy object considerably easier. First, tie the rope directly to the rafter. Then, attach a pulley to the top of the bookcase and run the rope through it. If you can then stand so that you are above the bookcase, you will have a much easier time lifting this heavy object. This is because the weight of the bookcase is now being distributed: half of it is acting on the rafter, and half of it is acting on you. In other words, this arrangement allows you to lift an object with half the force. This simple pulley system, therefore, has a mechanical advantage of 2. Note that in this arrangement, the unfixed pulley is acting like a second-class lever. The price you pay for your mechanical advantage is that whatever distance you raise your end of the rope, the bookcase will only be lifted half as much.

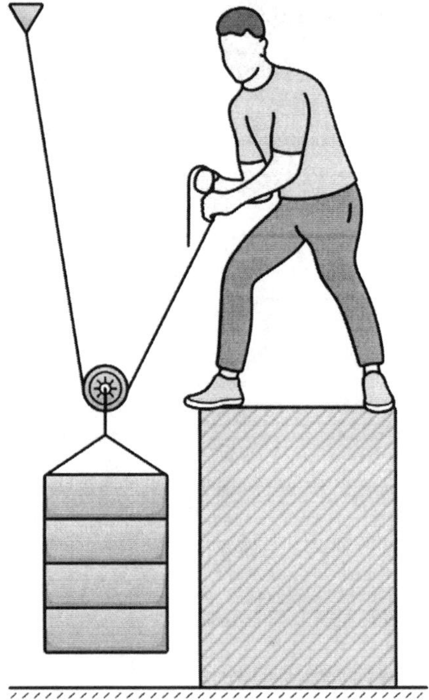

Of course, it might be difficult for you to find a place high enough to enact this system. If this is the case, you can always tie another pulley to the rafter and run the rope through it and back down to the floor. Since this second pulley is fixed, the mechanical advantage will remain the same.

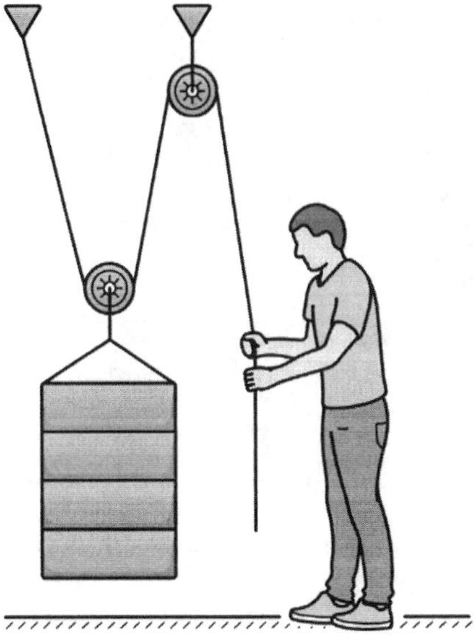

INCLINED PLANE

The inclined plane is perhaps the most common of the simple machines. It is simply a flat surface that elevates as you move from one end to the other. Consider how much easier it is for a person to walk up a long ramp than to climb a shorter but steeper flight of stairs; this is because the force required is diminished as the distance increases. Indeed, the longer the ramp, the easier it is to ascend.

Inclined planes often used to move heavy objects. For instance, moving a heavy box onto the back of a truck requires less force when pushing it up a ramp than when lifting it directly onto the truck bed. The longer the ramp, the greater the mechanical advantage, and the easier it will be to move the box. The mechanical advantage of an inclined plane is equal to the slant length divided by the rise of the plane.

$$\textbf{Mechanical Advantage} = \frac{\textbf{slant length}}{\textbf{rise}}$$

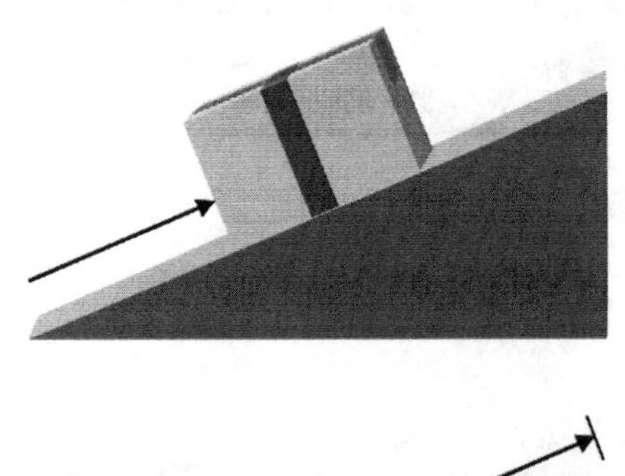

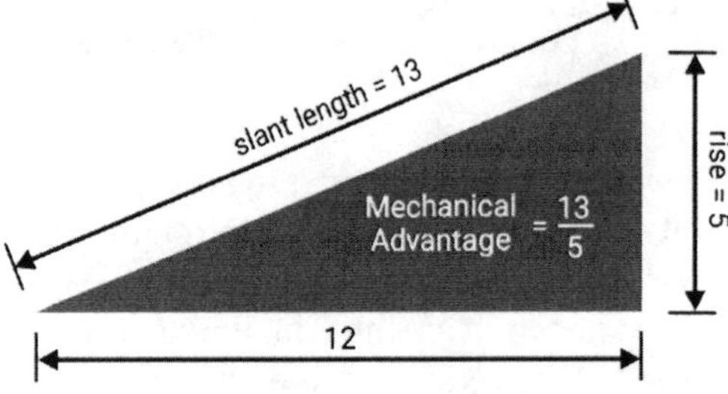

SCREW

A screw is simply an inclined plane that has been wound around a cylinder so that it forms a sort of spiral.

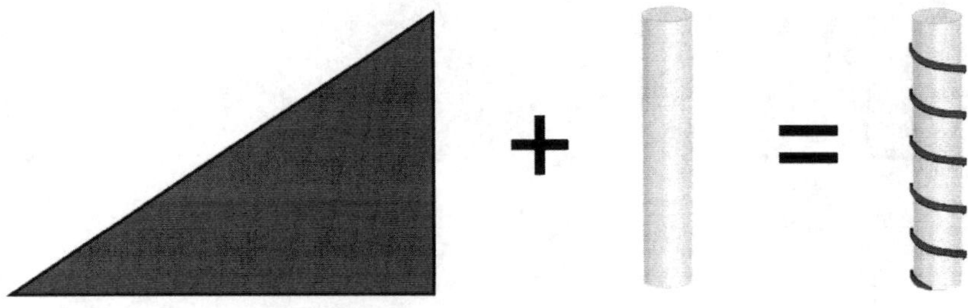

When it is placed into some medium, as for instance wood, the screw will move either forward or backward when it is rotated. The principle of the screw is used in a number of different objects, from jar lids to flashlights. The equation for the mechanical advantage is a modification of the inclined plane's equation.

Because the rise of the inclined plane is the length along a screw, length between rotations is the rise. The slant length is equal the circumference of one rotation ($2\pi r$).

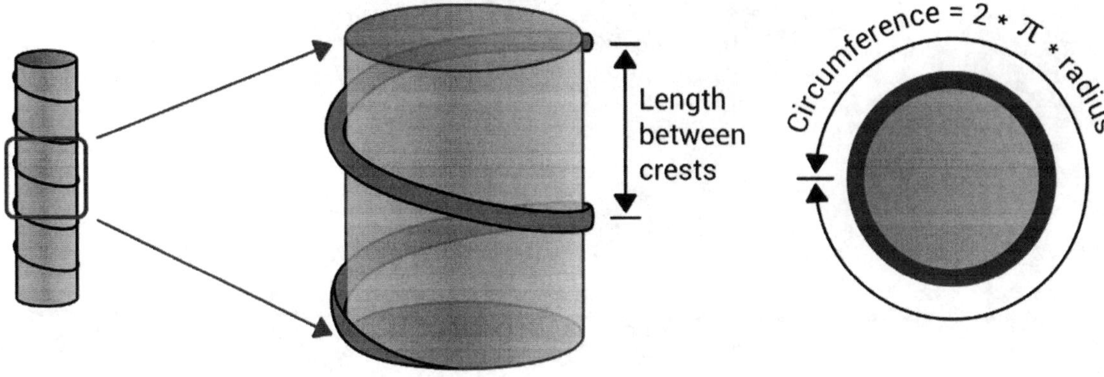

$$\textbf{Mechanical Advantage} = \frac{\mathbf{2 \times \pi \times radius}}{\textbf{length between crests}}$$

WEDGE

A wedge is a variation on the inclined plane, in which the wedge moves between objects or parts and forces them apart. The unique characteristic of a wedge is that, unlike an inclined plane, it is designed to move. Perhaps the most familiar use of the wedge is in splitting wood. A wedge is driven into the wood by hitting the flat back end. The thin end of a wedge is easier to drive into the wood since it has less surface area and, therefore, transmits more force per area. As the wedge is driven in, the increased width helps to split the wood.

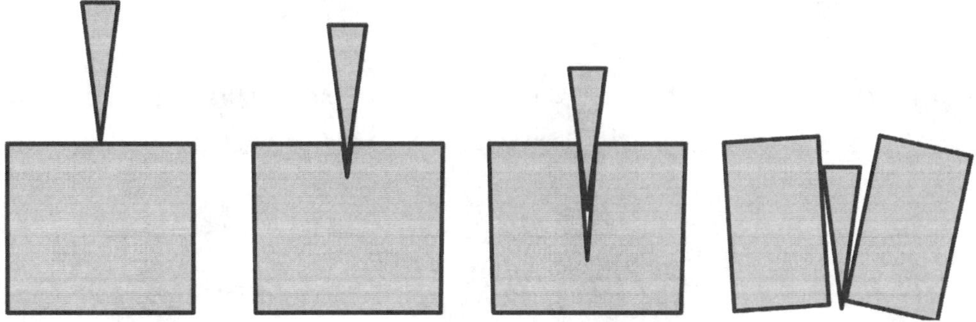

The longer and thinner the wedge, the greater the mechanical advantage. The equation for mechanical advantage of a wedge is:

$$\textbf{Mechanical Advantage} = \frac{\textbf{length}}{\textbf{width}}$$

GEARS

Gears are a system of interlocking wheels that can create immense mechanical advantages. The amount of mechanical advantage, however, will depend on the gear ratio; that is, on the relation in size between the gears.

When a small gear is driving a big gear, the speed of the big gear is relatively slow; when a big gear is driving a small gear, the speed of the small gear is relatively fast.

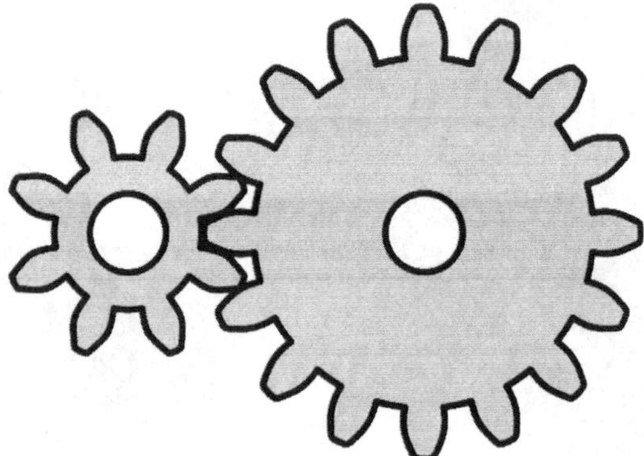

The equation for the mechanical advantage is:

$$\textbf{Mechanical Advantage} = \frac{\text{torque}_{\text{output}}}{\text{torque}_{\text{input}}} = \frac{r_{\text{output}}}{r_{\text{input}}} = \frac{\#\text{ of teeth}_{\text{output}}}{\#\text{ of teeth}_{\text{input}}}$$

Note that mechanical advantage is greater than 1 when the output gear is larger. In these cases, the output velocity (ω) will be lower. The equation for the relative speed of a gear system is:

$$\frac{\omega_{\text{input}}}{\omega_{\text{output}}} = \frac{r_{\text{output}}}{r_{\text{input}}}$$

Gear Ratios

A gear ratio is a measure of how much the speed and torque are changing in a gear system. It is the ratio of output speed to input speed. Because the number of teeth is directly proportional to the speed in meshing gears, a gear ratio can also be calculated using the number of teeth on the gears. When the driving gear has 30 teeth and the driven gear has 10 teeth, the gear ratio is 3:1.

$$\text{Gear Ratio} = \frac{\#\text{ of teeth}_{\text{driving}}}{\#\text{ of teeth}_{\text{driven}}} = \frac{30}{10} = \frac{3}{1} = 3:1$$

This means that the smaller, driven gear rotates 3 times for every 1 rotation of the driving gear.

Uses of Gears

Gears are used to change the direction, location, and amount of output torque, as well as change the angular velocity of output.

Change output direction

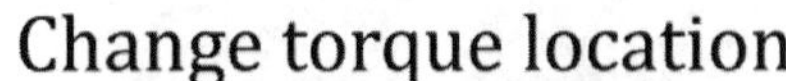

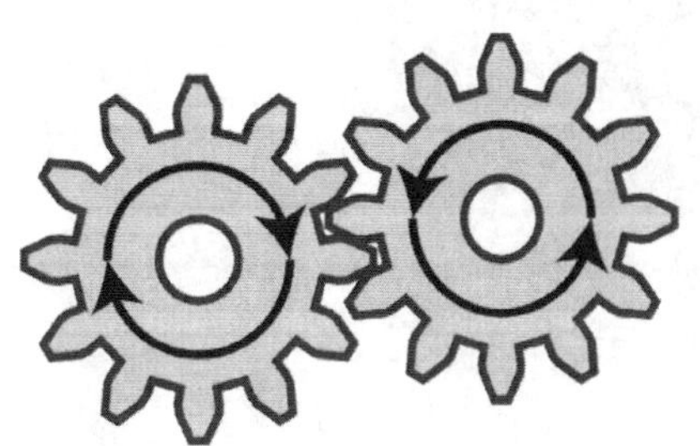

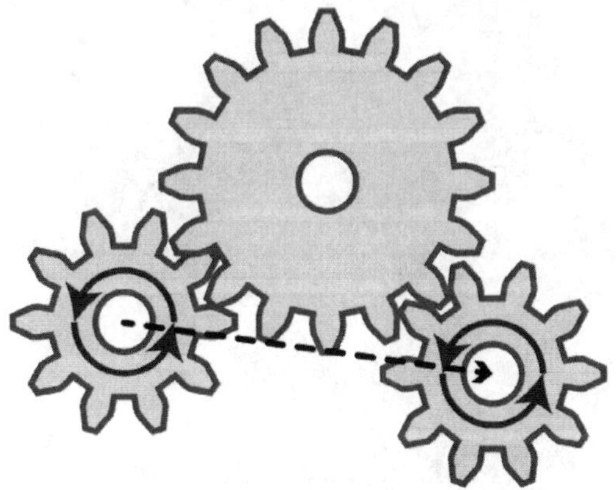

Change torque amount

Change output velocity

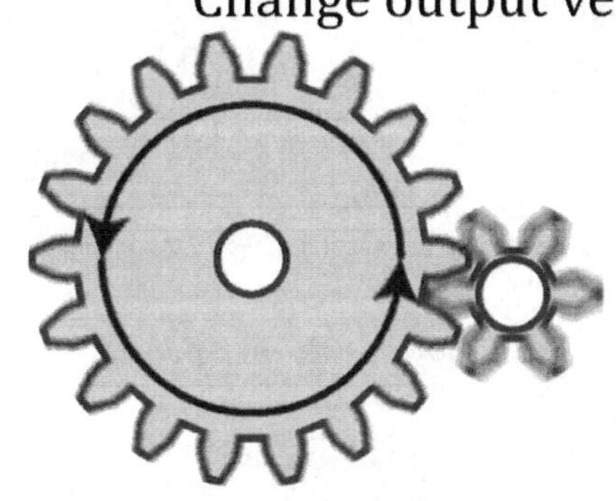

Energy

Energy is a word that has developed several different meanings in the English language, but in physics, it refers to the measure of a body's ability to do work. In physics, energy may not have a million meanings, but it does have many forms. Each of these forms, such as chemical, electric, and nuclear, is the capability of an object to perform work. However, the most commonly used concepts are mechanical energy and mechanical work. **Mechanical energy** is the sum of an object's kinetic and potential energies. While kinetic energy is linked to an object's motion, potential energy can be in a few different forms. The common forms of potential energy are gravitational and elastic.

Kinetic Energy

The **kinetic energy of an object** is that quality of its motion that can be related in a qualitative way to the amount of work performed on the object. Kinetic energy can be defined as $KE = \frac{mv^2}{2}$, in which m is the mass of an object and v is the magnitude of its velocity. Kinetic energy cannot be negative, since it depends on the square of velocity. Units for kinetic energy are the same as those for work: joules. Kinetic energy is a scalar quantity.

Changes in kinetic energy occur when a force does work on an object, such that the speed of the object is altered. This change in kinetic energy is equal to the amount of work that is done, and can be expressed as $W =$

$KE_f - KE_i = \Delta KE$. This equation is commonly referred to as the work-kinetic energy theorem. If there are several different forces acting on the object, then W in this equation is the total work done by all the forces, or by the net force. This equation can be very helpful in solving some problems that would otherwise rely solely on Newton's laws of motion.

Potential Energy

Potential energy is the amount of energy that can be ascribed to a body or bodies based on configuration. There are a couple of different kinds of potential energy. **Gravitational potential energy** is the energy associated with the separation of bodies that are attracted to one another gravitationally. Any time you lift an object, you are increasing its gravitational potential energy. Gravitational potential energy can be found by the equation $PE = mgh$, where m is the mass of an object, g is the gravitational acceleration, and h is its height above a reference point, most often the ground.

Another kind of potential energy is **elastic potential energy**; elastic potential energy is associated with the compression or expansion of an elastic, or spring-like, object. Physicists will often refer to potential energy as being stored within a body, the implication being that it could emerge in the future.

Review Video: Potential and Kinetic Energy
Visit mometrix.com/academy and enter code: 491502

Conservative and Non-Conservative Forces

Forces that change the state of a system by changing kinetic energy into potential energy, or vice versa, are called **conservative forces**. This name arises because these forces conserve the total amount of kinetic and potential energy. Every other kind of force is considered non-conservative. One example of a conservative force is gravity. Consider the path of a ball thrown straight up into the air. Since the ball has the same amount of kinetic energy when it is thrown as it does when it returns to its original location (known as completing a closed path), gravity can be said to be a conservative force. More generally, a force can be said to be conservative if the work it does on an object through a closed path is zero. Frictional force would not meet this standard, of course, because it is only capable of performing negative work.

For example, imagine a ball moving perpendicular to the surface of the Earth, in other words straight up and down, with its weight being the only force acting on it. As the ball rises, the weight will be doing work on the ball, decreasing its speed and its kinetic energy and slowing it down until it momentarily stops. During this ascent, the potential energy of the ball will be rising. Once the ball begins to fall back down, it will lose potential energy as it gains kinetic energy. Mechanical energy is conserved throughout; the potential energy of the ball at its highest point is equal to the kinetic energy of the ball at its lowest point, just before to impact.

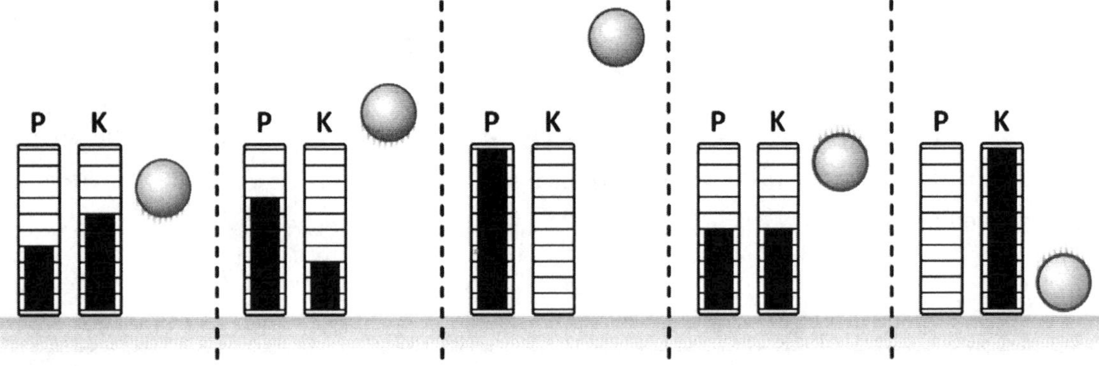

In systems where friction and air resistance are not negligible, we observe a different sort of result. For example, imagine a block sliding across the floor until it comes to a stop due to friction. Unlike a compressed spring or a ball flung into the air, there is no way for this block to regain its energy with a return trip.

Therefore, we cannot say that the lost kinetic energy is being stored as potential energy. Instead, it has been dissipated and cannot be recovered. The total mechanical energy of the block-floor system has been not conserved in this case but rather reduced. The total energy of the system has not decreased, since the kinetic energy has been converted into thermal energy, but that energy is no longer useful for work.

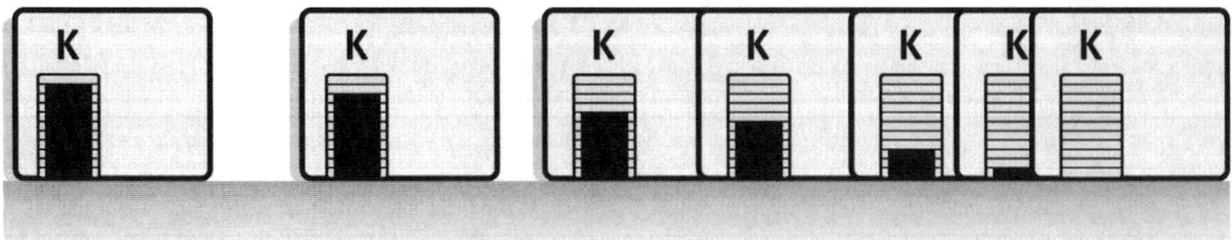

One-Dimensional Analysis of Work Done By a Variable Force

If the force on an object varies across the distance the object is moved, then a simple product will not yield the work. If we consider the work performed by a variable force in one dimension, then we are assuming that the directions of the force and the displacement are the same. The magnitude of the force will depend on the position of the particle. In order to calculate the amount of work performed by a variable force over a given distance, we should first divide the total displacement into a number of intervals, each with a width of Δx. We may then say that the amount of work performed during any one interval is $\Delta W = \boldsymbol{F}_{avg}\Delta x$, where $\boldsymbol{F}_{avg}$ is the average force over the interval Δx. We can then say that the total amount of work performed is the sum of all work performed during the various intervals. By reducing the interval to an infinitesimal length, we obtain the integral:

$$W = \int_{x_1}^{x_2} \boldsymbol{F}_x dx$$

This integral requires that the force be a known function of x.

Work Performed by a Spring

If we move a block attached to a spring from point x_i to point x_f, we are doing work on the block, and the spring is also doing work on the block. To determine the work done by the spring on the block, we can substitute $\boldsymbol{F}$ from Hooke's law into our equation for work performed by a variable force, and arrive at this measure: $W = \frac{k(x_i{}^2 - x_f{}^2)}{2}$. This work will be positive if $x_i{}^2 > x_f{}^2$, and negative if the opposite is true. If $x_i = 0$ and we decide to call the final position x, then we may change our equation: $W = \frac{-kx^2}{2}$. It is important to keep in mind that this is the work done by the spring. The work done by the force that moves the block to its final position will be a positive quantity.

Like all simple harmonic oscillators, springs operate by **storing and releasing potential energy**. The amount of energy being stored or released by a spring is equal to the magnitude of the work done by the spring during that same operation. The total potential energy stored in a spring can be calculated as $PE = \frac{kx^2}{2}$. Neglecting the effects of friction and drag, an object oscillating on a spring will continue to do so indefinitely, since total mechanical energy (kinetic and potential) is conserved. In such a situation, the period of oscillation can be calculated as $T = 2\pi \times \sqrt{\frac{m}{k}}$.

DISPLACEMENT, VELOCITY, AND ACCELERATION

DISPLACEMENT

When something changes its location from one place to another, it is said to have undergone **displacement**. If we can determine the original and final position of the object, then we can determine the total displacement with the equation $\Delta \boldsymbol{x} = x_f - x_i$, where x_f is the final position and x_i is the initial position.

If the object has moved in the positive direction, then the final position will be greater than the original position, so we can say that the change was positive. If the final position is less than the original, however, displacement will be negative. Displacement along a straight line is an example of a vector quantity; it has both a magnitude and a direction. If an object travels from position $x = -5$ cm to $x = 5$ cm, it has undergone a displacement of 10 cm. If it traverses the same path in the opposite direction, its displacement is −10 cm. A vector that spans the object's displacement in the direction of travel is known as a displacement vector, with units of length.

Review Video: Displacement in Physics
Visit mometrix.com/academy and enter code: 236197

DETERMINING POSITION

In order to determine anything about the motion of an object, we must first locate it. In other words, we must be able to describe its position relative to some reference point, often called an **origin**. If we consider the origin as the zero point of an axis, then positive values correspond to the location of an object one direction, and negative values are locations in the exact opposite direction. If a particle is located 5 cm from the origin in the positive direction of the x-axis, its location is said to be $x = 5$ cm. If another particle is 5 cm from the origin in the negative direction of the x-axis, its position is $x = -5$ cm. These two particles are 10 cm apart. A vector whose starting point is the origin and whose endpoint is the location of an object is that object's position vector, with units of length.

VELOCITY

INSTANTANEOUS VELOCITY

There are two types of velocity that are commonly considered in physics: average velocity and instantaneous velocity. In order to obtain the **instantaneous velocity** of an object, we must find its average velocity and then try to decrease Δt as close as possible to zero. As Δt decreases, it approaches what is known as a limiting value, bringing the average velocity very close to the instantaneous velocity. Instantaneous velocity is most easily discussed in the context of calculus-based physics.

AVERAGE VELOCITY

If we want to calculate the **average velocity** of an object, we must know two things. First, we must know its **displacement**, or the distance it has covered relative to a starting point. Second, we must know the **time it took to cover this distance**. Once we have this information, the formula for average velocity is: $\boldsymbol{v}_{avg} = \frac{(x_f - x_i)}{(t_f - t_i)}$, where the subscripts i and f denote the initial and final values of the position and time. In other words, the average velocity is equal to the change in position divided by the change in time. This calculation will indicate the average distance that was covered per unit of time. Average velocity is a vector and will always point in the same direction as the displacement vector (since time is a scalar and always positive).

ACCELERATION

Acceleration is the **change in the velocity** of an object. Like velocity, acceleration may be computed as an average or an instantaneous quantity. To calculate average acceleration, we may use the equation $\boldsymbol{a}_{avg} = \frac{v_f - v_i}{t_f - t_i}$, where the subscripts i and f denote the initial and final values of the velocity and time. The so-called instantaneous acceleration of an object can be found by reducing the time component to the limiting value until instantaneous velocity is approached. Acceleration will be expressed in units of distance divided by time squared; for instance, meters per second squared. Like position and velocity, acceleration is a vector quantity and will therefore have both magnitude and direction.

Review Video: Velocity and Acceleration
Visit mometrix.com/academy and enter code: 671849

Kinematics

Kinematic Equations

The phenomenon of constant acceleration allows physicists to construct a number of helpful equations. Perhaps the most fundamental equation of an object's motion is the **position equation**:

$$x_f = x_i + \boldsymbol{v}_i t + \frac{1}{2}\boldsymbol{a}t^2$$

If the object is starting from rest at the origin, this equation reduces to $x_f = \frac{at^2}{2}$. The position equation can be rearranged to give the **displacement equation**:

$$\Delta \boldsymbol{x} = \boldsymbol{v}_i t + \frac{1}{2}\boldsymbol{a}t^2$$

If the object's acceleration is unknown, the position or displacement may be found by the equation:

$$\Delta \boldsymbol{x} = \frac{(\boldsymbol{v}_f + \boldsymbol{v}_i)t}{2}$$

If the position of an object is unknown, the velocity may be found by the equation:

$$\boldsymbol{v}_f = \boldsymbol{v}_i + \boldsymbol{a}t$$

Similarly, if the time is unknown, the velocity after a given displacement may be found by the equation:

$$\boldsymbol{v}_f = \sqrt{(\boldsymbol{v}_i{}^2 + 2\boldsymbol{a}\Delta \boldsymbol{x})}$$

Projectile Motion

When we discuss **projectile motion**, we are referring to the movement of an object through two dimensions during a free fall. Two-dimensional motion may be described using the same equations as one-dimensional motion, but two equations must be considered simultaneously. For basic equations for projectile motion, it is often assumed that the rate of gravitational acceleration on the Earth is $\boldsymbol{g} = 9.8 \text{ m/s}^2$, and that the effect of air resistance can be ignored (Note: take care with the sign on gravitational acceleration make sure that it always points toward the Earth). If a projectile is launched under such ideal conditions, we may say that its initial velocity is $\boldsymbol{v}_0 = v_0 \cos\theta\, \mathbf{i} + v_0 \sin\theta\, \mathbf{j}$. These two velocity components are sometimes written as $\boldsymbol{v}_{0x}$ and $\boldsymbol{v}_{0y}$, respectively.

Example: If a cannon located at a height of 5 m above ground level fires a cannonball 250 m/s at an angle of $\frac{\pi}{6}$ from the horizontal, how far will the cannonball travel before hitting the ground?

When the cannonball hits the ground, it has been displaced by –5 m in the y-direction. Solving for the components of initial velocity yields $\boldsymbol{v}_{0x} = 216.5 \text{ m/s}$ and $\boldsymbol{v}_{0y} = 125 \text{ m/s}$. Setting up the y-direction displacement equation results in the following: $-5 = 125t_f - 4.9t_f{}^2$. Solving for t_f yields an impact time of around 25.5 seconds. To find the horizontal distance covered, set up the displacement equation for the

x-direction: $\Delta \boldsymbol{x} = \boldsymbol{v}_{0x} t_f + \frac{1}{2} \boldsymbol{a}_x (t_f)^2$. Since we ignore the effects of air resistance, acceleration in the x-direction is zero, yielding a flight distance of 5,530 m.

Review Video: Projectile Motion
Visit mometrix.com/academy and enter code: 719700

Uniform Circular Motion

We may say that a particle is in **uniform circular motion** when it is traveling in a circle, or circular arc, and at a constant speed. Crucially, we must note that such a particle is accelerating, even though the magnitude of its velocity does not change. This is because velocity is a vector, and consequently, any change in its direction is an acceleration. So, if we take two points on an arc of radius, r, separated by an angle, θ, and want to determine the time it will take a particle to move between these two points at a constant speed, $|\boldsymbol{v}|$, we can use the equation: $\Delta t = \frac{r\theta}{|\boldsymbol{v}|}$. The quantity $\frac{|\boldsymbol{v}|}{r}$ is often written as $\boldsymbol{\omega}$, or angular velocity, having units of radians per second, so the time may also be computed as $\Delta t = \frac{\theta}{\boldsymbol{\omega}}$. The speed, or absolute value of the velocity, of an object in uniform circular motion is also called the tangential speed, because the object is always moving in a direction tangent to the circle. Similarly, an increase in the magnitude of this velocity is called **tangential acceleration**.

A very important component of uniform motion is the centripetal acceleration. This is the acceleration that changes the direction of the velocity vector to follow the circular arc. It is directed toward the center of the circle or arc and is described by $\boldsymbol{a}_c = \frac{|\boldsymbol{v}|^2}{r} = r\boldsymbol{\omega}^2$.

Relative Motion and Inertial Reference Frames

When we describe motion as being **relative**, we mean that it can only be measured in relation to something else. If a moving object is considered as it relates to some stationary object or arbitrary location, it will have a different measured velocity than it would if it were compared to some other object that is itself in motion. In other words, the measure of an object's velocity depends entirely on the reference frame from which the measurement is taken. When performing measurements of this kind, we may use any reference point we like. However, once we have decided on a reference point, we must be consistent in using it as the basis for all of our measurements, or else we will go astray. Additionally, if we want to be able to apply Newton's laws of motion or Galilean principles of relativity, we must select an **inertial reference frame**: that is, a reference frame that is not accelerating or rotating. A car traveling at a constant speed in a straight line is an inertial reference frame. A car moving in uniform circular motion is not.

An object's velocity with respect to a frame fixed to the Earth can be computed by measuring its velocity from any inertial reference frame and combining that velocity by vector addition with the velocity of the inertial frame with respect to the Earth. For instance, if a man is traveling in the x-direction at 20 m/s, and he throws a rock out the window at a relative velocity of 15 m/s in the y-direction, the rock's velocity with respect to the Earth is found by adding the two vectors:

$$\boldsymbol{v}_r = 20\mathbf{i} + 15\mathbf{j} \text{ m/s}$$

Laws of Motion

Newton's Laws

Newton's First Law

Before Newton formulated his laws of mechanics, it was generally assumed that some force had to act on an object continuously in order to make the object move at a **constant velocity**. Newton, however, determined that unless some other force acted on the object (most notably friction or air resistance), it would continue in the direction it was pushed at the same velocity forever.

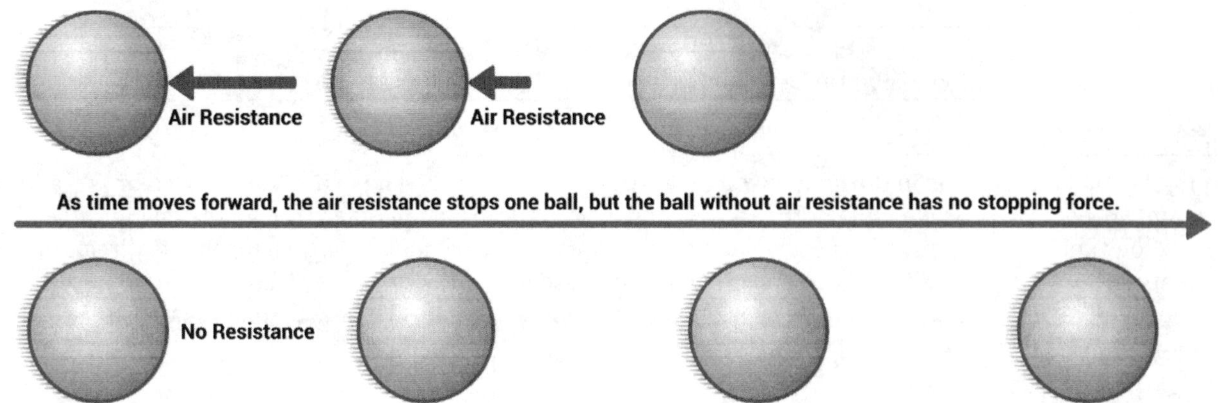

In this light, a body at rest and a body in motion are not all that different, and Newton's first law makes little distinction. It states that a body at rest will tend to remain at rest, while a body in motion will tend to remain in motion. This tendency of a body to remain in its present state of motion is referred to as **inertia**. In order for the body's state of motion to change, it must be acted on by a non-zero net force. **Net force** is the vector sum of all forces acting on a body. If this vector sum is zero, then there is no unbalanced force, and the body will remain in its present state of motion. It is important to remember that this law only holds in inertial reference frames.

Review Video: Newton's First Law of Motion
Visit mometrix.com/academy and enter code: 590367

NEWTON'S SECOND LAW

Newton's second law states that an **object's acceleration** is directly proportional to the net force acting on the object, and inversely proportional to the object's mass. It is generally written in equation form $\boldsymbol{F} = m\boldsymbol{a}$, where $\boldsymbol{F}$ is the net force acting on a body, m is the mass of the body, and $\boldsymbol{a}$ is its acceleration. It is important to note from this equation that since the mass is always a positive quantity, the acceleration vector is always pointed in the same direction as the net force vector. Of course, in order to apply this equation correctly, one must clearly identify the body to which it is being applied. Once this is done, we may say that $\boldsymbol{F}$ is the vector sum of all forces acting on that body, or the net force. This measure includes only those forces that are external to the body; any internal forces, in which one part of the body exerts force on another, are discounted.

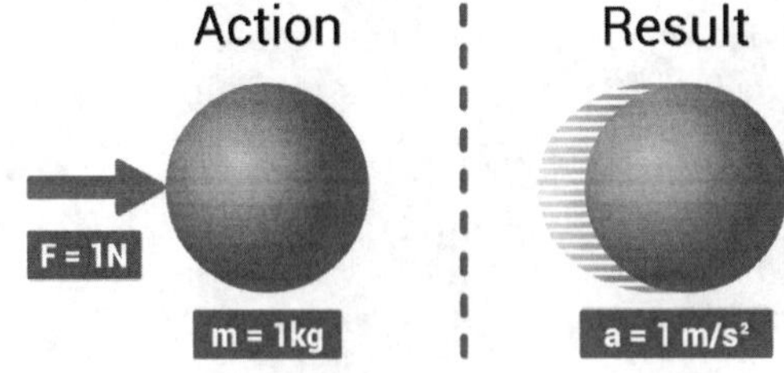

Newton's second law somewhat encapsulates his first, because it includes the principle that if no net force is acting on a body, the body will not accelerate. As was the case with his first law, Newton's second law may only be applied in inertial reference frames.

Review Video: Newton's Second Law of Motion
Visit mometrix.com/academy and enter code: 737975

NEWTON'S THIRD LAW

Newton's third law of motion can be stated as: **for every force, there is an equal and opposite force**. When a hammer strikes a nail, the nail hits the hammer just as hard. If we consider two objects, *A* and *B*, then we may express any contact between these two bodies with the equation $\boldsymbol{F}_{AB} = -\boldsymbol{F}_{BA}$. It is important to note in this kind of equation that the order of the subscripts denotes which body is exerting the force. Although the two forces are often referred to as the **action** and **reaction** forces, in physics there is really no such thing. There is no implication of cause and effect in the equation for Newton's third law. At first glance, this law might seem to forbid any movement at all. We must remember, however, that these equal, opposite forces are exerted on different bodies with different masses, so they will not cancel each other out.

As an example, consider two spring-based scales, both tipped on their sides, with the weighing surfaces facing each other. If scale #1 is pressing scale #2 into the wall, it exerts a force on scale #2, measurable by the reading on scale #2. However, because scale #1 is exerting a force on scale #2, scale #2 is exerting a force on scale #1 with an opposite direction, but the same magnitude.

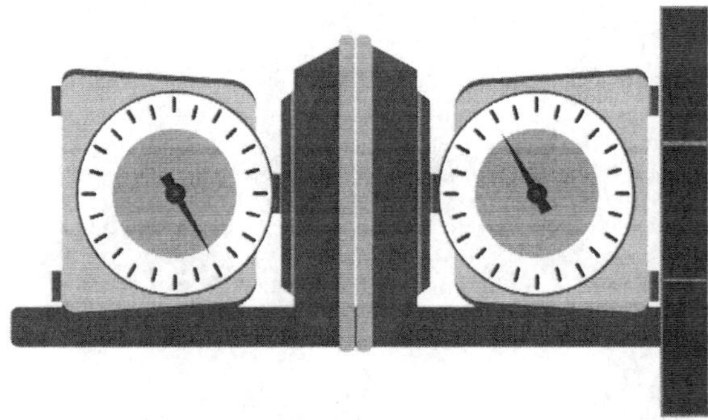

Review Video: Newton's Third Law of Motion
Visit mometrix.com/academy and enter code: 838401

EQUILIBRIUM AND FRICTION

NORMAL FORCE

The word *normal* is used in mathematics to mean perpendicular, and so the force known as normal force should be remembered as the perpendicular force exerted on an object that is resting on some other surface. For instance, if a box is resting on a horizontal surface, we may say that the normal force is directed upwards through the box (the opposite, downward force is the weight of the box). If the box is resting on a wedge, the normal force from the wedge is not vertical but is perpendicular to the surface.

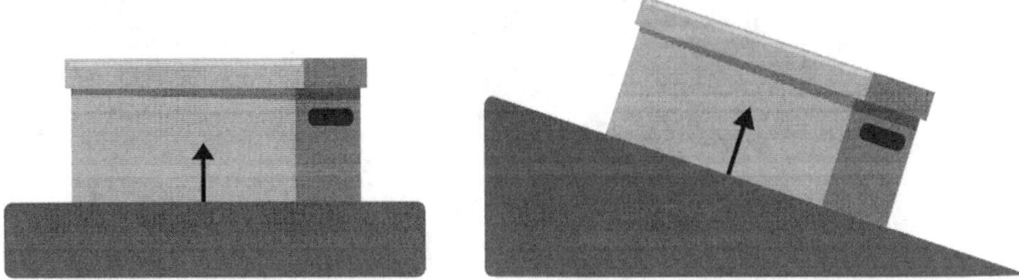

Static and Kinetic Frictional Forces

In order to illustrate the concept of friction, let us imagine a book resting on a table. As it sits there, the force of its weight ($\boldsymbol{W}$) is equal and opposite to the normal force ($\boldsymbol{N}$). If, however, we were to exert a force ($\boldsymbol{F}$) on the book, attempting to push it to one side, a frictional force ($\boldsymbol{f}$) would arise, equal and opposite to our force. This kind of frictional force is known as **static frictional force**.

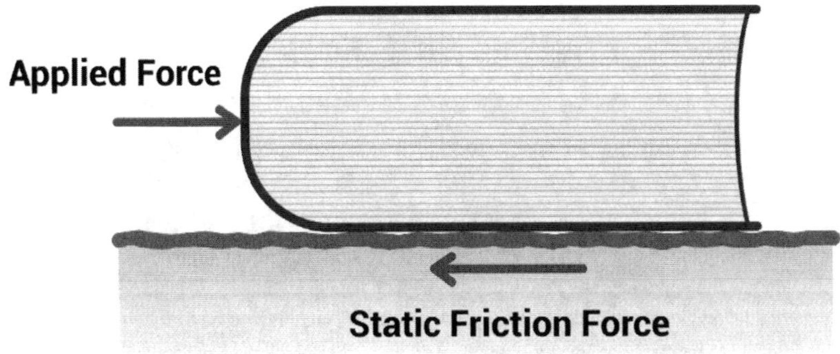

As we increase our force on the book, however, we will eventually cause it to accelerate in the direction of our force. At this point, the frictional force opposing us will be known as **kinetic frictional force**.

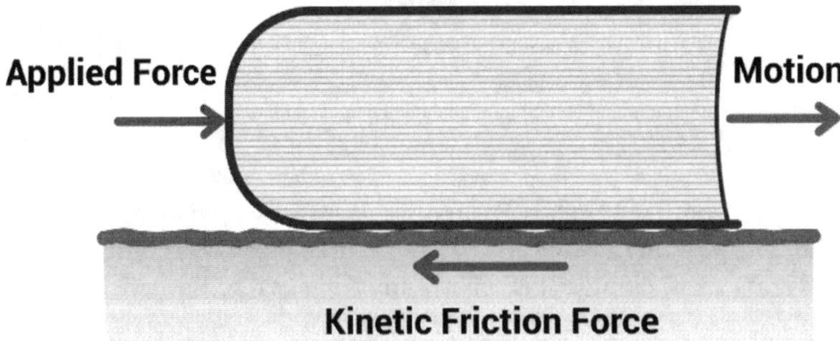

For the most part, kinetic frictional force is lower than static frictional force, and so the amount of force needed to maintain the movement of the book will be less than that needed to initiate movement. For wheels and spherical objects on a surface, static friction at the point of contact allows them to roll, but there is a frictional force that resists the rolling motion as well, due primarily to deformation effects in the rolling material. This is known as rolling friction, and tends to be much smaller than either static or kinetic friction.

COEFFICIENT OF FRICTION

If an object does not move when a horizontal force $\boldsymbol{F}$ is applied, then the **static frictional force** ($\boldsymbol{f_s}$) is exactly equal and opposite to $\boldsymbol{F}$, i.e., $\boldsymbol{f_s} = -\boldsymbol{F}$. Static frictional force has a maximum value, however, which is expressed as $\boldsymbol{f}_{s,max} = \mu_s N$, in which μ_s is the coefficient of static friction, and N is the magnitude of the normal force. If the magnitude of horizontal force applied to an object exceeds the maximum value of static friction, the object will begin to move. Once the object has begun to slide, the frictional force will generally decrease. The value to which the frictional force will diminish is expressed as $\boldsymbol{f}_k = \mu_k N$, in which μ_k is the coefficient of kinetic friction. For objects inclined to roll, such as balls or wheels, there is a rolling frictional force that resists the continued rolling of such an object. This force is expressed by $\boldsymbol{f}_r = \mu_r N$, in which μ_r is the coefficient of rolling friction. All of these frictional coefficients are dimensionless. Since the value of the frictional force depends on the interaction of the body and the surface, it is usually described as friction between the two.

Review Video: Friction
Visit mometrix.com/academy and enter code: 716782

EQUILIBRIUM

We may say that an object is in a **state of equilibrium** when it has a **constant linear momentum** ($\boldsymbol{p}$) at its center of mass, or when **angular momentum** ($\boldsymbol{L}$) **is also constant about the center of mass**. In other words, a wheel may be in equilibrium when it is spinning at a constant speed, and a hockey puck may be in equilibrium as it slides across ice. These are both examples of **dynamic equilibrium**. The phrase **static equilibrium**, however, is reserved for objects in which both linear and angular momentum are at zero. An object sitting on a table could be considered as being in static equilibrium.

USING EQUILIBRIUM CONDITIONS

For a **body in equilibrium**, the net force vector and the net torque vector will both be equal to zero. For the most common cases, two-dimensional systems, these conditions can be fully expressed by one or two force summation equations and one torque summation equation. Torque summations may be taken about any point on the body, though strategic placement can make calculations simpler. To determine the **torque exerted by a force**, multiply the magnitude of the force by the perpendicular distance to the point of interest. It will be necessary to decide in advance which direction of torque (clockwise or counterclockwise) will be considered positive.

For example, if we have a bar of known mass, m, that is suspended by cables at each end and whose center of mass is two thirds of the way along its length, L, we can use the equilibrium conditions to determine the tension in each cable. Gravity exerts a force of $-\boldsymbol{mg}$ on the bar's center of mass. Translational equilibrium conditions tell us that $\boldsymbol{T}_1 + \boldsymbol{T}_2 - \boldsymbol{mg} = 0$. Setting the total torque about the center of mass equal to zero, considering counterclockwise torque to be positive, yields the equation $\boldsymbol{T}_2\left(\frac{L}{3}\right) - \boldsymbol{T}_1\left(\frac{2L}{3}\right) = 0$. Solving these equations results in $\boldsymbol{T}_1 = \frac{mg}{3}$ and $\boldsymbol{T}_2 = \frac{2mg}{3}$. This result makes sense since the center of mass is closer to the second cable.

TRANSLATIONAL AND ROTATIONAL EQUILIBRIUM

If a body is in **translational equilibrium**, then its linear momentum will be constant, and there will be a net force of zero. Likewise, a body in rotational equilibrium will have a constant angular momentum, and again there will be a net torque of zero. Both of these equations are vector equations, and as such are both equivalent to three scalar equations for the three dimensions of motion, though in most instances, only one or two dimensions will be considered at a time. We may say that the two requirements for a body to be in equilibrium are that the vector sum of all the external forces acting on the body must be zero, and the vector sum of all the external torques acting on the body must also be zero. Conversely, if we are told that a body is in equilibrium, we may assume that both of these conditions will hold, and that we can use them to find unknown forces or torques.

CONSERVATION OF ENERGY AND MOMENTUM

APPLYING CONSERVATION OF ROTATIONAL ENERGY AND ANGULAR MOMENTUM

A metal hoop of mass m and radius r is released from rest at the top of a hill of height h. Assuming that it rolls without sliding and does not lose energy to friction or drag, what will be the hoop's angular and linear velocities upon reaching the bottom of the hill?

The hoop's initial energy is all potential energy, $PE = mgh$. As the hoop rolls down, all of its energy is converted to **translational** and **rotational kinetic energy**. Thus, $mgh = \frac{1}{2}m\boldsymbol{v}^2 + \frac{1}{2}I\boldsymbol{\omega}^2$. Since the moment for a hoop is $I = mr^2$, and $\boldsymbol{\omega} = \frac{\boldsymbol{v}}{r}$, the equation becomes $mgh = \frac{1}{2}m\boldsymbol{v}^2 + \frac{1}{2}mr^2\left(\frac{\boldsymbol{v}^2}{r^2}\right)$, which further simplifies to $gh = \boldsymbol{v}^2$. Thus, the resulting velocity of the hoop is $\boldsymbol{v}_f = \sqrt{gh}$, with an angular velocity of $\boldsymbol{\omega}_f = \frac{\boldsymbol{v}_f}{r}$. Note that if you were to forget about the energy converted to rotational motion, you would calculate a final velocity of $\boldsymbol{v}_f = \sqrt{2gh}$, which is the **impact velocity** of an object dropped from height h.

Angular momentum, $\boldsymbol{L}$, of an object is defined as its moment of inertia multiplied by its angular velocity, or $\boldsymbol{L} = I\boldsymbol{\omega}$. Consider a planet orbiting the sun with an elliptical orbit where the small radius is r_S and large radius is r_L. Find the angular velocity of the planet when it is at distance r_S from the sun if its velocity at r_L is $\boldsymbol{\omega}_L$.

Since the size of a planet is almost insignificant compared to the interplanetary distances, the planet may be treated as a single particle of mass m, giving it a moment about the sun of $I = mr^2$. Since the gravitational force is incapable of exerting a net torque on an object, we can assume that the planet's angular momentum about the sun is a constant, $\boldsymbol{L}_L = \boldsymbol{L}_S$. Thus, $m{r_L}^2\boldsymbol{\omega}_L = m{r_S}^2\boldsymbol{\omega}_S$. Solving this equation for $\boldsymbol{\omega}_S$ yields $\boldsymbol{\omega}_S = \boldsymbol{\omega}_L\left(\frac{r_L}{r_S}\right)^2$.

MASS-ENERGY RELATIONSHIP

Because mass consists of atoms, which are themselves formed of subatomic particles, there is an energy inherent in the composition of all mass. In other words, it would require a significant input of energy to form all the atoms in a given mass from their most basic particles. This rest energy is the energy that Einstein refers to in his famous mass-energy relation $E = mc^2$, where c is the speed of light in a vacuum. In theory, if all the subatomic particles in a given mass were to spontaneously split apart, it would give off energy $E = mc^2$. For example, if this were to happen to a single gram of mass, the resulting outburst of energy would be $E = 9 \times 10^{13}$ J, enough energy to provide power for over 2,000 average households for a whole year.

In some nuclear reactions, small amounts of mass are converted to energy. The amount of energy released can be calculated through the same relation, $E = mc^2$. Most such reactions involve mass losses on the order of 10^{-30} kg.

WEIGHT AND MASS

WEIGHT

Not to be confused with mass (quantity of matter), weight the term for the force due to the gravitational attraction between the masses of the two bodies. This force is described by the expression $\frac{Gm_1m_2}{r^2}$, where G is the gravitational constant, m_1 and m_2 are the masses of the two objects, and r is the distance between the centers of mass. Since the majority of humans are concerned with events close to the surface of the Earth, one of the masses (M_E) and the distance (R_E) are essentially constant and are combined into $\boldsymbol{g}$, which is the acceleration due to gravity near the surface of the Earth $\left(\boldsymbol{g} = \frac{GM_E}{(\boldsymbol{R}_E)^2}\right)$. Thus, we can express weight as $\boldsymbol{W} = m\boldsymbol{g}$.

Since it is a force, the SI unit for weight is the Newton. As a vector, $\boldsymbol{W}$ can be expressed as either $-mg\mathbf{j}$ or $-W\mathbf{j}$, in which $\mathbf{j}$ is the direction on the axis pointing away from the Earth.

> **Review Video: Mass, Weight, Volume, Density, and Specific Gravity**
> Visit mometrix.com/academy and enter code: 920570

Electrical Properties of Materials

Common Means of Transferring Electrical Charge

Charge is transferred in three common ways: conduction, induction, and friction. **Conduction**, as the name implies, takes place between conductive materials. There must be a point of contact between the two materials and a potential difference, such as when a battery is connected to a circuit. **Induction also requires conductive materials. It occurs when a conductive material encounters a changing magnetic field**. The change can be the result of a changing magnetic field or the material moving within a constant magnetic field. Charge transfer due to **friction** does not require conductive materials. When two materials are rubbed together, electrons may be transferred from one to the other, leaving the two materials with equal and opposite charges. This is observed when shoes are dragged across a carpeted floor.

> **Review Video: Charging by Conduction**
> Visit mometrix.com/academy and enter code: 502661

Conductors, Insulators, and Semiconductors

In many materials, electrons are able to move freely; these are known as **conductors**. Due to their atomic structure and delocalized electrons, **metals** tend to be the best conductors, particularly copper and silver. Highly conductive wires are instrumental in creating low-resistance pathways for electrons to travel along within a circuit.

Other materials naturally inhibit the movement of charge and are known as **insulators**. Their electrons are tightly held by the individual constituent atoms. Glass, pure water, wood, and plastic are all insulators. Insulators are necessary in circuits to prevent charge from escaping to undesirable places, such as an operator's hand. For this reason, most highly conductive materials are covered by insulators.

Semiconductors, as the name suggests, are materials that only partially conduct electrical charge. The elements silicon and germanium are both common semiconductors, and are frequently used in microelectronic devices because they allow for tight control of the rate of conduction. In many cases, the conduction ability of semiconductors can be controlled by adjusting the temperature of the material.

Doping Semiconductors

Resistivity is the physical property of resistance of different materials: metals, which easily conduct electricity, have low resistivity; insulators have high resistivity; and the resistivity of **semiconductors** falls in between (example: silicon). **Doping** is the process of mixing different semiconductor atoms in order to control conductivity of the material. **N-type semiconductors** have an excess of electrons as a result of the doping process; when an electric field is applied, a negative pole forms due to the buildup of negatively charged electrons (example: silicon doped with antimony). **P-type semiconductors** have a shortage of electrons; when an electric field is applied, a positive pole forms (example: silicon doped with boron).

Introduction to Circuits and Current

Electric Current

Charge is a physical property of particles. For the particles of an atom, protons have a positive charge of +1, neutrons have no charge, and **electrons** have a negative charge of –1. Like charges repel each other (positive and positive or negative and negative), and opposite charges attract (negative and positive). The **net charge** of an atom or molecule can be found by adding up all the protons and electrons that it contains. When dealing with charge on the macro level, it is helpful to aggregate the charges in a material with different units. The coulomb is the SI unit for charge and is equivalent to about 6.24×10^{18} charged particles.

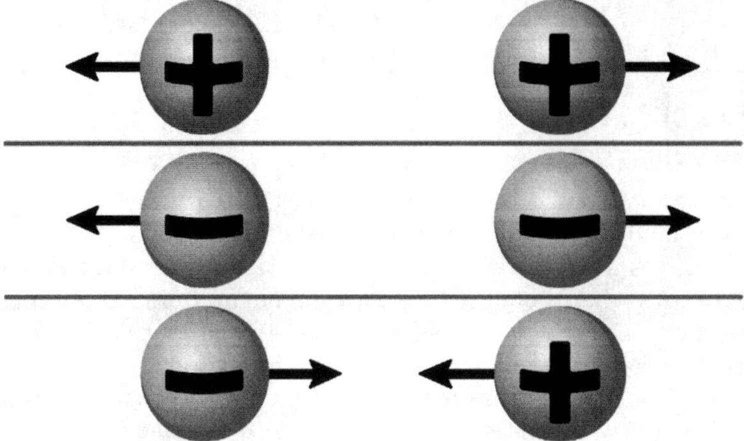

Electric current is the net rate of flow of charge (electrons) past a specific point, as in a wire or circuit. Current (represented by I in equations) is measured in amperes or amps (A). An ampere is equal to one coulomb per second $\left(\mathrm{A} = \frac{\mathrm{C}}{\mathrm{s}}\right)$. Ammeters are tools that can be used to measure current.

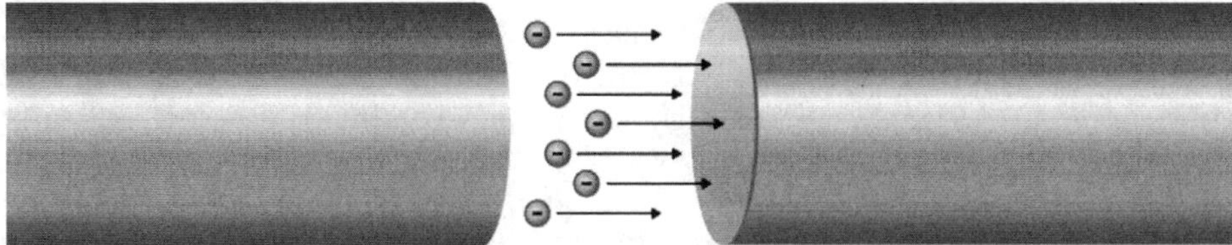

Electric current carries energy much like moving balls carry energy.

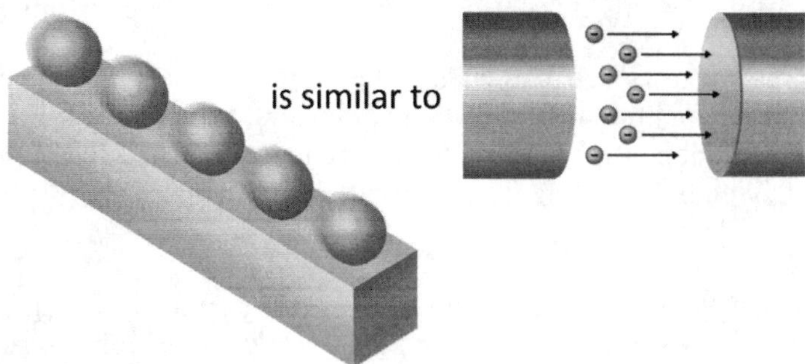

Electron flow theory states that electrons (e^-) flow from the negative terminal to the positive terminal. **Electricity** is the form of energy that exists statically (potential energy) with an accumulation of protons or electrons or dynamically with their movement (current).

> **Review Video: Electric Charge**
> Visit mometrix.com/academy and enter code: 323587

Alternating and Direct Current

For circuits with **direct current** (DC), when current flows in only one direction, the voltage and current are constant. Direct current is supplied by batteries and is used in cell phones, ships, and planes. **Alternating current** (AC), in which current periodically reverses direction, can be produced using generators and is used for land-based applications (including in homes) because less power is lost when electricity travels long distances. In the United States, AC electricity is supplied most commonly at 120 V and 240 V.

Electric Potential

Electric potential energy is the energy stored in a charge by virtue of its proximity to other charged regions. It can be calculated in the same way as calculating the amount of work required to move it to that location from an infinite distance away. The work required to move a charge of magnitude q from infinity to a distance r from another charge of magnitude Q is calculated to be $PE_e = W = \frac{kQq}{r}$, where k is the **electrostatic constant**.

Electric potential, V, is closely related to electric potential energy. The potential due to a charge Q can be found by dividing the electric potential energy of another charge q by its magnitude, $V = \frac{PE_e}{q}$, or by the equation $V = \frac{kQ}{r}$.

The difference between the electric potential of two points is known as **voltage**. It is measured in volts, or joules per coulomb. Since it is impractical to find a point of zero absolute electric potential, for each system a reference point or ground is defined, to which all other points in the system may be related. Voltage is similar to gravitational potential energy.

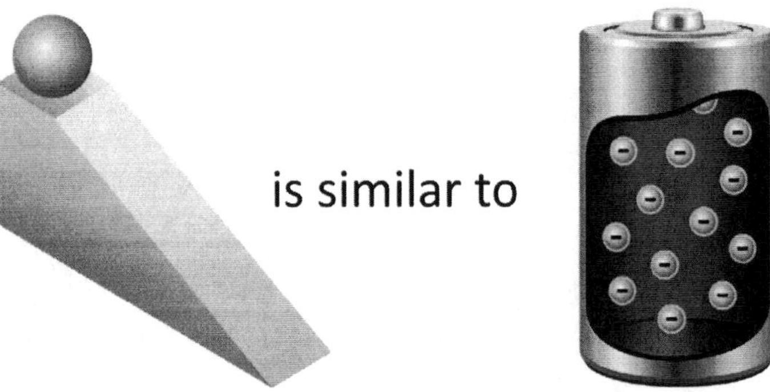

Electromotive Force and Common EMF Devices

A force that maintains a potential difference between two locations in a circuit is known as an **electromotive force (emf).** A device that creates this force is referred to as an **emf device**. The most common emf device is the battery. **Batteries** operate by converting chemical energy stored in the electrolyte, the internal chemical material, into electrical energy. The reaction causes a lack of electrons on the cathode, and when the circuit is connected, they flow from the anode, creating a flow of current. The electrolyte's composition also determines whether the battery is classified as acidic or alkaline, and wet or dry. Another emf device is the **photocell**, also commonly called the solar cell, since most photocells are powered by the sun. These operate by absorbing photons, which cause the electrons to be excited and flow in a current, a process of converting light energy into electrical energy. A third type of emf device is the **generator**. This device converts mechanical energy to electrical energy. A generator may be powered by such diverse sources as gasoline engines, flowing water, or even manually powered cranks. These devices utilize a rotating shaft to spin a coil within a magnetic field, creating a potential difference by induction.

Ohm's Law

If we were to apply the exact same potential difference between the ends of two geometrically similar rods, one made of copper and one made of glass, we would create vastly different currents. This is because these two substances have different **resistances. Ohm's Law** describes the relation between applied voltage and induced current, $V = IR$. This is one of the most important tools of circuit analysis. Resistance, then, can be calculated as $R = \frac{V}{I}$. The SI unit for resistance is the **ohm** (Ω), equal to a volt per ampere. When a component is placed into a circuit to provide a specific resistance, it is known as a **resistor**. For a given potential difference, the greater the resistance is to the current, the smaller the current will be. Electrical resistance is much like friction, resisting flow and dissipating energy.

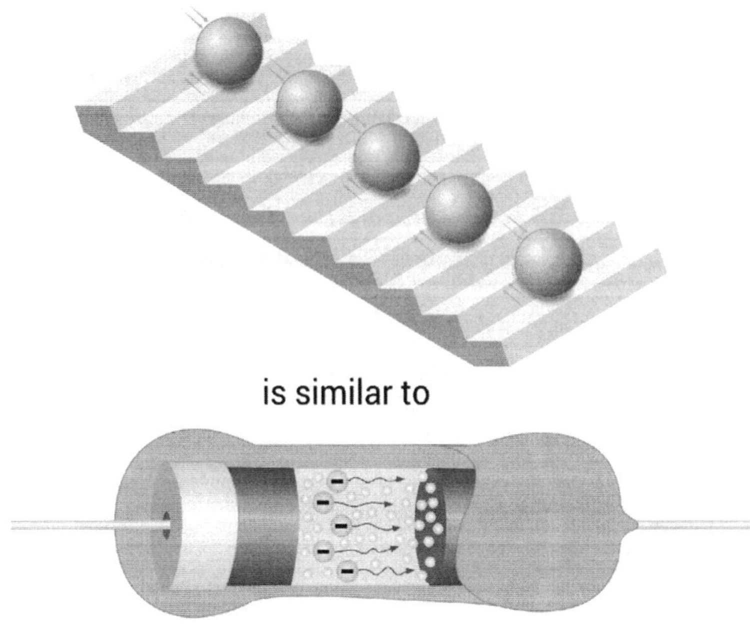

If we wish to look instead at the quality of the material of which the resistor is made, then we must consider resistivity. **Resistivity**, ρ, is a physical property of every material, which, if known, can be used to size a resistor for a specific resistance. Resistance is dictated by both the material and the dimensions of the resistor, given by the relation $R = \frac{\rho L}{A}$, where L is the effective length of the resistor and A is the effective cross-section. Alternatively, an unknown resistivity may be calculated by rearranging the equation as $\rho = \frac{RA}{L}$.

Resistivity will often change with temperature. In these cases, the relevant resistivity may be calculated $\rho = p_{ref}\left(1 + \alpha(T - T_{ref})\right)$, where α is the resistivity proportionality constant and T is the material temperature.

Review Video: Resistance of Electric Currents
Visit mometrix.com/academy and enter code: 668423

Ground

Grounding is the process of neutralizing the charge of an object by removal of excess electrons to or donation of additional electrons by a much larger object (example: the Earth). This ground or large object can seemingly infinitely donate or accept electrons without mathematically significant changes to its net voltage. Examples of grounds include lighting rods and the round component of a three-pronged plug, as used for home appliances. Current does not usually flow through air, but lightning is the visible current that results when charge builds up in clouds; lightning rods provide a safe, low-resistance ground so the high-voltage current is less likely to be destructive. The round component of three-pronged plugs serves as one of the residential applications of this concept.

Energy and Power

Electric circuits operate by **transferring** electrical energy from one location in the circuit to another. Some devices in a circuit can store and release energy while other devices, like resistors, dissipate energy. **Power** is a measure of the rate at which energy is stored, released, transferred, or dissipated. It is measured in watts (W), or joules per second. Power is calculated by $P = VI$. The amount of power being released by a 9-V battery producing a current of 5 A is 45 W. When calculating the amount of power dissipated by a resistor, Ohm's Law can be combined with the power equation to form two other equations for power, $P = I^2R$ and $P = \frac{V^2}{R}$.

When power consumption over long periods of time needs to be measured, it will often be measured in units of kilowatt-hours, which is the amount of energy consumed at a rate of 1 kW over the course of an hour. One kilowatt-hour is equal to 3,600 kJ.

Capacitors and Dielectrics

Capacitors are devices used in circuits to store energy in the form of electric fields. They are most often composed of two oppositely charged parallel plates separated by a medium, generally air. This medium is referred to as the capacitor's **dielectric**.

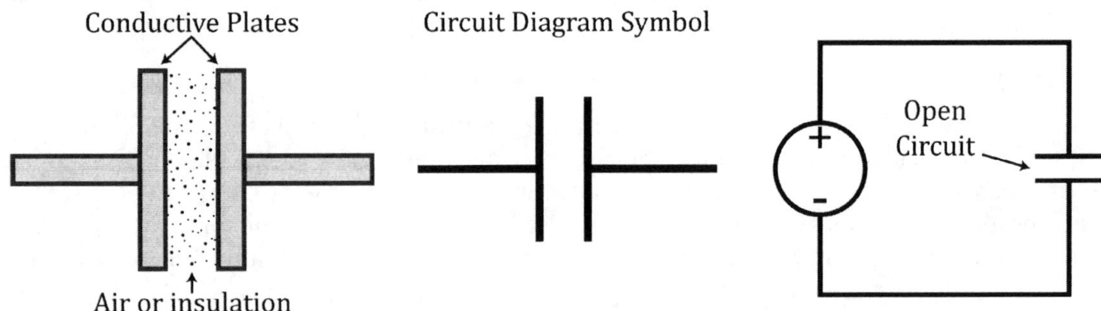

The dielectric material dictates the amount of energy in the electric field and, consequently, the amount of energy that can be stored by the capacitor. The measurable quality of a capacitor is known as its **capacitance**, which is defined as the amount of charge that it can store per volt of potential difference. This is given by the equation $C = \frac{Q}{V}$, with capacitance having units of farads or coulombs per volt. Physically, the capacitance depends on three things: the **area** of the parallel plates, the **separation distance** between them, and the **dielectric** material. For cases in which the separation distance is insignificant compared to the area, the capacitance can be found by the equation $C = \frac{\varepsilon A}{d}$, where ε is the permittivity of the dielectric material. Often, instead of being given the permittivity, we will be given the dielectric constant, κ, which is the ratio of the permittivities of the material and air, $\kappa = \frac{\varepsilon}{\varepsilon_{air}}$. This yields an obvious result of $\kappa_{air} = 1$.

The energy stored in a capacitor can be calculated in three different ways: $E = \frac{CV^2}{2} = \frac{Q^2}{2C} = \frac{VQ}{2}$. Another quantity associated with capacitors is the electric field energy density, η. This energy density is found by $\eta = \frac{\varepsilon E^2}{2}$.

Inductors

When current passes through a wire coil, a magnetic field develops. An **inductor** is an electrical component made of a coil of wire that can store energy and opposes the rate of change of alternating current flowing through it; however, direct current passes through easily. They can be used as filters, sensors, motors, and transformers.

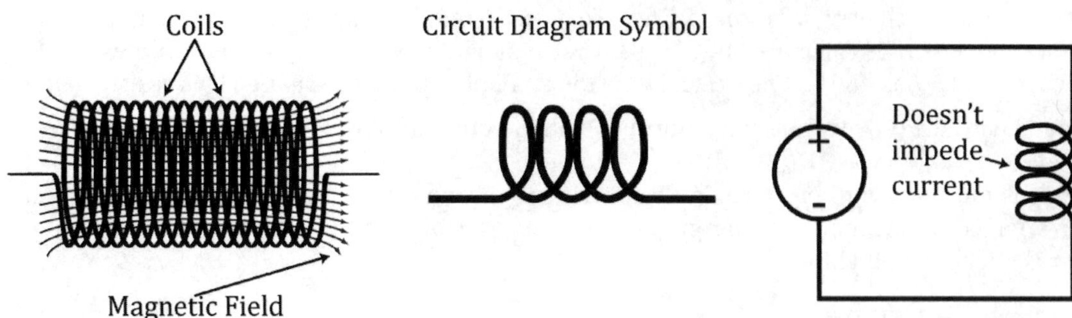

Inductance is the measure of ability of an inductor to resist changes in current. **Faraday's Law of Induction** describes the ways voltage or electromagnetic frequency can be generated by changing the magnetic environment in a coil of wire by moving a magnet within it, changing the external magnetic field of the magnet, or changing the area of the coil.

Capacitors and Inductors in AC Circuits

Capacitors and inductors both oppose immediate acceptance of the flow reversal of alternating current. This opposition is referred to as **impedance** and is similar to resistance, also having units of ohms, but unlike resistance, impedance is a complex value, meaning that it may have an **imaginary component** as well as a **real component**. For ideal capacitors and inductors, impedance is purely imaginary, and for ideal resistors, impedance is purely real. It is only when combining the effects of these devices that the full expression for impedance, Z, is necessary: $Z = R + X_i$, where $i = \sqrt{(-1)}$. X is a quantity known as reactance. For capacitors, $X_c = \frac{1}{\omega C}$, where ω is the angular frequency of the current, and for inductors, $X_L = \omega L$.

Other Electrical Components

Diodes

Diodes are a basic component of circuits, but they can't be described using Ohm's law; they operate as an electrical "valve", only allowing current to pass in one direction. This allows them to rectify alternating current by converting it to direct current, which is preferred or necessary for some applications. A common example is the light-emitting diode (LED) bulb, which emits light when powered more efficiently than regular light bulbs.

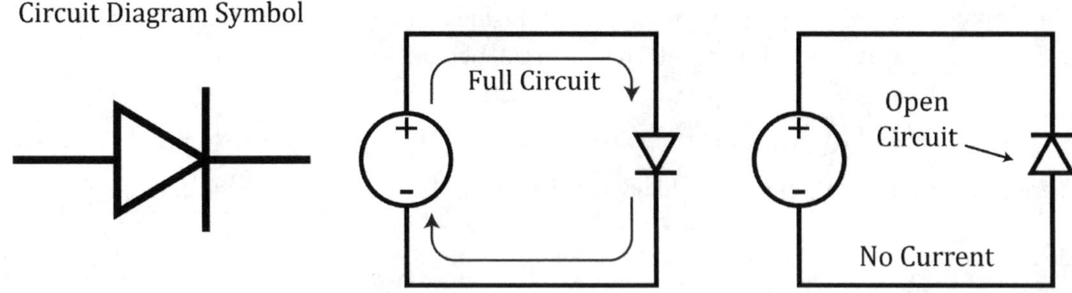

A **p-n junction diode** is formed by fusing a p-type semiconductor and an n-type semiconductor and is considered a solid-state device, because electricity flows through solid material rather than a vacuum tube. The p-region of the junction is positively charged and the n-region is negatively charged. Reverse bias occurs when the diode is connected such that the positive voltage is applied to the n-region; forward bias occurs when the positive voltage is applied to the p-region.

Transistors

Bipolar junction **transistors**, p-n-p or n-p-n, are two p-n junction diodes arranged back-to-back with three electrical leads or terminals: the emitter, the collector, and the base. Transistors are used to boost electrical signals or switch them on or off at high speeds. A large current flows from the emitter to the collector, and a smaller current entering through the base lead can be used to control the larger collector current.

Transformers

Transformers are devices made of two or more coils of wire that use induction to transfer electricity between circuits. A **step-up transformer**'s input (primary) voltage is lower than its output (secondary) voltage; and a **step-down transformer**'s input voltage is higher than its output voltage. This allows for electricity to be to be generated safely at a lower voltage (example: 12 kV), passed through a step-up transformer for transport through power lines at high voltage (example: 400 kV), and passed through step-down transformers for distribution and use (example: 240 V residential use).

Motors and Generators

Motors use electromagnetic induction to convert electrical energy (electricity) to mechanical energy (motion). In a **DC motor**, torque is produced by magnetic force, which results from current passing through coil located in a magnetic field. They have been around for more than 100 years and are simple, inexpensive, and easy to maintain. In **AC (synchronous) motors**, torque is produced the same way as in DC motors, but much higher current is required, and they are inefficient. **Induction (asynchronous) motors** are more common, and they rotate a magnetic field in order to induce alternating current.

Generators use electromagnetic induction to convert mechanical energy to electrical energy. **AC generators** mechanically turn a coil in a magnetic field to produce voltage output and induce alternating current.

Properties of Magnets

Magnets and Magnetism

A **magnet** is a piece of metal, such as iron, steel, or magnetite (lodestone) that can affect another substance within its field of force that has like characteristics. Magnets can either attract or repel other substances.

Magnets have two **poles**: north and south. Like poles repel and opposite poles (pairs of north and south) attract. The magnetic field is a set of invisible lines representing the paths of attraction and repulsion.

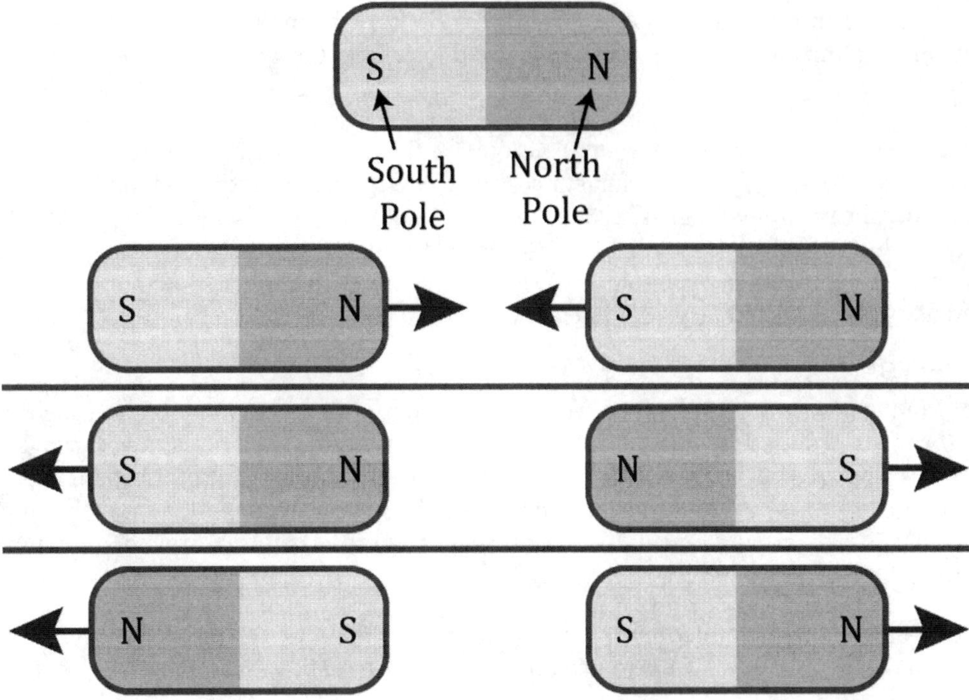

Magnetism can occur naturally, or ferromagnetic materials can be magnetized. Certain matter that is magnetized can retain its magnetic properties indefinitely and become a permanent magnet. Other matter can lose its magnetic properties. For example, an iron nail can be temporarily magnetized by stroking it repeatedly in the same direction using one pole of another magnet. Once magnetized, it can attract or repel other magnetically inclined materials, such as paper clips. Dropping the nail repeatedly will cause it to lose its magnetic properties.

Review Video: Magnets
Visit mometrix.com/academy and enter code: 570803

Magnetic Fields and Atomic Structure

Motion of a charge produces a **magnetic field**. Within an atom, the negatively-charged electrons moving around the nucleus each generate a magnetic field. In most materials, these fields all perfectly oppose and cancel each other, but in certain elements (e.g., iron, cobalt, nickel) the fields are not completely canceled, which makes each atom a tiny magnet. The strength and direction of a magnetic field is known as the magnetic moment.

Pairs of electrons moving in opposite directions cancel each other out, creating a **net magnetic field** of zero. Materials that have an unpaired electron are magnetic. Those with a weak attractive force are referred to as **paramagnetic materials**, while **ferromagnetic materials** have a strong attractive force. A **diamagnetic material** has electrons that are paired, and therefore does not typically have a magnetic moment. There are, however, some diamagnetic materials that have a weak magnetic field.

A magnetic field can be formed not only by a magnetic material, but also by electric current flowing through a wire. When a coiled wire is attached to the two ends of a battery, for example, an **electromagnet** can be formed by inserting a ferromagnetic material such as an iron bar within the coil. When electric current flows through the wire, the bar becomes a magnet. If there is no current, the magnetism is lost. A **magnetic domain** occurs when the magnetic fields of atoms are grouped and aligned. These groups form what can be thought of as miniature magnets within a material. This is what happens when an object like an iron nail is temporarily magnetized. Prior to magnetization, the organization of atoms and their various polarities are somewhat random with respect to where the north and south poles are pointing. After magnetization, a significant percentage of the poles are lined up in one direction, which is what causes the magnetic force exerted by the material.

Types of Waves and Their Characteristics

Transverse and Longitudinal Waves

Transverse waves have oscillations that are **perpendicular** to the direction of motion. A light wave is an example of a transverse wave. A group of light waves traveling in the same direction will be oscillating in several different planes. Light waves are said to be polarized when they are filtered such that only waves oscillating in a particular plane are allowed to pass, with the remainder being absorbed by the filter. If two such polarizing filters are employed successively and aligned to allow different planes of oscillation, they will block all light waves.

Longitudinal waves are waves that oscillate in the **same direction** as their primary motion. Their motion is restricted to a single axis, so they may not be polarized. A sound wave is an example of a longitudinal wave.

Velocity, Amplitude, Wavelength, and Frequency

The **velocity of a wave**, v, is the rate at which it travels in a given medium. It is defined in the same way that velocity of physical objects is defined, a change in position divided by a change in time. A single wave may have a different velocity for every medium in which it travels. Some types of waves, such as light waves, do not require a medium.

Amplitude, A, is one measure of a wave's strength. It is half the verticle distance between the highest and lowest points on the wave, the crest and trough, respectively. The vertical midpoint, halfway between the crest and trough, is sometimes called an equilibrium point, or a node.

The **wavelength**, λ, is the horizontal distance between successive crests or troughs, or the distance between the first and third of three successive nodes.

Frequency, f, is the number of crests or troughs that pass a particular point in a given period of time. It is the inverse of the period, the time required for the wave to cycle from one crest or trough to the next. Frequency is generally measured in hertz, or cycles per second.

Velocity, wavelength, and frequency are not independent quantities. They are related by the expression $v = \lambda f$. Note that amplitude, however, is independent from these quantities.

Intensity

The **intensity** I of a wave is equivalent to the flux through a given area over a period of time. It may also be defined as the energy density of a wave times its velocity. Intensity has units of watts per square meter. This can be seen in light waves as well. The intensity of light decreases as the distance from the light source increases. The inverse square law states that the intensity is inversely proportional to the square of the distance from the source. It is also directly proportional to the power P of the light source. This is shown mathematically by the expression $I = \frac{CP}{r^2}$, where C is the proportionality constant. This may be better understood by imagining the light waves emanating from a source as an expanding sphere. As their distance r from the source increases, the area over which they must divide themselves increases at a rate of $4\pi r^2$.

Standing Waves

A **standing wave** is the result of **interference** between two waves of the same frequency moving in opposite directions. These waves, although in constant motion, have certain points on the path where the amplitude is zero referred to as **nodes**. One example of a standing wave is a plucked guitar string. Since the string is attached at both ends, the fixed ends will be nodes. The primary tone will be that of the fundamental, or first harmonic, shown in the first figure below. It has a wavelength of twice the length of the string, L. The other three pictures below are those of the second through fourth harmonics. The nth harmonic has wavelength and frequency of $\lambda_n = \frac{2L}{n}$ and $f_n = \frac{nv}{2L}$, where v is wave velocity.

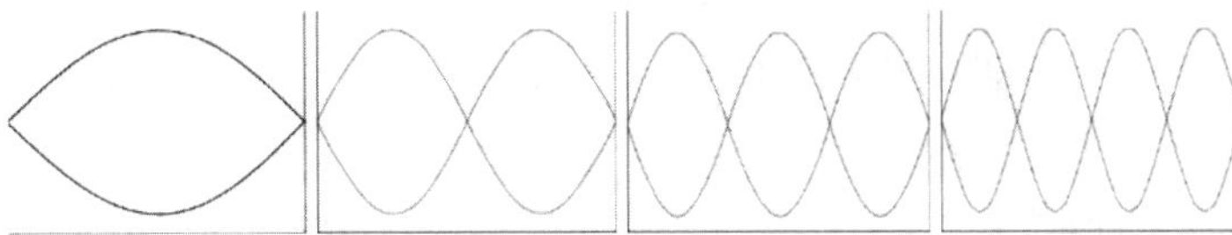

This same phenomenon occurs inside the tubes of wind instruments, though it is much more difficult to visualize. With a tube, however, there will be one or two open ends. Rather than a node, each open end will coincide with an **antinode**: that is, a crest or trough. For waves in a tube with two open ends, the wavelength and frequency calculations are the same as those for the plucked string. For the case with one open end, only the odd harmonics will be seen. The frequency of the nth harmonic becomes $f_n = \frac{nv}{4L}$, where n is odd.

Reflection, Refraction, Interference, and Diffraction of Waves

Reflection, Transmission, and Absorption

When light waves make contact with matter, they are either reflected, transmitted, or absorbed. If the light is **reflected** from the surface of the matter, the **angle** at which it hits the surface will be the same as the angle at which it leaves. If the ray of light is perpendicular to the surface, it will be reflected back in the direction from which it came.

When light is **transmitted** from one medium to another, its direction may be **altered** upon entering the new medium. This is known as **refraction**. The degree to which the light is refracted depends on the index of refraction, n, for each medium.

Light that is neither reflected nor transmitted will be **absorbed** by the surface and **stored as heat** energy. Because there are no ideal surfaces, most light and matter interaction will be a combination of two or even all three of these. Another result of imperfect surfaces is **scattering**, which occurs when waves are reflected in multiple directions. Rayleigh scattering is the specific case of a light wave being scattered by tiny particles that single out particular wavelengths. Dust particles in the atmosphere scatter primarily the blue wavelength of sunlight to give our sky a predominantly blue hue.

Review Video: Reflection, Transmission, and Absorption of Light
Visit mometrix.com/academy and enter code: 109410

Snell's Law

When light is transmitted from one medium to another, its direction may be altered upon entering the new medium. This is known as **refraction**. The degree to which the light is refracted depends on the index of refraction, n, for each medium. The **index of refraction** is a ratio of the speed of light in a vacuum to the speed of light in the medium in question, $n = \frac{c}{v_m}$. Since light can never travel faster than it does in a vacuum, the index of refraction is always greater than one. Snell's law gives the equation for determining the angle of refraction: $n_1 \sin(\theta_1) = n_2 \sin(\theta_2)$, where n is the index of refraction for each medium, and θ is the angle the light makes with the normal vector on each side of the interface between the two media.

We will examine a special case by trying to determine the angle of refraction for light traveling from a medium with $n_1 = 3$ to another medium with $n_2 = 1.5$. The light makes an angle $\theta_1 = 35°$ with the normal. Using Snell's law, we find that $\sin(\theta_2) = 1.15$. Since this is not mathematically possible, we conclude that the light cannot be refracted. This case is known as total internal reflection. When light travels from a more dense medium to a less dense medium, there is a minimum angle of incidence, beyond which all light will be reflected. This critical angle is $\theta_1 = \sin^{-1}\left(\frac{n_2}{n_1}\right)$. Fiber-optic cables make use of this phenomenon to ensure that the signal is fully reflected internally when it veers into the outer walls of the fiber.

Resonance and Natural Frequency

Every physical object has one or more **natural frequencies**, or frequencies at which it will naturally vibrate. The natural frequency is based on the object's dimensions, density, orientation, and other factors. If the object is acted on by a periodic force, it will vibrate at its natural frequency, regardless of the forcing frequency. If the excitation force is operating at the object's natural frequency, the object will experience **resonance**, in which the object receives all of the energy exerted by the excitation force. The amplitude of the vibration will increase rapidly and without bound until either the excitation force changes frequency or the natural frequency of the object is altered.

Diffraction and Dispersion

Diffraction occurs when a wave encounters a physical object. It includes phenomena such as bending, diverging, and other aperture effects. When light emerges from a single small slit, a rippling effect may be observed. The results of Young's double-slit experiment are due to diffraction as the light waves from these slits diverge. Similarly, light emerging from a circular aperture will project concentric light and dark rings due to diffraction. Diffraction grating is an arrangement of material whose reflective properties are intentionally varied at equally spaced intervals. Due to the arrangement, incident light is reflected in specific directions, known as diffraction orders, based on its wavelength.

Dispersion occurs when light consisting of multiple wavelengths enters a medium whose propagation behavior depends on the wavelength of transmitted light. This is what is observed when light passes through a prism, splitting it into its component colors.

Review Video: Diffraction of Light Waves
Visit mometrix.com/academy and enter code: 785494

Young's Double-Slit Experiment

Thomas Young's **double-slit experiment** visually demonstrated the interference between two sets of light waves. It consisted of shining light through two thin, closely spaced parallel slits and onto a screen. The interference between light waves from the two slits caused a pattern of alternately light and dark bands to appear on the screen, due to constructive and destructive interference, respectively. The dimensions of the experimental setup can be used to determine the wavelength of the light being projected onto the screen. This is given by the equation $\lambda = y\frac{d}{x}$, where y is the distance between the centers of two light bands, d is the distance between the slits, and x is the distance from the slits to the screen. Thin-film interference is caused when incident light is reflected both by a partially reflective thin layer on a surface and by the surface itself. This interference may be constructive or destructive.

Wave Superposition and Interference

The principle of **linear superposition** states that two or more waves occupying the same space create an effect equal to the sum of their individual amplitudes at that location. This is known as interference. If the resultant amplitude is larger than either individual amplitude, it is constructive interference. Similarly, if the interference reduces the effect, it is considered destructive.

Some special cases of interference are standing waves and beats, in which two waves having the same and nearly the same frequency, respectively, interfere with one another. Another concept related to interference is phase. If two waves with the same frequency are in phase, then they have perfectly constructive interference. The nodes in each wave will line up, as will the respective crests and troughs. If those same two waves are 180 degrees out of phase, they will experience perfectly destructive interference. The nodes will still line up, but each crest will be aligned with a trough, and vice versa. From this it can be seen that constructive interference results in a larger wave amplitude than destructive interference. If two identical waves are 180 degrees out of phase, the resultant wave will have zero amplitude. This effect is the design impetus for some noise-cancellation technology.

HEAT TRANSFER

HEAT TRANSFER

Heat transfer is the flow of thermal energy, which is measured by temperature. Heat will flow from warmer objects to cooler objects until an **equilibrium** is reached in which both objects are at the same temperature. Because the particles of warmer objects possess a higher kinetic energy than the particles of cooler objects, the particles of the warmer objects are vibrating more quickly and collide more often, transferring energy to the cooler objects in which the particles have less kinetic energy and are moving more slowly. Heat may be transferred by conduction, convection, or radiation. In **conduction**, heat is transferred by direct contact between two objects. In **convection**, heat is transferred by moving currents. In **radiation**, heat is transferred by electromagnetic waves.

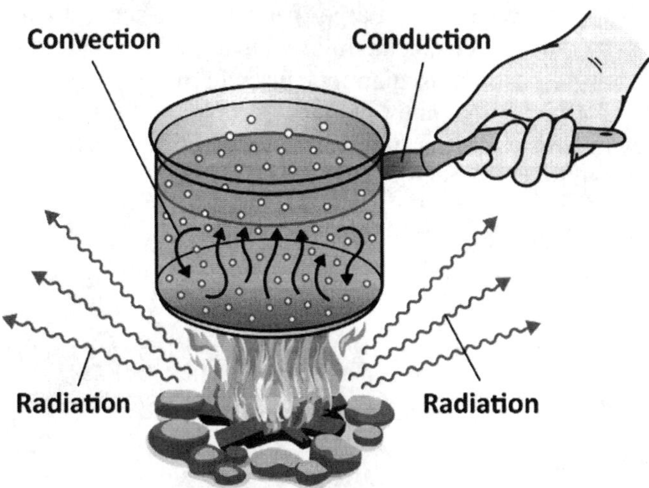

Review Video: Heat Transfer at the Molecular Level
Visit mometrix.com/academy and enter code: 451646

CONVECTION

Heat always flows from a region of higher temperature to a region of lower temperature. If two regions are at the same temperature, there is a thermal equilibrium between them and there will be no net heat transfer between them. Convection is a mode of heat transfer in which a surface in contact with a fluid experiences a heat flow. The heat rate for convection is given as $q = hA\Delta T$, where h is the convection coefficient, and q is the heat transferred per unit of time. The convection coefficient is dependent on a number of factors, including the configuration of the surface and the nature and velocity of the fluid. For complicated configurations, it often has to be determined experimentally.

Convection may be classified as either free or forced. In free convection, when a surface transfers heat to the surrounding air, the heated air becomes less dense and rises, allowing cooler air to descend and come into contact with the surface. Free convection may also be called natural convection. Forced convection in this example would involve forcibly cycling the air: for instance, with a fan. While this does generally require an additional input of work, the convection coefficient is always greater for forced convection.

Conduction

Conduction is a form of heat transfer that requires contact. Since heat is a measure of kinetic energy, most commonly vibration, at the atomic level, it may be transferred from one location to another or one object to another by contact. The rate at which heat is transferred is proportional to the material's thermal conductivity k, cross-sectional area A, and temperature gradient $\frac{\Delta T}{\Delta x}$:

$$q = kA\left(\frac{\Delta T}{\Delta x}\right)$$

If two ends of a rod are each held at a constant temperature, the heat transfer through the rod will be given as $q = k\mathrm{A}\left(\frac{T_H - T_L}{d}\right)$, where d is the length of the rod. The heat will flow from the hot end to the cold end. The thermal conductivity is generally given in units of $\frac{\mathrm{W}}{\mathrm{m\,K}}$. Metals are some of the best conductors, many having a thermal conductivity around 400 $\frac{\mathrm{W}}{\mathrm{m\,K}}$. The thermal conductivity of wood is very small, generally less than 0.5 $\frac{\mathrm{W}}{\mathrm{m\,K}}$. Diamond is extremely thermally conductive and may have a conductivity of over 2,000 $\frac{\mathrm{W}}{\mathrm{m\,K}}$. Although fluids also have thermal conductivity, they will tend to transfer heat primarily through convection.

Radiation

Radiation heat transfer occurs via electromagnetic radiation between two bodies. Unlike conduction and convection, radiation requires no medium in which to take place. Indeed, the heat we receive from the sun is entirely radiation since it must pass through a vacuum to reach us. Every body at a temperature above absolute zero emits heat radiation at a rate of $q = e\sigma AT^4$, where e is the surface emissivity and σ is the Stefan-Boltzmann constant. The net radiation heat-transfer rate for a body is given by $q = e\sigma A(T^4 - T_0^4)$, where T_0 is the temperature of the surroundings. Emissivity, which has a value between 0 and 1, is a measure of how well a surface absorbs and emits radiation. Dark-colored surfaces tend to have high emissivity, while shiny or reflective surfaces have low emissivity. In the radiation heat-rate equation, it is important to remember to use absolute temperature units, since the temperature value is being raised to a power.

Types of Energy

Chemical, Electrical, Electromagnetic, Nuclear, and Thermal Energy

Different types of energy may be associated with systems:

- **Chemical energy** is the energy that is stored in chemical bonds and intermolecular forces.
- **Electrical energy** is the energy associated with the movement of electrons or ions through a material.
- **Electromagnetic energy** is the energy of electromagnetic waves of several frequencies including radio waves, microwaves, infrared light, visible light, ultraviolet light, x-rays, and gamma rays.
- **Nuclear energy** is the binding energy that is stored within an atom's nucleus.
- **Thermal energy** is the total internal kinetic energy of a system due to the random motions of the particles.

Basics of Radioactivity

Radioactivity

Radioisotopes: Also known as radionuclides or radioactive isotopes, radioisotopes are atoms that have an unstable nucleus. This is a nucleus that has excess energy and the potential to undergo radioactive decay, which most often results in the emission of alpha, beta, or gamma radiation. Many radionuclides occur naturally but others have only been produced artificially.

Radioactive decay: This occurs when an unstable atomic nucleus spontaneously loses energy by emitting ionizing particles and radiation. Decay is a form of energy transfer, as the energy lost by the nucleus is given to the particles or radiation emitted. It also results in products that are different from the initial atoms. Before decay there is one type of atom, called the **parent nuclide**. After decay there are one or more different products, called the **daughter nuclide(s)**.

Radioactivity: This refers to particles or energy that are emitted from nuclei as a result of nuclear instability.

Review Video: Radioactivity
Visit mometrix.com/academy and enter code: 537142

Radiation is the term for energy emitted or transmitted as waves or particles. Radiation is classified as either ionizing (able to detach an electron from an atom) or non-ionizing. Nuclear weapons, nuclear reactors, and radioactive substances are all examples of things that involve ionizing radiation. Acoustic radiation and electromagnetic radiation (with wavelength greater than 125 nm) are types of non-ionizing radiation.

Radioactive half-life is the time it takes for half of the radioactive nuclei in a sample to undergo radioactive decay. Radioactive decay rates are usually expressed in terms of half-lives. The different types of radioactivity lead to different decay paths, which transmute the nuclei into other chemical elements. **Decay products** (or daughter nuclides) make radioactive dating possible. **Decay chains** are a series of decays that result in different products. For example, uranium-238 is often found in granite. Its decay chain includes 14 daughter products. It eventually becomes a stable isotope of lead, which is why lead is often found with deposits of uranium ore. Its first half-life is equivalent to the approximate age of the earth, about 4.5 billion years. One of its products is radon, a radioactive gas.

Isotopes that have not been observed to decay are **stable**, or non-radioactive, isotopes. It is not known whether some stable isotopes may have such long decay times that observing decay is not possible. Currently, 80 elements have one or more stable isotopes. There are 256 known stable isotopes in total. Carbon, for example, has three isotopes. Two (carbon-12 and carbon-13) are stable and one (carbon-14) is radioactive.

Ionizing radiation comes in three types: alpha (α), beta (β), and gamma (γ). Alpha particles are positive, beta particles are negative, and gamma rays are neutral. **Alpha particles** are larger than beta particles and can cause severe damage if a source of alpha particles is ingested. Because of their large mass, however, they can be easily stopped. Even paper can protect against this type of radiation. **Beta particles** can be beta-minus or beta-plus. Beta-minus particles contain an energetic electron, while beta-plus particles are emitted by positrons. Beta particles can be stopped with a thin sheet of metal. **Gamma rays** are a type of high energy electromagnetic radiation. Gamma radiation is one of the ways a decaying nucleus emits excess energy after it has emitted either alpha or beta radiation. Gamma rays can cause serious damage when absorbed by living tissue, and it takes a lot of shielding (typically lead) to stop them. Alpha, beta, and gamma radiation can also have positive applications.

Nuclear fission and nuclear fusion are similar in that they occur in the nucleus of an atom, can release great amounts of energy, and result in the formation of different elements (nuclear transmutation). They are different in that **nuclear fission** is the splitting of a nucleus into smaller particles, and **nuclear fusion** is the joining of nuclei to form a heavier nucleus. It requires immense pressures and temperatures, but when fusion occurs, energy can either be absorbed or released, depending on the resultant nucleus. Fusion occurs naturally in stars, and is thought to be the process responsible for the generation of all naturally occurring elements (stellar nucleosynthesis).

Radioactive waste is a waste product that is considered dangerous because of either low levels or high levels of radioactivity. Radioactive waste could include discarded clothing that was used as protection against radiation or decay products of substances used to create electricity through nuclear fission. Small amounts of radioactive material can be ingested as a method of tracing how the body distributes certain elements. Other radioactive materials are used as light sources because they glow when heated. Uncontrolled radiation or even small amounts of radioactive material can cause sickness and cancer in humans. **Gamma radiation** is fast moving radiation that can cause cancer and damage genetic information by crashing into DNA molecules or other cells. Low-level radiation also occurs naturally. When related to everyday occurrences, radiation is measured in millirems per hour (mrem/hr). Humans can be exposed to radiation from stone used to build houses, cosmic rays from space, x-rays and other medical devices, and nuclear energy products.

Health

Factors that Affect Health and Development

Heredity, Environment, and Behavior

Heredity, environment, and behavior contribute to overall health:

- **Hereditary** factors are traits passed within a family that can impact one's health in both negative and positive ways. For example, a family history of heart disease and cancer can negatively impact risk of disease, and a family history of long life can positively affect longevity.
- Environment refers to the **physical environment** (i.e., polluted air and water, unsafe home, etc.) and the social environment (i.e., substance abuse in the home, partner abuse, etc.). Both can impact health.
- **Behavior** refers to **personal** choices that impact health. These behaviors include decisions on tobacco and alcohol use, drinking and driving, and dietary choices.

These elements interact to positively and negatively impact health. For example, a person with a family history of cancer (**hereditary factor**) should avoid excessive sun exposure, eat a high-fiber/low-fat diet, and receive more frequent cancer screenings (**behaviors**) than a person without the hereditary risk. As another example, one who is aware of a family history of heart disease (**hereditary factor**) and therefore chooses to eat a balanced, low-fat, high-protein diet and exercise (**behavior**) can reduce their risk. As a final example, a person with a family history of lung disease (**hereditary factor**) may decide to live in an area with reduced air pollution (**environment**) and choose not to smoke tobacco (**behaviors**).

Effect of Nutrition on Growth and Development

An adequate and **balanced diet** is a key element in proper growth and development. A balance of carbohydrates, proteins, fats, fiber, and minerals is necessary for the growth, development, functioning, and repair of the body. **Dietary deficiencies** of these nutritional building blocks can lead to health problems early in life with some that can extend into adulthood. For example, a diet consisting of whole grains with carbohydrates, fibers, and vitamins, etc. not only provides proper nutrition to growing bodies, but also provides energy allowing for increased exercise tolerance. A quality, balanced diet goes hand-in-hand with **physical activity** to maintain desired body weight and regulate blood sugars. Good dietary habits established early in life, when combined with physical activity, often extend into adulthood to maintain health as one ages.

Effect of Exercise on Growth and Development

Early development of bones and muscles are the foundation of proper growth. **Exercise** helps develop necessary bone mass and density which can reduce the likelihood of osteoporosis and other bone diseases. Proper exercise also reduces the risk of heart disease and diabetes later in life. In addition to **disease prevention**, proper levels of exercise/physical activity increase coordination, balance, posture, and flexibility. It is recommended children aged 6-17 perform 60 minutes of aerobic exercise per day, combined with muscle strengthening exercises (i.e., pushups, rope climbing, etc.) and bone strengthening exercises (i.e., jumping, running, etc.) at least three times per week.

Effect of Sleep on Growth and Development

Proper sleep directly impacts growth, stress hormones, the immune system, respiration, and cardiovascular function. **Lack of sleep** is linked to obesity, heart disease, and increased infections later in life. **Adequate sleep** is linked to improved exercise outcomes because of the increased time given for muscle recovery. In addition, **growth hormones** which are critical to proper growth and development are released during sleep. It is recommended that:

- **Preschool children** (3-5 years) should sleep 10-13 hours during each 24-hour period.
- **Elementary school children** (6-12) should sleep 9-12 hours during the same 24-hour period.
- **Teenagers** (13-18) should sleep 8-10 hours each 24-hour period.
- **Adults** (18-60) should sleep 7 or more hours each 24-hour period.

Key signs that one is receiving **enough sleep** include the ability to sleep through the night with minimal interruption, and awakening rested and alert.

Relationship Between Diet and Exercise

Personal health behaviors often have the greatest impact upon lifetime health, and many of these behaviors begin early in life. One of these key behaviors is eating a **balanced diet,** like one based on the **Healthy Plate Model**. A healthy diet combined with adequate, regular exercise have a cumulative effect on reducing obesity, the leading cause of **morbidity and mortality** (i.e., disease and death) in the U.S. It is recommended that one participate in at least 150 minutes of moderate physical activity or 75 minutes of vigorous activity each week. This should include a balance between **aerobic** exercise (i.e., activities that make a person breath hard and sweat), and **strengthening** exercises (i.e., activities that focus on increasing muscle mass and flexibility).

Common Changes Occurring in Puberty

The onset of **puberty** can occur as early as elementary school (8-12 years of age) or as late as high school (13-15 years of age) and can create a host of **physical and emotional** responses. Often these include changes in **personal hygiene** (i.e., increased showering due to body odor, use of feminine hygiene products in response to the start of the menstrual cycle, etc.) For females, puberty typically consists of beginning of the **menstrual cycle**, changes in body shape, breast tenderness, and hair growth. In males, puberty is characterized by acne, genital growth, hair growth, deepening of the voice, height and muscle growth, erections, and nocturnal emissions. Though the physical changes are the most obvious, the **emotional and social** impacts on personal health can be profound. Youth going through puberty often become more self-conscious, experience dramatic mood swings, develop a sexual interest in others, and experience changes in sleep patterns and energy levels. Given that sexuality is an uncomfortable topic for many parents, it is not uncommon for students to have little to no information about puberty. This creates further anxiety and confusion among many students.

Human Physical Development

Human Physical Development

Physical development is characterized by milestones for physical growth at various ages (i.e., newborn infant, 18-month-old toddler, etc.). Many milestones indicate the child is developing appropriate developmental tasks, including **fine and gross motor skills.**

- **Fine motor skills** refer to small movements in the hand, wrist, and fingers. Examples include grasping eating utensils and writing instruments.
- **Gross motor skills** involve the development of larger muscle groups that allow a developing infant to sit, crawl, and eventually walk. As the child ages, more complex tasks are accomplished through development of physical coordination and balance.

Much of physical growth and development is tied to the development and functioning of the various **body systems** (i.e., skeletal, neuromuscular, nervous system, etc.) used to regulate these behaviors.

Physical Development for Newborns to Six Months of Age

Developmental milestones are characterized by skills at least 75% of children can accomplish by a specific age. In the first **six months** of life a baby should exhibit specific **gross motor** physical developmental markers, such as using large muscle groups (i.e., arms, legs, neck, abdomen, etc.) to kick their feet when on their back, control head bobbing, lift their head when placed on their stomach, hold all of their body weight when supported in a standing position, and push up with the arms from a stomach position. **Fine motor skill**

milestones include being able to hold objects placed in their hands, reaching for and grabbing objects, and drawing these objects closer to the body.

Physical Development for Children 6 to 12 Months of Age

By **9 months of age**, a child should be able to move into a sitting position unassisted and maintain that position without support, switch objects from one hand to the other, use their fingers to move food closer to the mouth, and be able to stop and pivot to pick up an object. A child may begin crawling at this age, though that may not occur until later. A **12-month-old** baby should be able to pull up on another object (i.e., chair) to stand unassisted, walk with support from other objects (i.e., furniture), drink from a cup with adult assistance, be able to point and poke with their fingers, and bang items together. They can also begin to feed themselves in a high chair, but often squeeze and squish food as they learn about texture and eating solid food.

Physical Development for Children 12 to 18 Months of Age

Children at this age are often known as **toddlers.** They advance from infancy towards greater independence in many functions. Children in the **12–18-month** range develop **gross motor** skills include unassisted standing, walking independently, squatting to pick up items, development of a gait for stiff running, crawling up stairs, and seating themselves on low-profile chairs. They often use their bodies to express their needs by shaking/nodding their heads, pointing, and grunting. **Fine motor** skills include pointing to pictures in a book, scribbling with a crayon, stacking items on top of each other, feeding themselves with more precision, and drinking from a cup with some spillage.

Physical Development for Children 18 Months to Three Years of Age

Children in this age group are known as older toddlers and demonstrate increased **gross** and **fine motor** skills. Children in this age group can usually run well, walk up and down stairs with minimal assistance, remove shirts and pants without assistance, stack multiple blocks on top of each other, and feed themselves with less assistance. In addition, it is common for children in this age range to help bathe themselves. They demonstrate improved skill in catching, throwing, and kicking balls. They may also be able to jump and land on a spot, turn pages in a book, ride a tricycle, and unscrew lids. These tasks are directly related to improved hand/eye coordination.

Physical Development for Children 3 to 5 Years of Age

Most children in this age group are very **physically active** and develop increased **independence**. Milestones include walking backwards easily, easily climbing up and down stairs, interchanging their feet without assistance, tumbling, skipping, hopping with balance, and easily catching a thrown ball. They can also stay balanced on one foot with their eyes closed. It is common for these children to show more skill using simple tools and eating utensils. They also use the toilet independently and feed themselves with minimal spills. Children demonstrate a **hand preference** and can hold crayons/writing instruments between the thumb and first two fingers. They can independently cut paper with scissors and can imitate a variety of shapes when drawing (i.e., triangles, squares, and circles, etc.).

Physical Development for Youth 6 to 12 Years of Age

Adolescents in this age group typically demonstrate increased muscle strength and dexterity as hand/eye coordination continues to be refined. The **gross motor** skills of increased large group muscle mass leads to skill development in sports and other physically-demanding activities. The **fine motor** skills of increased small muscle development leads to the ability to complete complex tasks such as typing on a computer, bowling, playing golf, solving multi-piece puzzles, and working closely with other small, detailed tasks. It is during this phase that involvement in team sports increases as physical abilities continuously improve with maturation. Increases in the **sex hormones** estrogen and testosterone during puberty is also responsible for much of the rapid growth of weight and muscle mass, leading to increased strength, endurance, and dexterity.

Physical Development for Adolescents Ages 13 to 18 Years of Age

As **puberty** (a period of rapid physical development) heightens in the teenage years, the **sex hormones** testosterone and estrogen begin to play a more prominent role in physical development. In **males**, the voice deepens, genitals become larger, facial hair may begin to appear, muscle mass increases dramatically, sweat glands become more active, and acne develops. In **females**, acne becomes more common, breasts become larger, body hair increases, body fat increases, and the menstrual cycle begins. Due to the **idiosyncratic** (individualized) nature of the release of testosterone and estrogen, physical developments may come earlier or later for each individual teen. Hormones also often lead to dramatic mood swings. changes in temperament, and differing emotional responses.

Individual Variation in Patterns of Physical Development

Individual variations in developmental patterns are normal. **Physical changes** can be impacted by a variety of factors including environment, heredity, sex, exercise, nutrition, hormones, and familial influence.

The most common delay in physical development in infants is **motor delay** (i.e., rates in sitting, crawling, and walking independently). When there is no identifiable underlying cause for the delay, most children eventually "catch up" with their peer group. **Diseases** such as Down's Syndrome and Autism can result in mild to profound physical development variation. Along with a number of cognitive developmental issues, these diseases can create a spectrum of **developmental delays** that vary from person to person.

Human Cognitive Development

Cognitive development refers to the way children experience the world and make sense of it. The steps of cognitive development include **reasoning**, **intelligence**, **language**, and **memory**.

- **Reasoning** refers to thinking about things in a logical and rational manner.
- **Intelligence** refers to the ability to obtain, interpret, and apply knowledge and skills in common daily interactions.
- **Language** refers to the emergence of words and communication through symbols.
- **Memory** refers to the ability to encode, store, and retrieve information so that once novel concepts/situations become routine and recognizable.

Cognition involves recognizing familiar scenarios and reacting in an appropriate manner based on past behaviors. Age-appropriate cognitive development is characterized by children gaining knowledge through interactions with the world at-large and building upon stored knowledge

Piaget's Stages of Cognitive Development

Jean Piaget's **Theory of Cognitive Development** divides cognition into phases within approximate age ranges.

- **Sensorimotor Intelligence** (approximately birth to 2 years of age) is marked by the infant interacting with the world through movements and sensations, along with looking, reaching, grasping, and sucking.
- The **Preoperational Phase** (approximately 2- 7 years of age) is marked by the use of language and pictures to represent objects. In addition, children in this phase are egocentric and only think of the world from their perspective. Preoperational children struggle **object constancy**, the concept that things exist even though they may not be visually apparent.
- The **Concrete Operational Stage** (approximately 7-11 years of age) is marked by the use of logical thinking and the development of reasoning ability.
- The **Formal Operational Stage** (approximately 12 years of age and older) is marked by the development and use of abstract thought, reasoning through hypothetical situations, and the development and refinement of moral, philosophical, ethical, and moral reasoning.

Individual Variation in Patterns of cognitive Development

Cognitive development refers to how children perceive, think, and respond to different aspects of their world. **Cognitive delays** are conditions in which children lag significantly behind their peer group in cognitive development. Depending on the severity, these delays may be classified as intellectual disabilities or a cognitive/intellectual disorder. With appropriate therapy, many of these cognitive delays can be remediated. **Speech/language delays** are those in which the child is not developing an age-appropriate vocabulary and lags behind their peers in developing speech patterns, such as with pronunciation and grammar. Language and cognitive skills are linked in that stronger language skills often means stronger cognitive skills (i.e., language as a programming tool for cognition). Therefore, early, consistent therapy to remediate delayed language skills is essential to improving eventual cognitive function.

Social/Emotional Development

Social/emotional development refers to a person's ability to experience, regulate, and express emotions, and to communicate and interact with others. It also includes the recognition of and adherence to social norms and mores. These skills develop as the child interacts with others, and lay the foundation for other, more advanced, cognitive skills like literacy and numeracy. Self-awareness, self-management, social awareness, relationship skills, and responsible decision-making are all components of social/emotional learning. **Empathy** is a key milestone in social/emotional development.

Patterns and Processes

Social/emotional development begins at birth when children **bond** with parents and other adults by understanding emotions through facial expressions and voice patterns. Infants are particularly sensitive to social and emotional stimulation. As the child ages, maintaining positive relationships with parents and other nurturing caregivers leads to increased social/emotional development. This development is characterized by:

- **Interactions and relationships with adults**: cooperative activities with caregivers
- **Interactions and relationships with peers**: cooperative activities with same-age children
- **Identity of self in relation to peers**: responding to own name, body parts, etc.
- **Recognition of ability**: understanding they make things happen
- **Expression of emotions**: using facial expressions and vocalization
- **Regulation of emotion**: exhibiting voluntary control over emotion
- **Development of empathy:** recognizing and experiencing the emotional states of others
- **Impulse control**: exhibiting voluntary control over behaviors
- **Social understanding:** relating to others' reactions and life experiences

Individual Variation and Risk Patterns

Age-appropriate social and emotional development is impacted by several factors.

- **Family risk factors** include maternal depression or mental illness in the family, parental substance abuse, parental incarceration, family violence, poverty, and parental unemployment.
- **Environmental factors** include unsafe or unhealthy living conditions, low-quality childcare, and lack of resources in the community to support the child and their family.

These and other factors can result in developmental delays marked by changes in **temperament** (i.e., the way a child experiences and reacts to the world) and **behavior** (i.e., control of behavior in response to specific situations.) Common signs of social/emotional delays are delayed empathy for others and difficulty making social/emotional connections with peers.

Prenatal Care

A Healthy Embryo and Fetus

Practices that promote **development** of a healthy embryo and fetus include early and consistent **prenatal care**, avoiding tobacco or alcohol use, taking vitamin supplements such as folic acid, following a healthy diet, exercising with the guidance of a physician, avoiding exposure to toxic substances, limiting caffeine intake, and maintaining a healthy weight.

Avoiding **maternal disease** can also improve fetal outcomes. Pregnant women should maintain all vaccinations and avoid contact with people carrying infectious diseases (i.e., measles, mumps, etc.) **Fetal development** can be measured through ultrasound and amniocentesis procedures.

Poor fetal development can lead to a lifetime of **physical, mental, and emotional challenges**. It is therefore important to detect pregnancy at its earliest stages in order to begin a medically supervised **prenatal program,** which can reduce the risk to the developing fetus.

Physical, Mental, and Emotional Health Problems as a Result of Restricted Prenatal Growth

Poor prenatal growth is often referred to as **Intrauterine Growth Restriction** (IUG) and can impact the developing infant in a variety of ways. The key marker for IUG is when the developing fetus is not as big as expected given the **stage of pregnancy** (i.e., "gestational age"). The typical cause of IUG is a lack of proper nutrients to the developing fetus. **Low birth weight** (less than 5.5 pounds) is often tied to **prematurity** (birth before the 37th week of pregnancy) which can lead to trouble eating, difficulty gaining weight, and difficulty fighting infections. **Neurodevelopmental challenges** for IUG infants can include reduced responsiveness, delayed bonding with the mother, and lack of engagement with adult faces. Some IUG infants show increased cognitive and developmental delays later in life. The vast majority of IUG cases can be prevented by improved maternal diet, increased maternal sleep, and avoidance of alcohol and other drugs.

Personal Health Plans

Developing and Following a Personal Health Plan

Maintaining adequate nutrition, exercise, and an appropriate body weight are key parts of improving overall wellness. A **personal health plan** (PHP) is a personalized roadmap to achieve health and wellness goals. To develop a personal health plan, one should complete a **personal health inventory** to evaluate their overall health and find their starting point. For example, an individual can assess whether they are at a healthy weight by calculating their **body mass index** (BMI) and their **waist circumference**. Regularly reflecting on and assessing nutritional habits is a crucial component of developing a personal health plan. Keeping a food and beverage diary that tracks daily food and beverage consumption can help one identify their current intake patterns. An activity log can track physical activity throughout the day. Pedometers, fitness watches, or smartphone fitness applications can also be used to track activity levels. **SMART goals** (specific, measurable, attainable, realistic, and time-bound) can help an individual create actionable steps to achieve their health and wellness goals based on their personal health inventory. Finally, **new habits** can be reinforced and unhealthy behaviors replaced through regular **reflection and positive self-talk**.

Overview of Disease and Illness

Communicable Diseases

Diseases are divided into two types: communicable and noncommunicable. **Communicable diseases** are illnesses caused by infectious agents transmitted from an infected person or animal to other people or animals. They are caused by **pathogens** like bacteria, viruses, and fungi. Transmission can be **direct contact**, which occurs through contact with an infected person via blood or bodily fluids, touching (e.g. staphylococcus), kissing or sexual contact (e.g. gonorrhea, HIV), or contact with fecal or oral secretions (e.g. hepatitis A), or **indirect contact**, which occurs without human-to-human contact but through contact with contaminated surfaces or objects (e.g. Norwalk virus), food (e.g. salmonella, E. coli), water (e.g. cholera), insect bites (e.g. malaria, yellow fever, and plague), or air (e.g. tuberculosis, measles). Most communicable diseases are acute—which means the disease and symptoms appear over a short period of time—and occur seasonally.

NONCOMMUNICABLE DISEASES

Noncommunicable diseases (NCDs) are diseases that are not contagious or transmittable to other people. They contribute to far more deaths worldwide than communicable diseases—approximately 70% of all deaths. Unlike communicable diseases, NCDs are long-lasting, slow progressing **chronic illnesses** that are often a result of poor lifestyle choices (e.g., type 2 diabetes, emphysema, and cardiovascular disease) or genetic mutation (e.g., cystic fibrosis, sickle cell anemia, lupus, and cancer). They are not the result of a pathogen; rather, they result from multiple risk factors that are further divided into modifiable risk factors, environmental risk factors, and non-modifiable risk factors. **Modifiable risk factors** are personal behavior or lifestyle choices that can be reduced or controlled by intervention like diet, physical activity, smoking, and alcohol or drug use. **Environmental risk factors** result from the physical environment and contribute to health outcomes like pollution, radiation, noise, and climate change. **Non-modifiable risk factors** cannot be reduced or changed like age, gender, family history, and race.

Review Video: Gene Mutation
Visit mometrix.com/academy and enter code: 955485

VIRUSES AND HOW THEY ARE TRANSMITTED

A **virus** is a microscopic entity that uses living organisms like animals, plants, or bacteria to replicate. Viruses **reproduce** by attaching themselves to their host's cells and reprogramming them to make new copies of the virus, effectively spreading as they go. The most common virus **transmission** methods are through droplets generated from coughing and sneezing, fecal contamination of food or water, contact with skin rashes or lesions, contact with contaminated surfaces, and bites from an infected animal vector. Once infected, the virus can cause damage to one or multiple body systems.

BACTERIA AND HOW THEY ARE TRANSMITTED

Bacteria are single-cell microorganisms that can live inside and outside of the body. They are larger and more complex than viruses and can **reproduce** on their own. Although most bacteria are harmless and even beneficial, those that cause illness in humans are called pathogenic bacteria. **Pathogenic bacteria** are infectious but not always contagious, which means that they cause sickness when they enter the body but are not always spread from person to person. Bacteria are **classified** by their gram-negative or gram-positive status—the ability to produce an **endotoxin** that causes tissue damage or death— and their need for oxygen, genus, and shape (spheres, rods, and spirals). Similar to viruses, bacteria can be **transmitted** through coughing and sneezing (e.g., pertussis), contact with infected people (e.g., impetigo, chlamydia), animals or insects (e.g., Lyme disease), contact with contaminated surfaces (e.g., cellulitis), and food or water (e.g., salmonella).

FUNGI AND HOW THEY ARE TRANSMITTED

A **fungus** is an organism that feeds on **decaying organic matter**. Although fungi are often found outdoors in soil and plants, they can also be found on and inside of the body. Fungi **reproduces** through the spread of microscopic spores. When an individual inhales or touches fungal spores, they may contract a lung and skin infection. Fungal infections are rarely transmitted from one person to another. There are two types of fungal infections: opportunistic and primary.

- **Opportunistic fungal infections** spread aggressively, but typically only impact individuals with weak immune systems.
- **Primary fungal infections** can develop in individuals with functioning immune systems, but are slow to develop. and usually emerge once a person has inhaled fungal spores.

Fungal infections can be local or systemic.

- **Local** infections only affect one area of the body. For example, a local fungal infection may only show up on the nail that was infected–not any other part of the body. Common locales for local infections also include the skin, genitals, and mouth.

- **Systemic** infections can affect many areas of the body or multiple organs at one time.

Parasites and How They Are Transmitted

Parasites are organisms that live in or on their host and feed on their host while causing it harm. There are three main types of parasites that cause disease in humans: protozoa, helminths, and ectoparasites.

- **Protozoa** are rapidly reproducing microscopic single-celled organisms that invade the body's tissues to obtain nourishment. They are spread through a variety of ways, but are most often transmitted by contact with human feces (e.g., giardia, cryptosporidium).
- **Helminths** (worms) are macroscopic multi-celled organisms that live in and outside of the body and cause infection. They are transmitted by eggs spread through fecal contamination and are most common in tropical and subtropical regions. Examples of parasitic diseases include Guinea worm disease, Chagas disease, and trichomoniasis.
- **Ectoparasites** are large multi-celled organisms that live on or feed off of skin (e.g., ticks, mosquitos, fleas, lice). They are vectors of infectious viral and bacterial diseases like Lyme disease, typhus, encephalitis, malaria, etc.

Communicable Diseases

Risk Factors for Contracting Communicable Diseases

An individual's **risk** of contracting a **communicable disease** varies based on their overall health, vaccination status, personal hygiene, number of people they live and work with, socioeconomic status, and condition of their housing. Those who frequently come into contact with wildlife and other potential vectors (e.g., mosquitos) are at **higher risk** of contracting a communicable disease. Certain populations are at **higher risk** of becoming severely ill (i.e., hospitalization, ventilator, death) once they are infected. This includes individuals who are 65+ years old or under 2 years old, individuals experiencing health and social inequities (e.g., racial and ethnic minorities, low socioeconomic status), and people with medical conditions like cancer, chronic lung disease, diabetes, and heart conditions. Individuals living in communities with poor water and sanitation, insufficient public health surveillance, poor waste management, and inadequate government regulations regarding food and water safety are at higher risk of contracting a communicable disease. Communities with high exposure to climate-related catastrophes and few health professionals or medications are more susceptible to disease outbreak and inadequate disease management.

Methods for Treating Different Types of Communicable Diseases

- **Bacterial diseases** are treated with **antibiotics**, which kill bacteria or slow their development to allow for the immune system to respond.
- **Viral infections** can be prevented with **vaccines**. When given a vaccine which contains an agent (e.g., weakened forms of the microbe, proteins) that resembles the virus, the body mounts an **immune response** and produces **antibodies** that will terminate the active form of the virus in the future. If already infected with a virus, **antiviral medications** can be used to treat the infections. They do not destroy the pathogen, but inhibit further development of the virus.
- **Fungal infections** are treated with **antifungal medications** that attack the fungal cell membrane to either kill fungal cells or prevent them from reproducing.
- **Parasites** are treated with **antiparasitic drugs** that kill the parasite.

Preventative Measures Reducing Spread of Communicable Disease

The most effective way to **limit the spread** of many communicable diseases is through **quarantine** and **physical distancing**. **Vaccines** also prevent many infectious diseases. Keeping up to date on vaccinations, getting vaccinated before traveling, and getting the recommended vaccinations during childhood are important for reducing transmission. **Practicing good hygiene** (i.e., hand washing after using the bathroom, before and after eating, treating a wound, touching others' hands or an animal, or coughing/sneezing) can prevent the spread of bacteria, viruses, and parasites. **Safe food handling and preparation**, such as washing utensils and surfaces during food preparation, washing fruits and vegetables before eating, and cooking/storing food at proper temperatures, are also effective strategies for preventing the spread of many foodborne illnesses. **Cleaning surfaces** regularly with soap and water, especially the bathroom and kitchen, can reduce the spread of many diseases that are transmitted indirectly. Finally, **reducing stress** can prevent disease transmission as chronic stress can suppress the immune system and make a person more susceptible to infection.

Non-Communicable Diseases

Asthma

Asthma is a noncommunicable disease. While the exact **cause** of asthma is unknown, genetics, allergies, respiratory infections, and contact with allergens or environmental irritants are likely to contribute to the development of asthma. Those with asthma experience **recurring symptoms** like chest pain, chest tightness, and shortness of breath. Individuals with an **asthmatic parent** are more likely to develop asthma. A **childhood respiratory infection and allergies** can increase the risk of asthma. Working or living in **environments** in which one comes into contact with **irritants** like industrial or wood dust, chemical fumes, and solvents can lead to the development of asthma. Smoking, secondhand smoke, and air pollution can also lead to asthma. Additional **social factors** like poverty and poor access to health care can exacerbate asthma symptoms.

Diabetes

Diabetes is a noncommunicable disease that affects how the body uses a sugar called glucose. There are three types of diabetes: type 1 diabetes, type 2 diabetes, and gestational diabetes.

- **Type 1 diabetes** is caused by an autoimmune reaction which causes the body to destroy cells in the pancreas that make **insulin**. The pancreas is unable to produce insulin, and glucose is unable to move out of the blood and into the cells which results in **very high blood sugar levels**. **Risk factors** for type 1 diabetes include family history of diabetes and exposure to a viral infection that triggers the autoimmune disease.
- In **type 2 diabetes**, cells become **resistant** to insulin and sugar builds up in the blood. **Risk factors** for type 2 diabetes are being overweight or obese, family history of diabetes, physical inactivity, race and ethnicity, older age, gestational diabetes, abnormal cholesterol, and high blood pressure.
- **Gestational diabetes** is a pregnancy-induced condition in which the pancreas is unable to produce enough extra insulin to overcome the hormone-induced insulin resistance. This must be a new-onset condition that presents in the second or third trimester of pregnancy to be diagnosed.

Cancer

Cancer is a noncommunicable disease that occurs when there are **DNA mutations** within a cell that inhibits growth and replication. The new cancerous cells crowd out non-cancerous cells and damage body tissues. The most common **causes** and **risk factors** are related to environmental exposure, radiation exposure, infections, age, family history, and various lifestyle factors. Exposure to carcinogens, asbestos, and benzene in the home and workplace environment can lead to cancer. As people age, they are exposed to more **carcinogens** and the body loses its ability to find and destroy cancerous cells, which can lead to the development of cancer. **Radiation** from the sun or medical treatment, viral infections that affect the DNA or suppress the immune system (e.g., HIV, human papillomavirus), and **genetic susceptibility** can also cause cancer. **Major lifestyle risk factors** like tobacco use, alcohol use, physical inactivity, obesity, diets high in processed and red meats, sun exposure, and unsafe sex can increase the risk of cancer.

Heart Disease

Heart disease refers to numerous conditions that affect heart health (e.g., coronary artery disease, arrhythmias, congenital heart defects, heart valve disease, heart infection). The causes of heart disease depend on what kind of heart disease a person has. For example, **coronary artery disease** is caused by a buildup of plaque in arteries. **Heart infection**—also called endocarditis—is caused by bacteria, viruses, and parasites. **Cardiomyopathy**—the thickening of heart muscle—can be caused by damage from heart attacks, drugs, or genetics. **Risk factors** for heart disease include old age, sex, family history, smoking, poor diet, high blood pressure and cholesterol, diabetes, obesity and overweight status, physical inactivity, stress, and poor dental health.

Methods for Preventing Noncommunicable Diseases

Primary disease prevention seeks to prevent disease or injury before it occurs through restricting exposure, modifying existing risk factors, and increasing resistance to disease before exposure. Examples of noncommunicable primary disease prevention include adjusting poor eating habits, tobacco cessation, exercising and weight loss, using legislation to ban substances associated with a disease or health condition (e.g., asbestos, lead paint), and implementing legislation to mandate safe and healthy practices (e.g., workplace health standards, restrictions on air pollution emissions, tobacco regulations).

Methods for Early Detection of Noncommunicable Diseases

Secondary prevention aims to reduce the impact of existing disease or injury through early disease detection and treatment and developing strategies to prevent reinjury or reoccurrence of disease. A common secondary prevention method is the implementation of regular **cancer screening tests** to detect early-stage disease (e.g., regular mammograms to detect breast cancer, colonoscopies to detect colorectal cancer, and pap smears to check for cervical cancer). Another method is **genetic counseling** to assess the likelihood of a person or their relative developing a genetic condition or disease and help them explore treatment options. Genetic counseling can be conducted before and during pregnancy to address concerns that can affect infant health (i.e., birth defects, genetic conditions, abnormal test results, maternal infections). It can also be used to address concerns about genetic disorders in childhood like abnormal newborn screening results, birth defects, or intellectual and developmental disabilities. Genetic counseling is often used in adulthood to assess symptoms of a condition or family history of a hereditary condition (e.g., hereditary breast and ovarian cancer, Huntington's disease, sickle cell disease, muscular dystrophy).

Immune Responses

Immune System Response to an Antigen

Many different organs, cells, and proteins make up the **immune system**. The immune system defends the body from **pathogens** and removes harmful substances from the body. When a foreign substance—called an **antigen**—enters the body and attaches to immune system cells, the immune system begins mounting a response. Examples of **common antigens** include bacteria, fungi, viruses, allergens, and pollutants. Once eliminated, the immune system stores information about the pathogen and how to eliminate it to maintain protection for future encounters.

Fevers

A **fever** is a temporary rise in body temperature above the **normal range**, which is within 1 degree above or below 98.6 degrees Fahrenheit. Although commonly thought to be bad for the body, a fever is an example of one of the many **helpful defense mechanisms** that the body employs to respond to disease. When the immune system identifies an antigen, it sends biochemical substances called **pyrogens** to a part of the brain called the **hypothalamus**. In response, the hypothalamus commands the body to produce and retain more heat. An elevated body temperature creates an **inhospitable environment** for pathogens like viruses to replicate or temperature-sensitive bacteria to survive. Fevers also speed up and strengthen immune cell response by altering their surface proteins to improve their ability to reach the infection site. Since fevers help the immune system fight disease, it is not always necessary to suppress them. However, if a fever exceeds the safe temperature threshold or is accompanied by unusual behavior, medical attention should be sought.

Antibody Formation

Antibody formation is an example of a process that the immune system uses to respond to disease. **Antibodies**—also referred to as immunoglobulins—are proteins that the immune system manufactures when it identifies an antigen in the body. Antibodies are created by **white blood cells** called B lymphocytes or **B cells**. B cells bind to antigens and produce antibodies that are circulated throughout the body. The released antibodies ambush all antigens like the one that prompted the body to mount an immune response. The body continues to produce antibodies until it eliminates all detected antigens, but antibodies may remain in the body for up to several months.

The white blood cells of the immune system include the following:

WBC	Type	% of WBCs	Causes of Increase	Causes of Decrease
Basophils (black or purple)	Granulocyte	1%	Asthma, chronic myelocytic leukemia, Crohn's disease, dermatitis, estrogen, hemolytic anemia, Hodgkin's disease, hypothyroidism, polycythemia vera, and viruses	Allergies, corticosteroids, hyperthyroidism, pregnancy, and stress.
Eosinophils (orange-red, double-lobed nucleus)	Granulocyte	1-3%	Allergy, asthma, or parasitic infestation	Cushing's disease or glucocorticoids use
Lymphocytes (dark, large nucleus surrounded by thin cytoplasm rim)	Agranulocyte	15-40%	Antigens or chronic irritation	AIDS
Monocytes (lavender)	Agranulocyte	2-8%	Myeloproliferative process, like an inflammatory response or chronic myelomonocytic leukemia (CMML)	Hairy cell leukemia
Neutrophils (pink cytoplasm, dark nucleus)	Granulocyte	50-70%	Burns, kidney failure, heart attack, cancer, hemolytic anemia	Leukemia and abscess

Autoimmune Responses and the Immune System

Occasionally, the body mistakes its own cells as antigens during an immune response and attacks healthy, harmless cells in the body. This process is called an **autoimmune response**. When an individual has an **autoimmune disease**, their immune system is unable to distinguish between foreign cells and healthy cells and releases proteins called autoantibodies to attack parts of the body (e.g., the pancreas attacked in type 1 diabetes) or the whole body (e.g., lupus). The exact cause of autoimmune responses is unknown, but scientists theorize that family history, sex, diet, prior infections, and exposure to chemicals may contribute to developing an autoimmune disease. Examples of **common autoimmune diseases** are rheumatoid arthritis, psoriasis, ulcerative colitis, and psoriatic arthritis.

Review Video: Immune System
Visit mometrix.com/academy and enter code: 622899

Factors Influencing Disease Risk

Environmental Factors Affecting Health and Disease

Environmental factors have a significant impact on health and disease. In fact, 70-90% of chronic disease risk can be attributed to **environmental factors** like air, water, and soil pollution, exposure to harmful chemicals, metals, and nanomaterials, climate change and natural disasters, and ultraviolet radiation. Exposure can **disrupt bodily function** and cause health problems like respiratory diseases, cardiovascular diseases, and certain types of cancer. The health impacts of and exposure to the previously mentioned environmental factors can be exacerbated by an individual's **socioeconomic** and **biological characteristics**. This places people with low incomes, those living or working in heavily polluted or poorly environmentally-regulated areas, children, pregnant women, and immunocompromised individuals at increased risk of poor health and/or disease due to environmental factors.

Influence of Laws and Policies on Disease Prevention

Health laws and policies are important preventative measures to address health-related issues.

- **Health policies** are plans, decisions, and actions that achieve health goals. They can be implemented at the local, state, and national level or codified within a clinical environment.
- **Health laws** are legally binding regulations that can lead to consequences if not followed. Local, state, and national legislation are necessary for eliciting changes that reduce disease.

When legislation to address factors contributing to disease is enacted at each level, it can have a **profound impact** on disease prevention. For example, local smoke-free restaurant and business ordinances, state-wide tobacco tax increases, and a national program like the National Tobacco Control Program influence the ease with which individuals can acquire tobacco and consume it and limits broad exposure to harmful pollutants that tobacco contains.

Stages of Prevention and Intervention Along the Continuum of Care

The continuum of care includes all aspects of care that influence outcomes. The primary components are prevention, intervention, and recovery/maintenance during which the person is monitored for compliance.

Prevention	Intervention
May be aimed universally at the entire population, at selected groups, or at-risk individuals, and it usually involves long-term goals. Primary: Aims to prevent disease occurrence and may include educational campaigns (no smoking, use seatbelts), vaccinations. Secondary: Aims to identify and reduce impact (screening mammograms, BP checks). Tertiary: Aims to prevent/delay disease progression (support programs).	Usually aimed at specific groups or individuals and often involves specific treatments (such as surgery, chemotherapy, medications) to alleviate a problem or disorder. Goals may be long term, or they may be time limited with the aim to resolve the problem as quickly as possible.

Health Hazards and Factors that Contribute to Safety Concerns

Biological and Chemical Hazards to Health and Safety

Biological hazards (e.g., viruses, bacteria) and chemical hazards (e.g., non-biological substances like acids) can be found in the home, school, and community. **Biological hazards** like bacteria and viruses are **transmitted** through contaminated objects, droplets, or contact and can spread disease among the residents of a school, home, or community. Poor or dated building infrastructure may contribute to **exposure** to various molds or materials like asbestos and lead, which can cause moderate to severe **allergic reactions** and the development or exacerbation of **asthma**. The risk of exposure to biological hazards increases in communities with high population density and high contact potential with wild animals or insects (e.g., ticks, bats, rodents). **Chemical hazards** may arise from use of **cleaning supplies**, **chemical agents** used in science labs, **mishandling of medications**, **lead exposure** from contaminated pipes or paint, **rodent control supplies** (e.g., super warfarin), or **carbon monoxide** leaks. If ingested or inhaled, chemical hazards can cause serious health problems.

Environmental and Equipment Hazards to Health and Safety

Environmental hazards refer to natural conditions that cause adverse health effects and can impact the health and safety of a home, school, or community. These include **extreme weather** events like earthquakes, hurricanes, heat waves, freezes, blizzards, and floods. Environmental hazards can also result from **pollution** (e.g., oil spills, sewage leaks). **Equipment hazards** result from misuse or malfunctioning of a machine or device. Fires, electric shock, or drowning are unfortunate outcomes of equipment hazards. Fires may be caused by heat generating appliances (e.g., ovens, dryers) or electronics used for an extended amount of time, cooking mishaps (e.g., oil fires), faulty electrical wires, unattended candles or fires, and smoking. **Improper use of pool equipment or poor supervision** at pools and in bathtubs can lead to drownings, especially among those who are unable to swim or those who are incapacitated in or near water.

Avoiding and Preventing Unintentional Injuries

Driving an Automobile

Unintentional injuries refer to those that are not deliberate and are typically accidental. They can often be prevented by adherence to safety rules and precautions.

- **Following all traffic laws** pertaining to automobile safety can prevent unintentional injuries.
- **Staying alert and cautious** while driving can ensure that other drivers, bicyclists, or pedestrians who may not be attentive remain safe and free from injury.
- Proper and consistent **use of seatbelts and car seats** can protect all passengers from car accident-related injuries or fatalities.
- Practicing safe driving measures (e.g., maintaining a **safe speed**, keeping a **safe distance between cars**) and abstaining from erratic driving behavior can prevent unintentional injuries while driving an automobile. Additionally, avoiding alcohol or substance use before/while driving can prevent injury or death.
- **Limiting distracted driving**—any activity that limits the driver's focus and attention (e.g., texting or talking on the phone, eating or drinking, using a music player or navigation device)—can help keep all passengers safe from unintentional injury.

Bicycling

Similar to drivers, it is imperative that all bicyclists **adhere to local traffic laws** to prevent unintentional injury or fatality. Individuals should:

- Use hand signals, hand bells, or electronic devices to **signal their intention** to turn, pass, or brake.
- **Bike in a predictable manner** (e.g., no weaving or abrupt stops) and avoid substance use while biking.
- Since bicycles are often harder for automobile drivers to see, it is important that riders **exercise caution** on shared roads and **stay alert**. To stay alert, bicyclists should refrain from using cellular or navigation devices and listening to music. Staying alert while riding can also prevent injury that may occur from objects in the road, stationary objects, potholes, uneven surfaces, etc., that can cause a rider to lose control of their bicycle.
- **Using traffic lanes designated for bicycles** or sidewalks can prevent injury that may occur from sharing lanes with motor vehicles.
- **Wear protective gear** (e.g., helmets, protective glasses) and reflective gear to protect themselves and maximize their visibility while on the road.
- Bicycles should be appropriate for the rider's height and weight, and should receive regular maintenance to prevent unintentional injury.

Swimming

Prior to entering the water, it is important that one **learns how to swim** and/or properly wears a well-fitted **floatation device**. Individuals should:

- **Swim in supervised areas** patrolled by a lifeguard, and swim with or around another person whenever possible.
- **Obey all rules and safety regulations** and always make sure that it is safe to swim. Regardless of the location, swimmers should prepare to exit the water if thunder or lightning occurs. When at a natural body of water, swimmers should avoid swimming in fast-moving water or choppy waves. They should also practice caution when walking in the water as there may be submerged objects.
- **Enter water feet first** will protect swimmers from head or neck injuries associated with diving.

- **Refrain from alcohol or substance use** and swimming after eating to prevent unintentional drowning.
- Learn **resuscitation techniques** to prevent unintentional injury or death from drowning.

Fatigue

Fatigue refers to drowsiness or tiredness; it can significantly impair one's motor functioning, concentration, and psychological health. It can result from reduced sleep duration and quality, strenuous or stressful work conditions, and long or demanding work hours. Those who are fatigued **may experience** mood changes, communication and processing delays, irritability, reduced concentration, diminished memory, and impaired decision making. Each of these traits can **increase the risk of injury** as a person may exhibit irrational behavior and make poor or uncharacteristic choices. Fatigue is associated with **greater accident and injury rates** in fields like health care, emergency response, military, education, and manufacturing. Fatigue is also associated with **higher risk** of motor vehicle accidents, job error, poor productivity, and illness.

Use of Alcohol and Drugs

An individual who engages in **risk-taking behavior** makes potentially harmful or hazardous choices that can endanger themselves or others. Examples of risk-taking behavior include substance use, dangerous or impaired driving, or unsafe sex. Those who make risky behaviors often make **impulsive**, thrill-seeking choices that place them at **high risk** of sustaining injury or injuring others. Use of alcohol and drugs **impairs** a person's **decision-making abilities** and **psychomotor functioning**, which can cause an individual to engage in risk-taking behavior and have poor control over their physical motions. Research shows that as alcohol consumption increases, an individual's function and inhibitions decrease while their tendency toward risky behavior increases. For example, an inebriated person may lack the ability to recognize how impaired they are and become increasingly confident that they can return home safely. While driving, they will likely experience delayed reaction time, poor concentration, and an inclination to drive erratically. Their behaviors increase their risk of self-injury or injury to others.

Personal Responsibility in Avoiding Risky Behaviors

Personal Responsibility in Preventing Injury

Although **unintentional injuries** may occur due to others' poor or risky choices, individuals should act responsibly to minimize and prevent the risk of injury. One should always try to understand and respect the **safety rules and expectations** of their school, workplace, etc. In doing so, they can **maximize safety** for all and prevent potential hazards that result from non-adherence. Each person has a right to **opt out** of unsafe or risky behavior, and it is the responsibility of all to ensure that everyone involved has the ability to **communicate their concerns or refusal**. Maintaining effective communication with others can ensure that all feel confident and comfortable to speak up when they feel their safety is threatened. An individual should **utilize refusal skills** to establish boundaries or guidelines for what they will or will not do in order to maintain safety. **Peer pressure** is a powerful and coercive force, yet individuals should **always reject participation** in unsafe behavior—despite its real or perceived consequences—and maintain common sense to avoid situations that could result in unintentional injury. **Awareness of personal risk** is important for preventing injury. This involves being alert and aware of one's surroundings and being mindful of situations that may put others at risk.

Risky behaviors	Harmful behaviors
Critical—Public or private criticism, purposefully humiliating the person.	Aggressive/Abusive—Any type of hitting, shoving, pushing, or physical violence.
Irresponsible/Immature—Constant problems (social, financial) and discord.	Controlling/Possessive—Attempts to control another person's life and to isolate the person from others.
Noncommunicative—Difficulty expressing feelings and being open with others.	Volatility—Unpredictable bouts of anger and rage.
Self-centered—thinks only in terms of personal needs.	Manipulative—Pressuring someone to do something or using guilt or threats to get one's way.

SAFE AND UNSAFE BEHAVIORS

The **leading cause of death** for individuals under the age of 44 in the United States is unintentional injury. **Infants** are extremely curious but have little to no concept of danger and lack motor functioning. Thus, they are at higher risk of choking or falling and need constant supervision from a caregiver. From ages 4-9, **young children** begin to learn about the concept of danger from others or past experience and improve their self-control, yet they still **lack a mature ability** to recognize dangerous situations and employ strategies to prevent injury. They also begin to **gain confidence**, which makes them more likely to engage in risky behavior without the knowledge of their own limitations. During **adolescence**, teenagers begin to exhibit risk-taking behavior due to **peer pressure** and **lack a clear sense of mortality**. They are at far more **risk for injury**, and their behavior can have **lasting implications** for their adult health (e.g., adolescent substance abuse and increased risk of cancer, addiction, or permanent injury).

RECOGNIZING AND AVOIDING POTENTIALLY DANGEROUS SITUATIONS

Maintaining personal safety requires that one recognize and avoid **potentially dangerous situations**. A potentially dangerous situation is any event or experience in which a hazardous or harmful outcome is possible, and the individual(s) involved feel uncomfortable or unsafe. A person can protect themselves from potentially dangerous situations by **avoiding areas where criminal activity often occurs** or those who engage in criminal activity. **Maintaining situational awareness**—the awareness of the physical and social happenings around a person—at all times can ensure that an individual **recognizes possible threats to safety** before they happen and takes actions to prevent them. Avoiding situations or crowds in which others begin to act aggressively or erratically can prevent a potentially dangerous situation from occurring.

PREVENTING AND RESPONDING TO DATING VIOLENCE

Dating violence refers to physical, emotional, or sexual abuse within a romantic relationship. An important first step to preventing dating violence is to **understand the characteristics of healthy/unhealthy relationships** and the early warning signs of intimate partner violence (e.g., excessive communication, jealous or controlling behavior, gaslighting). **Learning and practicing skills** to communicate effectively, manage emotions, and refusing behaviors that make one feel uncomfortable can reduce the risk of dating violence. Developing **positive relationship-building skills** and **self-respect** during childhood and adolescence can prevent the victimization or perpetration of dating violence. **Assertiveness and boundary setting** are effective strategies to respond to dating violence. Both encourage an individual to **advocate** for their needs and **respectfully decline** any unwanted activity or behavior. Educating communities on **bystander intervention** can help individuals identify intimate partner violence and empower others to take action to support those affected.

PREVENTING AND RESPONDING TO GANG VIOLENCE

Gang violence refers to any violence—physical, emotional, sexual—committed by members of a gang (e.g., assault, rape, intimidation). Violence may be directed **internally** (e.g., initiation) or toward other gangs and innocent bystanders. The most effective way for a person to prevent gang violence is to **remove oneself from the threat of violence**. If possible, one should **avoid locations** where gangs have a strong presence and **avoid association** with gang members. They should **avoid engaging in criminal activity and exhibiting aggressive behavior** when in public or online that may incite violence. Establishing healthy relationships with others who are not affiliated with a gang or do not commit criminal acts can prevent an individual's exposure to gang violence. If inadvertently exposed to gang violence, one should respond by **leaving the situation** or **alerting emergency responders** or law enforcement. At the organizational and community-level, **early and collaborative intervention** by community groups, school staff, law enforcement, parents, and local government is necessary to address risk factors for gang initiation and violence.

Preventing and Responding to Hate Crimes

A **hate crime** is any violent act or criminal offense directed at a person because of their identity (e.g., race, ethnicity, religious affiliation, gender, sexuality, or disability). **Federal legislation** like the Matthew Shepard and James Byrd, Jr. Hate Crimes Prevention Act and the Emmett Till Anti-Lynching Act dictate that individuals who commit hate crimes may be liable to prosecution. Additionally, **state and local legislation** exists as a preventative and protective measure against hate crimes. If an individual experiences or witnesses a hate crime, it is important to **alert emergency responders and law enforcement** immediately. Victims and witnesses should respond with **caution** as offenders may exhibit violent behavior; however, it is important for bystanders to **de-escalate** the situation and support victims of hate crimes. **Education on hate crimes and its impacts** and **critical-thinking skills** are important preventative measures to address hate crimes. Those who are able to identify hate crimes and assess discriminatory speech, material, or actions may be better able to prevent and respond to it. Improving **media literacy** is also an important strategy for preventing hate crimes since they increasingly happen online.

Emergency Response Planning

Home Safety Plans

A **home safety plan** is a set of procedures and preventative measures intended to lower the risk of danger at home. Home safety plans can **minimize injuries or fatalities** and **provide a sense of security** among those who live in the home. When revisited and practiced routinely, home safety plans can **alleviate the confusion or chaos** that often accompanies breaches to home safety. A home safety plan typically includes an emergency contact list and a detailed checklist of what to do if an emergency happens. An **emergency contact list** may include numbers of caregivers, family members or friends, neighbors, and emergency responders; it is intended to improve communication in case of a safety concern. Home safety plans may also include a **detailed checklist** of what to do in response to an emergency or safety concern (e.g., fire, tornados, burglary, unknown visitors, injury, power outage). Home safety plans can also include a **list of important information** or tools located in the home. This list can include information regarding when to replace the batteries in smoke/carbon monoxide detectors, how to check home alarm systems, and the location of fire extinguishers and stockpiles of emergency supplies (e.g., extra food, water, first aid kit).

Emergency Response Plans

Emergency response plans include a set of procedures for unexpected threats to health and safety. It is similar to a home safety plan but includes **detailed information regarding emergency response and recovery**. Emergency response plans typically include an emergency contact list, a list of external emergency resources, responsibilities for each household member, evacuation plans, and important information about where to locate emergency supplies. An **emergency contact list** can include contact information for caregivers or other family members, friends, neighbors, and emergency response teams. It can also include a **list of resources** an individual can access in case of an emergency (e.g., natural disaster shelters). Emergency response plans can also include a **list of instructions** for responding to various emergencies (e.g., fires, sudden weather event, intruder). Emergency plans may also include **designated roles and responsibilities** necessary to ensure the safety of all (e.g., who will contact first responders, administer first aid, acquire the emergency supplies). Emergency response plans often include **evacuation plans**—diagrams of the safest and quickest exit routes—and emergency supplies information. The location and contents of emergency supplies (first aid kit, food, water, clothing) is often listed in an emergency response plan.

CPR

Cardiopulmonary Resuscitation (CPR) is a first aid procedure that is performed when an individual's heart stops beating—also known as **cardiac arrest**. CPR consists of continuous chest compressions that restore blood flow to the rest of the body. If administered correctly, a person's **chance of survival is 2-3 times higher** when they receive CPR. There are three CPR methods: 1) "hands only" CPR, 2) conventional CPR, and 3) automated external defibrillator (AED).

- **Hands only CPR** is the recommended method for the general public. Those performing hands only CPR should push hard and quickly on the person's chest—usually at a rate of 100-120 compressions per minute. The depth of the compression varies depending on the depth of the victim's chest.
- The **conventional method** consists of chest compressions and mouth-to-mouth breaths. Those administering conventional CPR administer 30 chest compressions and 2 rescue breaths, which push air and oxygen into the lungs.
- Portable machines called **AEDs** administer an electric shock to the heart to force it to beat again.

Use of conventional CPR and AEDs is only recommended for health care professionals and trained individuals.

Conscious Choking

A **conscious choking** person may be awake or reactive yet is unable to breathe, cough, or speak due to a foreign object lodged in their throat. Their skin and lips may begin to flush and turn blue. It is vital that first aid be administered immediately, since an **obstructed airway** can prevent oxygen from reaching the brain. If a person is no longer able to speak, cry, laugh, or cough forcefully, the rescuer can use the "five-and-five" method or the Heimlich maneuver to clear their airway. The **"five-and-five" method** consists of 5 back blows between the victim's shoulder blades with the palm of the hand and 5 abdominal thrusts. Back blows and abdominal thrusts should be repeated until the object is dislodged. The **Heimlich maneuver** is performed by a person standing behind the victim, administering quick abdominal thrusts with a closed fist, until the object is dislodged. Those providing **choking first aid to infants** should administer thrusts with two fingers on the breastbone in a seated position and with the infant resting on their forearm. If at any point the victim becomes **unconscious**, the rescuer should begin performing CPR immediately until help arrives.

Health Care Agencies, Programs, and Services

Primary Health Care

Primary health care describes the delivery of health services by entities that manage patients with acute and chronic conditions below a level of specialized care. **Primary care providers** (e.g., family doctors or general physicians, gynecologists, nurse practitioners) are often referred to as "gatekeepers" because they are often the first physician that individuals encounter in the health care system. Primary care providers may be the first physician visited when a person develops symptoms, and they are responsible for diagnosis, treatment, and management of illness or injury. They hold an **extensive breadth of medical knowledge** and frequently deliver patient education. Primary care providers may also **coordinate services** and **identify patient resources**. For example, if a patient requires specialized care or community resources (e.g., food assistance, reduced cost medication), primary care providers may refer them to a specialist or a community organization who provides wraparound services. Primary health care can be delivered at physician's offices or through community agencies (e.g., community health centers and free clinics, health departments).

Preventative Health Care

Preventative health care seeks to prevent disease before it develops and reduce the impact of an illness once it occurs. It is typically divided into primary, secondary, and tertiary prevention.

- **Primary preventative health care** seeks to prevent the onset of illness or injury through legislation, education, and immunization. Lawmakers and government agencies may **implement legislation to reduce risk of injury** (e.g., tobacco tax, seat belt mandate) or **ban hazardous substances and working conditions** (e.g., lead ban). It can also include **interventions** like immunization and mandatory vaccination, health education/promotion, and nutritional fortification.
- **Secondary preventative health care** reduces the impact of disease or injury on an individual by identifying and administering disease treatment as soon as it is detected (e.g., cancer screening, preventative drug therapy).
- **Tertiary preventative health care** describes programs and services that **minimize complications or disability** that result from **chronic disease** and improve quality of life. Examples include diabetes management programs and cardiac rehabilitation. Secondary and tertiary preventative health care may take place within a medical setting but are **frequently implemented in the community** (e.g., community diabetes management classes, free STD testing at health departments, community cancer screenings).

Emergency Health Care

Emergency health care describes the rapid treatment of acute illness or injury and the prevention of serious complications from disease or death. Emergency health care is typically administered at emergency health care centers (e.g., hospitals, urgent care centers) by trained and licensed physicians. They are responsible for providing **immediate care** to individuals with **serious, sometimes fatal, conditions**. Emergency mental health care programs exist outside of the medical health care system, too. Many community organizations provide mental health first aid to intervene when an individual experiences a mental health crisis to reduce the risk of resultant harm. Federal and state entities and non-profit organizations (e.g., FEMA, DHHS, American Red Cross, Salvation Army) may deploy emergency health practitioners and services when a community experiences a natural disaster or infectious disease outbreak. Their role is often to provide emergency aid and mitigate the damage caused by the emergency.

Community and National Health Care Needs and Goals

Community health care needs and goals are typically outlined in annual **community health assessments** (CHA). CHAs are often developed by state, local, or tribal government bodies to examine key health indicators within the communities they serve. Quantitative and qualitative data on risk factors, social determinants of health, and morbidity and mortality rates are collected and analyzed to identify health needs. Findings are paired with information on community assets, key partners, and essential services to establish health goals. National health care needs and goals are commonly identified through the US Department of Health and Human Services' (USDHHS) **Healthy People program**. Similar to local community health assessments, goals and objectives are identified through data collection, but needs and goals are redefined every ten years instead of annually. Both engage stakeholders and assets within their reach to address identified health needs.

Health-Related Social, Political, and Economic Issues

According the Bureau of Labor Statistics, medical costs have increased an average 2.1% annually over the past ten years. Over the same time period, the cost of commercial health insurance premiums rose 5.8% annually. **Rising medical costs** impact an individual's access to health care. Individuals may delay or avoid seeking care due to cost, which can have devastating impacts on their long-term health and wellbeing. **Uninsured and underinsured families**—who are often more likely to simultaneously experience poverty and poor health—are disproportionately affected by rising health care costs. Those who lack sufficient health care coverage are more likely to accumulate medical debt, delay or forgo treatment, utilize emergency health care instead of primary care services, or ration medical supplies and medication. Thus, health care delivery often transitions from primary care and prevention to late-stage treatment of injury and disease or emergency health care treatment.

Factors Influencing Cost, Availability, Accessibility, and Use of Health Care

Individual Factors

Social determinants of health (SDOH) describe the social and economic conditions that influence health outcomes (e.g., economic and housing stability, education, food access, the physical environment, social norms and attitudes, and culture). Those with low **socioeconomic status**—one's economic position compared to others—have diminished access to health care and worse health outcomes than their peers. **Low financial security** may influence their decision to seek care and the type of care they receive. A person's **cultural background** and **health attitudes** can impact their perception of health, as well as their accessibility to and use of health care. The cultural background of one delivering care can impact **how well health information is communicated** and the **patient's treatment adherence**. One's cultural background can influence their **understanding** of the causes, severity, and treatment regimen of illness or injury and may also influence their health attitudes. For example, historically marginalized groups who have experienced medical maltreatment and discrimination are often more reluctant to use health care services. **Age** can influence health care use. For example, youth may lack access to care since their caregivers are responsible for their medical decisions. Older adults may use health care more frequently, yet their mobility can impact access.

Societal Factors

Economic trends can impact an individual's access to health care. During **economic recessions** or downturns, employers may revise coverage and benefits to reduce costs. Economic downturns are also associated with **increased unemployment**. One's loss of financial security and employee-sponsored insurance can influence their **accessibility to services and their willingness to seek care**. Widescale unemployment and changes in coverage associated with economic downturn can impact health care delivery. Inability to pay for services can lead hospitals to avoid clinical and technological upgrades or avoid hiring new health care professionals, which can diminish the health care quality. Medicare and Medicaid are federal insurance programs for seniors and disabled individuals and those with low income, respectively. Government policies like **Medicaid expansion** increase coverage and affordability of health care. **Price regulation** (e.g., price caps on prescription drugs and hospital service costs) enforced through government policy can reduce health care costs, improve affordability and accessibility of care, and increase use of health care services.

Health Care Systems and Services

Hospitals

The **primary role of hospitals** is to provide patients with medical care and support. Hospitals provide **emergency or trauma health care to patrons and host a range of specialized services** (e.g., radiology, oncology, psychiatry, gynecology). At a hospital, an individual may also receive such medical treatments and procedures as a surgery, an MRI or X-ray, radiation, or dialysis, among many others. Depending on the level of care needed, patients may stay overnight or for longer durations. In addition to providing patient care, **some hospitals provide training to medical residents and conduct health research.** Hospital staff often assist patients in identifying community resources to maintain good health after discharge. Hospitals are quickly becoming hubs for wraparound services and primary care. Individuals experiencing rising inaccessibility to health care (e.g., uninsured or underinsured, low proximity to primary care providers, reduced capacity of practitioners to provide timely care) are increasingly relying on hospitals and emergency medicine practitioners for primary care.

Clinics

Clinics are health care facilities that provide routine outpatient care. At clinics, **primary care providers conduct health checkups, provide immunizations, and treat mild to moderate illnesses.** Clinics rarely allow overnight stays, and appointments with medical practitioners can be booked ahead of time. Patients may also have the option of walk-in appointments; however, clinic hours are usually limited to the standard workday. Whereas hospitals generally provide disease treatment, at clinics, physicians may provide preventative health care services (e.g., blood pressure measurements, cancer screenings, vaccinations, or health counseling). **Clinics may also refer to specialized care locations at which medical practitioners**

perform outpatient care. For example, a psychiatrist may conduct diagnostic tests, psychiatric treatment, and therapy at an outpatient psychiatry clinic. Some clinics—often referred to as free clinics—provide reduced or free services to the public. These clinics are managed by volunteer physicians, nurses, and administrative staff to serve community members experiencing financial hardship.

Health Care Professionals

Health care professionals are individuals who are licensed to perform medical services. Examples include primary care doctors, physician's assistants, dieticians, pharmacists, registered nurses, and specialty care physicians (e.g., pediatricians, obstetricians, dermatologists). The role of health care professionals varies by specialty, yet overall, they are responsible for **disease prevention, diagnosis, and treatment**. Health care professionals engage in **disease prevention** through health education and health counseling. For example, a primary care doctor whose patient was recently diagnosed with high cholesterol may explain the risks associated with the condition and assess modifiable lifestyle factors. The physician may also assist with drafting a personalized plan of action to prevent the onset of diseases like heart disease and stroke. Health care professionals, like dieticians and pharmacists, also provide disease treatment. For example, a dietician may provide medical nutrition therapy for a person with Crohn's disease to manage nutrient loss, while a pharmacist may supply immunosuppressants to control symptoms.

Benefits of Regular Medical Checkups

Medical checkups are annual comprehensive exams performed by a primary care provider. A medical checkup is a valuable preventative and diagnostic tool that can **delay the onset of disease, treat diseases early, and improve or prolong well-being**. It typically consists of a physical exam, a review of one's medical history, blood tests, and health counseling. Regular medical checkups can **reduce one's risk of developing an illness and can lead to the early detection of a disease**. Identifying a disease early can increase the success of treatment and reduce the risk of health complications. Patients with **existing health conditions** can be **monitored regularly** to track disease progression and adjust treatment strategies if needed. **Long-term benefits** of regular medical checkups include a longer lifespan, lower health care costs, and greater health knowledge.

Benefits of Regular Dental Checkups

Dental checkups are biannual exams conducted by a dentist and a dental hygienist. They typically consist of a **dental cleaning** (e.g., plaque and tartar removal, polishing) and an **oral exam**. Fluoride application and dental X-rays may also take place to prevent tooth decay, identify cavities or potential cavities, and monitor tooth migration. The dentist will also evaluate a patient's head and neck, soft tissue (e.g., tongue, cheeks), and gums to **identify possible oral health problems or diseases** like mouth cancer. Regular dental checkups can **prevent the onset or exacerbation of tooth decay or gum disease**. Both, if left untreated, can result in costly medical bills, infection, and tooth loss. The dentist can provide information on how to maintain proper dental hygiene and refer patients to other providers (e.g., orthodontists, prosthodontists, oral surgeons) for specialized care.

Advertising and Marketing in Healthcare

Advertising and Marketing Techniques Used

Testimonials and statistics are commonly used health product and health service promotion techniques. **Health testimonials** utilize an endorsement by a celebrity or a trusted individual (e.g., health care professional, current user of the health product or service) to convince the consumer to purchase the product or service. **Statistics** are used to appeal to a person's logic. People often trust numbers and research—even if the statistics are inaccurate or unclear. Advertisements may also utilize a **personal appeal** that is intended to evoke an **emotional response** (e.g., joy, sadness, fear) that inspires the consumer to select or purchase the health product or service. For example, many hospitals and health care-related organizations released advertisements that urged the public to get vaccinated during the COVID-19 pandemic. They used strong emotional imagery, such as footage of vaccinated individuals reuniting with their family members after a substantial social distancing period and/or speeches from nurses and doctors describing their experiences, to

evoke empathy. Most advertisements will use a combination of multiple techniques to enhance the consumer response and increase the likelihood that the public will purchase a product or service.

Determining If Advertising Claims Are Accurate

A consumer can **determine the accuracy** of an advertised service or product by **evaluating the legitimacy of its claims**. A review of a product's claims can be conducted through conversations with trusted peers or through independent research (e.g., examining consumer reviews, exploring available research about the product's or service's efficacy, reviewing similar products). For instance, a person seeking a personal trainer to lose weight might consult some fitness-related groups or his or her provider, friends, or family to determine the best service for his or her health goals or to identify possible trainers. **Feedback from trusted sources** can help someone determine if a trainer's advertised services are accurate and trustworthy. **Consumer reviews** often provide a spectrum of responses about various aspects of a health product, service, or provider. Consumers can assess desirable or undesirable attributes of a health care product by reviewing similar health products and doing so may **reveal inconsistent advertising claims** if a product promises results not achievable by similar products. Reviewing research about different health care goods can help **identify trustworthy products** and **reveal the legitimacy of claims**.

Determining If Advertising Claims Are Misleading or Deceptive

Consumers should **avoid products or services that claim to be a cure-all or quick fix**. Very few products can be used to cure a wide range of diseases or treat illnesses in a short period of time. Products or services that list a suspiciously long list of ailments they treat or promise unreasonable desirable outcomes (e.g., "lose 15 pounds in two weeks," "eliminate type 2 diabetes") are likely **misleading or deceptive**. Testimonials can also be used to make misleading or deceptive claims about a health product or service since they are difficult to dispute. **Endorsements from credible health care professionals** are often more trustworthy than a testimonial from a single product user. A person should **pay attention to websites or advertisements with sensational titles and quotes that have been shortened** (e.g., "this product helped me lose weight ...") as these may be used to garner attention and misrepresent the truth. **Reviewing the statistics cited and/or any graphs or diagrams** depicted in the health product advertisement can help a person determine whether a claim is accurate or misleading.

Evaluating Health-Related Products

Evaluating and Selecting Health-Related Products, Treatments, and Services

Criteria

When evaluating and selecting health-related products, treatments, and services, one should consider the following criteria: cost, insurance coverage, quality, and legitimacy.

- **Cost and insurance coverage** can often be prohibitive factors when selecting a health product, treatment, or service. **A review of one's budget and the funds necessary** to sustain the intended health outcomes can help one determine if the product or service is a good choice. **A review of one's health insurance coverage** is also necessary to determine affordability as some products, treatments, or services may not be covered.
- The **quality of a product** can reveal its **effectiveness** for treating a health condition or attaining a health goal. An **evaluation of the product's formula** can imply adequate quality. Oftentimes, **approval from a federal regulatory agency** like the Food and Drug Administration (FDA) is a good indicator of a product's reliability.
- The **legitimacy of a product** can be determined by **identifying the credentials and authority** of the seller and product. A **credible seller** is licensed by a legitimate certifying entity, such as the National Association of Boards of Pharmacy (NABP). Reviews or ratings from other consumer protection organizations, like the Better Business Bureau (BBB), can reveal the legitimacy of health-related businesses.

Skills

The following skills are important to use when **evaluating and selecting health-related products, treatments, and services**: health literacy, financial literacy, and negotiation skills.

- The Centers for Disease Control and Prevention describes **health literacy** as one's ability to locate, comprehend, and utilize health information and services. Health literacy is helpful for those evaluating and selecting health-related products, treatments, and services because those with high health literacy are **better at locating credible information and discerning between accurate and misleading claims**. They are also often **better at making informed health decisions** and **advocating for their health needs and goals**.
- Since cost is a significant factor when selecting a health product or service, high **financial literacy** can help an **individual budget** for his or her health care and **identify cost-effective solutions** to health care problems.
- **Negotiation skills** are important for **confidently communicating** one's health goals, one's service or product preferences, and one's health needs. Health literacy and a strong understanding of one's personal health status or needs can be beneficial when practicing negotiation skills in health care.

Criteria for Evaluating and Selecting Health Providers

Criteria for successfully evaluating and selecting health care providers includes staff medical knowledge, insurance coverage, cultural competence, and treatment management recommendations. These criteria can be used to **identify whether the physician is the right fit**; however, one should consider other important attributes prior to visiting. The extent of a **provider's medical knowledge** can be ascertained through a **review of his or her credentials** (e.g., licensing, certifications) and through **reviews by current or former patients**. There are many provider review websites that use overall patient satisfaction to rank or score health care professionals. These websites also often include information on licensing and certification, insurance coverage, and languages spoken. **Insurance coverage** can significantly lower the cost of health services. To determine whether a provider is in-network, one should consult his or her insurer directly. A provider's **cultural competence** can influence the type of care provided and impact the patient's overall experience. A physician who practices culturally competent care treats more than physical health; he or she meets the social, cultural, and linguistic needs of his or her patients.

Interpretation of Signs and Symbols

Sign/Symbol	Interpretation
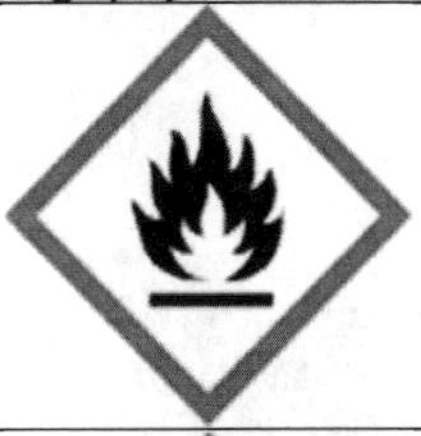	Flame: Includes flammable materials and gases and those that are self-heating or self-reactive.
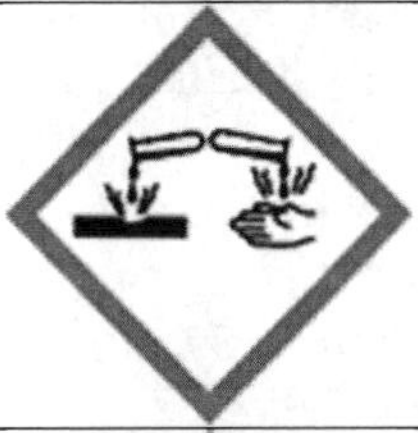	Corrosion: Includes substances that can cause skin burns, metal corrosion, and eye damage.
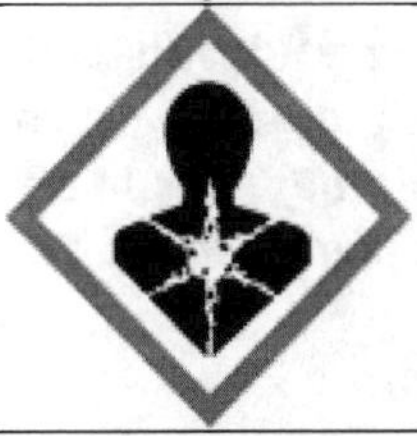	Health hazard: Includes carcinogens, toxic substances, and respiratory irritants.

Sign/Symbol	Interpretation
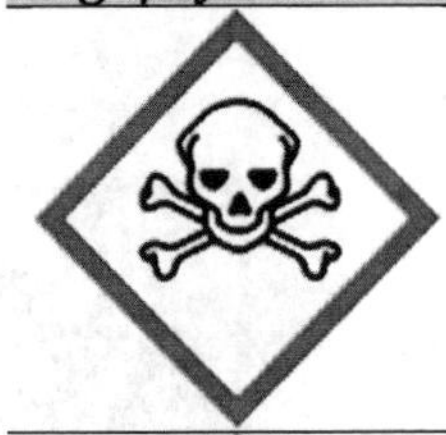	Poison: Includes materials, gases, or substances that are extremely toxic and may result in death or severe illness.
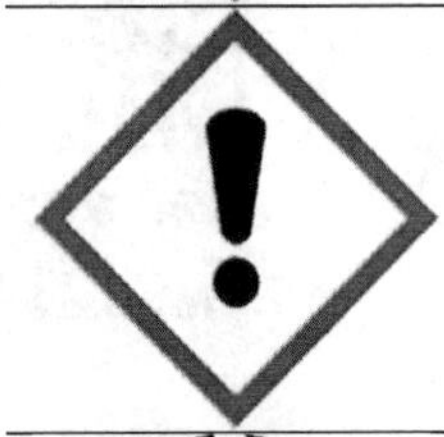	Irritant: Includes material, gases, or substances that are irritants to skin, eyes, and/or respiratory tract, acutely toxic, or have a narcotic effect.
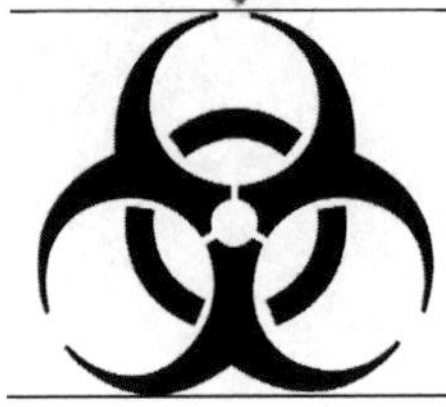	Biohazard: Includes biological substances, such as body fluids, that pose a threat to humans. Appears on sharps containers that hold contaminated needles.

PAX Practice Test #1

Want to take this practice test in an online interactive format?
Check out the bonus page, which includes interactive practice questions and much more: **mometrix.com/bonus948/pax**

Reading Comprehension

Refer to the following for questions 1 - 6:

The Bermuda Triangle

The area known as the Bermuda Triangle has become such a part of popular culture that it can be difficult to separate fact from fiction. The interest first began when five Navy planes vanished in 1945, officially resulting from "causes or reasons unknown." The explanations about other accidents in the Triangle range from the scientific to the supernatural. Researchers have never been able to find anything truly mysterious about what happens in the Bermuda Triangle, if there even is a Bermuda Triangle. What is more, one of the biggest challenges in considering the phenomenon is deciding how much area actually represents the Bermuda Triangle. Most consider the Triangle to stretch from Miami out to Puerto Rico and to include the island of Bermuda. Others expand the area to include all of the Caribbean islands and to extend eastward as far as the Azores, which are closer to Europe than they are to North America.

The problem with having a larger Bermuda Triangle is that it increases the odds of accidents. There is near-constant travel, by ship and by plane, across the Atlantic, and accidents are expected to occur. In fact, the Bermuda Triangle happens to fall within one of the busiest navigational regions in the world, and the reality of greater activity creates the possibility for more to go wrong. Shipping records suggest that there is not a greater than average loss of vessels within the Bermuda Triangle, and many researchers have argued that the reputation of the Triangle makes any accident seem out of the ordinary. In fact, most accidents fall within the expected margin of error. The increase in ships from East Asia no doubt contributes to an increase in accidents. And as for the story of the Navy planes that disappeared within the Triangle, many researchers now conclude that it was the result of mistakes on the part of the pilots who were flying into storm clouds and simply got lost.

1. Which of the following describes this type of writing?

a. Narrative
b. Persuasive
c. Expository
d. Technical

2. Which of the following sentences is most representative of a summary sentence for this passage?

a. The problem with having a larger Bermuda Triangle is that it increases the odds of accidents.
b. The area that is called the Bermuda Triangle happens to fall within one of the busiest navigational regions in the world, and the reality of greater activity creates the possibility for more to go wrong.
c. One of the biggest challenges in considering the phenomenon is deciding how much area actually represents the Bermuda Triangle.
d. Researchers have never been able to find anything truly mysterious about what happens in the Bermuda Triangle, if there even is a Bermuda Triangle.

3. With which of the following statements would the author most likely agree?

a. There is no real mystery about the Bermuda Triangle because most events have reasonable explanations.
b. Researchers are wrong to expand the focus of the Triangle to the Azores, because this increases the likelihood of accidents.
c. The official statement of "causes or reasons unknown" in the loss of the Navy planes was a deliberate concealment from the Navy.
d. Reducing the legends about the mysteries of the Bermuda Triangle will help to reduce the number of reported accidents or shipping losses in that region.

4. Which of the following represents an opinion statement on the part of the author?

a. The problem with having a larger Bermuda Triangle is that it increases the odds of accidents.
b. The area known as the Bermuda Triangle has become such a part of popular culture that it can be difficult to sort through the myth and locate the truth.
c. The increase in ships from East Asia no doubt contributes to an increase in accidents.
d. Most consider the Triangle to stretch from Miami to Puerto Rico and include the island of Bermuda.

5. Which of the following is a common argument that researchers make about the validity of the Bermuda Triangle's reputation?

a. It cannot be scientifically verified, since accidents happen for "causes or reasons unknown."
b. The boundaries of the area must be established and agreed upon before any test of the reputation would be possible.
c. The supernatural nature of the Bermuda Triangle is well established in popular culture.
d. Since the number of accidents attributed to the area is within a normal margin of error, there is nothing extraordinary about the Bermuda Triangle.

6. As it is used in the context of the passage, *discomposed* most nearly means:

a. Inverted
b. Forgetful
c. Broken down
d. Disoriented

Refer to the following for questions 7 - 12:

In the United States, the foreign language requirement for high school graduation is decided at the state level. This means the requirement varies, with some states deciding to forego a foreign language requirement altogether (www.ncssfl.org). It is necessary that these states reconsider their position and amend their requirements to reflect compulsory completion of a course of one or more foreign languages. Studying a foreign language has become increasingly important for the global economy. As technology continues to make international business relations increasingly easy, people need to keep up by increasing their communication capabilities. High school graduates with foreign language credits have been shown to have an increased college acceptance rate. In addition, students who have mastered more than one language typically find themselves in greater demand when they reach the job market. Students who did not study a foreign language often find themselves unable to obtain a job at all.

7. What is the main idea of this passage?

a. Studying a foreign language will help graduating students find jobs after high school.
b. Studying a foreign language should be a mandatory requirement for high school graduation.
c. Studying a foreign language helps students gain an understanding of other cultures.
d. Studying a foreign language is essential if a student hopes to get into college.

8. Which of the following statements represents the best summary of the claims made in this passage?

a. Studying a foreign language is important if you want to graduate from high school and get a job.
b. Studying a foreign language is important for the global economy because of the technological advances that have been made in international communications.
c. Studying a foreign language is important for the global economy, college acceptance rates, and becoming a sought-after candidate in the job market.
d. Studying a foreign language is important for college acceptance rates and obtaining a job after college.

9. Which of the following statements represents an exaggerated claim in support of the argument presented in this passage?

a. In the United States, the foreign language requirement for high school graduation is decided at the state level.
b. Studying a foreign language has become increasingly important for the global economy.
c. High school graduates with foreign language credits have been shown to have an increased college acceptance rate.
d. Students who did not study a foreign language often find themselves unable to obtain a job at all.

10. Which of the following would be a useful source of information to determine the validity of the argument presented in this passage?

a. A survey of high school students' preferences with regard to foreign language requirements
b. A comparison of the correlation between a second language introduced at home and subsequent college acceptance rates
c. A survey that asks parents to select the foreign language they would like their children to study in high school
d. A comparison of the correlation between high school students' study of a foreign language and subsequent college acceptance rates

11. Which of the following would be the best concluding statement for this passage?

a. States should consider how important foreign languages are for the global economy when making their policies regarding foreign language requirements for graduation from high school.
b. Policies regarding a foreign language requirement for graduation from high school should take into account the importance of foreign languages for the global economy and the correlation between foreign languages and increased college acceptance rates and employment opportunities.
c. High school graduation requirements should include a foreign language class because of the influence knowledge of a second language has on college acceptance rates.
d. Policies regarding a foreign language requirement for graduation from high school should take into account how difficult it is to obtain a job in today's economy for those who do not have knowledge of more than one language.

12. Based on this passage, the author would most likely agree with which of the following?

a. Learning a foreign language is only for fun and it should be up to the individual to decide whether or not they wish to learn one.
b. Learning a foreign language should be a basic requirement for all students, because studies have shown that it improves the local economy.
c. Learning a foreign language is an unreasonable expectation for the government to place upon students, since most people find no need to speak more than one language.
d. Learning a foreign language needs to be compulsory for all students in the United States.

Refer to the following for questions 13 - 18:

In 1603, Queen Elizabeth I of England died. She had never married and had no heir, so the throne passed to a distant relative: James Stuart, the son of Elizabeth's cousin and one-time rival for the throne, Mary, Queen of Scots. James was crowned King James I of England. At the time, he was also King James VI of Scotland, and the combination of roles would create a spirit of conflict that haunted the two nations for generations to come.

The conflict developed as a result of rising tensions among the people within the nations, as well as between them. Scholars in the 21st century are far too hasty in dismissing the role of religion in political disputes, but religion undoubtedly played a role in the problems that faced England and Scotland. By the time of James Stuart's succession to the English throne, the English people had firmly embraced the teachings of Protestant theology. Similarly, the Scottish Lowlands was decisively Protestant. In the Scottish Highlands, however, the clans retained their Catholic faith. James acknowledged the Church of England and still sanctioned the largely Protestant translation of the Bible that still bears his name.

James's son King Charles I proved himself to be less committed to the Protestant Church of England. Charles married the Catholic Princess Henrietta Maria of France, and there were suspicions among the English and the Lowland Scots that Charles was quietly a Catholic. Charles's own political troubles extended beyond religion in this case, and he was beheaded in 1649. Eventually, his son King Charles II would be crowned, and this Charles is believed to have converted secretly to the Catholic Church. Charles II died without a legitimate heir, and his brother James ascended to the throne as King James II.

James was recognized to be a practicing Catholic, and his commitment to Catholicism would prove to be his downfall. James's wife Mary Beatrice lost a number of children during their infancy, and when she became pregnant again in 1687 the public became concerned. If James had a son, that son would undoubtedly be raised a Catholic, and the English people would not stand for this. Mary gave birth to a son, but the story quickly circulated that the royal child had died and the child named James's heir was a foundling smuggled in. James, his wife, and his infant son were forced to flee; and James's Protestant daughter Mary was crowned the queen.

In spite of a strong resemblance to the king, the young James II was generally rejected among the English and the Lowland Scots, who referred to him as "the Pretender." But in the Highlands the Catholic princeling was welcomed. He inspired a group known as *Jacobites*, to reflect the Latin version of his name. His own son Charles, known affectionately as Bonnie Prince Charlie, would eventually raise an army and attempt to recapture what he believed to be his throne. The movement was soundly defeated at the Battle of Culloden in 1746, and England and Scotland have remained ostensibly Protestant ever since.

13. Which of the following sentences contains an opinion on the part of the author?

a. James was recognized to be a practicing Catholic, and his commitment to Catholicism would prove to be his downfall.
b. James' son King Charles I proved himself to be less committed to the Protestant Church of England.
c. The movement was soundly defeated at the Battle of Culloden in 1746, and England and Scotland have remained ostensibly Protestant ever since.
d. Scholars in the 21st century are far too hasty in dismissing the role of religion in political disputes, but religion undoubtedly played a role in the problems that faced England and Scotland.

14. Which of the following is a logical conclusion based on the information that is provided within the passage?

a. Like Elizabeth I, Charles II never married and thus never had children.
b. The English people were relieved each time that James II's wife Mary lost another child, as this prevented the chance of a Catholic monarch.
c. Charles I's beheading had less to do with religion than with other political problems that England was facing.
d. Unlike his son and grandsons, King James I had no Catholic leanings and was a faithful follower of the Protestant Church of England.

15. Based on the information that is provided within the passage, which of the following can be inferred about King James II's son?

a. Considering his resemblance to King James II, James Edward was very likely the legitimate child of the king and the queen.
b. Given the queen's previous inability to produce a healthy child, the English and the Lowland Scots were right in questioning the legitimacy of James Edward.
c. James Edward was not as popular among the Highland clans as his son Bonnie Prince Charlie.
d. James Edward was unable to acquire the resources needed to build the army and plan the invasion that his son succeeded in doing.

16. Which of the following best describes the organization of the information in the passage?

a. Cause-effect
b. Chronological sequence
c. Problem-solution
d. Comparison-contrast

17. Which of the following best describes the author's intent in the passage?

a. To persuade
b. To entertain
c. To express feeling
d. To inform

18. Who does the passage say ascended the throne because someone else did not have a legitimate heir?

a. King James Stuart
b. Queen Elizabeth I
c. King Charles II
d. King James II

Refer to the following for questions 19 - 24:

Global warming and the depletion of natural resources are constant threats to the future of our planet. All people have a responsibility to be proactive participants in the fight to save Earth by working now to conserve resources for later. Participation begins with our everyday choices. From what you buy to what you do to how much you use, your decisions affect the planet and everyone around you. Now is the time to take action.

When choosing what to buy, look for sustainable products made from renewable or recycled resources. The packaging of the products you buy is just as important as the products themselves. Is the item minimally packaged in a recycled container? How did the product reach the store? Locally grown food and other products manufactured within your community are the best choices. The fewer miles a product traveled to reach you, the fewer resources it required.

You can continue to make a difference for the planet in how you use what you bought and the resources you have available. Remember the locally grown food you purchased? Don't pile it on your plate at dinner. Food that remains on your plate is a wasted resource, and you can always go back for seconds. You should try to be aware of your consumption of water and energy. Turn off the water when you brush your teeth, and limit your showers to five minutes. Turn off the lights, and don't leave appliances or chargers plugged in when not in use.

Together, we can use less, waste less, recycle more, and make the right choices. It may be the only chance we have.

19. What is the author's tone?

a. The author's tone is optimistic.
b. The author's tone is pessimistic.
c. The author's tone is matter-of-fact.
d. The author's tone is angry.

20. Why does the author say it is important to buy locally grown food?

a. Buying locally grown food supports people in your community.
b. Locally grown food travels the least distance to reach you and therefore uses fewer resources.
c. Locally grown food uses less packaging.
d. Locally grown food is healthier for you because it has been exposed to fewer pesticides.

21. What does the author imply will happen if people do not follow his suggestions?

a. The author implies we will run out of resources in the next 10 years.
b. The author implies water and energy prices will rise sharply in the near future.
c. The author implies global warming and the depletion of natural resources will continue.
d. The author implies local farmers will lose their farms.

22. What is the best definition of the underlined word in the selection below, taken from the third paragraph of the passage?

You should try to be aware of your <u>consumption</u> of water and energy.

a. Using the greatest amount
b. Illness of the lungs
c. Using the least amount
d. Depletion of goods

23. Which of the following is one way the author specifies that a person can try to be aware of their consumption of water and energy?

a. Food that remains on your plate is a wasted resource, and you can always go back for a second helping.
b. Locally grown food and other products manufactured within your community are the best choices.
c. Don't leave appliances or chargers plugged in when not in use.
d. Participation begins with our everyday choices.

24. How does the author make a connection between the second and third paragraphs?

a. The author indicates he will make suggestions for how to tell other people what to buy.
b. The author indicates he will continue to give more examples of what you should buy.
c. The author indicates he will make suggestions for how to keep from buying more items.
d. The author indicates he will now make suggestions for how to use what you bought.

Refer to the following for questions 25 - 30:

In the United States, where we have more land than people, it is not at all difficult for persons in good health to make money. In this comparatively new field there are so many avenues of success open, so many vocations which are not crowded, that any person of either sex who is willing, at least for the time being, to engage in any respectable occupation that offers, may find lucrative employment.

Those who really desire to attain an independence, have only to set their minds upon it, and adopt the proper means, as they do in regard to any other object which they wish to accomplish, and the thing is easily done. But however easy it may be found to make money, I have no doubt many of my hearers will agree it is the most difficult thing in the world to keep it. The road to wealth is, as Dr. Franklin truly says, "as plain as the road to the mill." It consists simply in expending less than we earn; that seems to be a very simple problem. Mr. Micawber, one of those happy creations of the genial Dickens, puts the case in a strong light when he says that to have annual income of twenty pounds, per annum, and spend twenty pounds and sixpence, is to be the most miserable of men; whereas, to have an income of only twenty pounds, and spend but nineteen pounds and sixpence, is to be the happiest of mortals.

Many of my hearers may say, "we understand this; this is economy, and we know economy is wealth; we know we can't eat our cake and keep it also." Yet I beg to say that perhaps more cases of failure arise from mistakes on this point than almost any other. The fact is, many people think they understand economy when they really do not.

Excerpt from The Art of Money-Getting by P.T. Barnum

25. Which of the following statements best expresses the main idea of the passage?

a. Getting a job is easier now than it ever has been before.
b. Earning money is much less difficult than managing it properly.
c. Dr. Franklin advocated getting a job in a mill.
d. Spending money is the greatest temptation in the world.

26. What would this author's attitude likely be to a person unable to find employment?

a. Descriptive
b. Conciliatory
c. Ingenuous
d. Incredulous

27. According to the author, what is more difficult than making money?

a. managing money
b. traveling to a mill
c. reading Dickens
d. understanding the economy

28. Who is the most likely audience for this passage?

a. economists
b. general readers
c. teachers
d. philanthropists

29. Which word best describes the author's attitude towards those who believe they understand money?

a. supportive
b. incriminating
c. excessive
d. patronizing

30. This passage is most likely taken from a(n) ____.

a. self-help manual
b. autobiography
c. epistle
d. novel

Word Knowledge

1. The data in the graph exhibited an *aberration*.

***Aberration* means:**

a. Deviation from course
b. Linear appearance
c. Inverted appearance
d. Circular theme

2. The prince *abjured* the ambassador.

***Abjured* means:**

a. Congratulated
b. Renounced
c. Relieved
d. Fired

3. The chemist attempted to practice *alchemy*.

***Alchemy* means:**

a. Turning metal into gold
b. Separating ions
c. Fusion
d. Isolating chemical components

4. The man at the bar was *belligerent*.

***Belligerent* means:**

a. Friendly
b. Courteous
c. Angry
d. Talkative

5. The ships formed a *blockade* near the mouth of the Mississippi River.

***Blockade* means:**

a. Prevent passage
b. Fishing convoy
c. Whaling expedition
d. Zigzag formation

6. The men erected a *bulwark* near the opening.

***Bulwark* means:**

a. Trap
b. Obstacle
c. Barn
d. Runway

7. The group embarked on a *clandestine* operation.

***Clandestine* means:**

a. Environmental expedition
b. Shipping adventure
c. Scary
d. Secretive

8. The agent of the government was *choleric.*

***Choleric* means:**

a. Easily provoked
b. Undercover
c. Cooperative
d. Late

9. Some members of the organization broke away and created a grass roots *caucus.*

***Caucus* means:**

a. Group with political aims
b. Environmental group
c. Management organization
d. Religious movement

10. The circumstances were open to *conjecture.*

***Conjecture* means:**

a. Discussion
b. Guessing
c. Argument
d. Public

11. The news anchor attempted to *disseminate* the story.

***Disseminate* means:**

a. To convey
b. To deny
c. To rebuke
d. To review

12. The stockpiles for the occupation began to *dwindle*.

***Dwindle* means:**

a. To increase
b. To decrease
c. To rot
d. To be self-limiting

13. The chemicals began to *effervesce*.

***Effervesce* means:**

a. To combine
b. To catalyze
c. To break down
d. To bubble up

14. The witness began to *evince* critical details.

***Evince* means:**

a. To hide
b. To cover secretly
c. Exaggerate
d. To make manifest

15. The front line troops began to *extricate* from the enemy.

***Extricate* means:**

a. Confront
b. Surrender
c. Disentangle
d. Deploy

16. The congressman from Ohio started a *filibuster*.

***Filibuster* means:**

a. Bill
b. Congressional investigation
c. An attempt to disrupt legislation
d. Program related to welfare

17. The soldier showed *fortitude* during the engagement with the enemy.

***Fortitude* means:**

a. Patient courage
b. Willingness for action
c. Endurance
d. Professionalism

18. The southern lady was *genteel* when hosting northern businessmen.

***Genteel* means:**

a. Rude
b. Refined
c. Reserved
d. Resentful

19. The lawyer launched into a *harangue* when speaking to the witness.

***Harangue* means:**

a. Discussion
b. Monologue
c. Dialogue
d. Tirade

20. Some believe our destinies are *immutable*.

***Immutable* means:**

a. Professional
b. Conversational
c. Unchangeable
d. Unerring

21. The baby was diagnosed with *jaundice*.

***Jaundice* means:**

a. Yellowing condition
b. Condition of glucose intolerance
c. Condition of nutritional deficiency
d. Condition of dermatitis

22. The criminal was known for his *knavery*.

***Knavery* means:**

a. Quickness
b. Light-footedness
c. Burglary ability
d. Deceitfulness

23. The patient exhibited signs of *languor*.

***Languor* means:**

a. Confusion
b. Anxiety
c. Depression
d. Deceitfulness

24. The Romans were able to *macadamize* a large portion of the Italian peninsula.

***Macadamize* means:**

a. To pave
b. To supply
c. To connect
d. To protect

25. The patient's lower extremity began to show signs of *necrosis*.

***Necrosis* means:**

a. Maceration
b. Tissue death
c. Induration
d. Redness

26. The traffic official began to *obviate* the construction.

***Obviate* means:**

a. Clear away
b. Identify
c. Reproduce
d. Delegate

27. The general *presaged* the battle plan to his subordinate officers.

***Presaged* means:**

a. Delegated
b. Clarified
c. Foretold
d. Introduced

28. The orange grove was under *quarantine*, because of a local virus.

***Quarantine* means:**

a. Pressure
b. Demolition
c. Reconstruction
d. Isolation

29. The defendant was asked to *remunerate* the damage he caused during the robbery.

***Remunerate* means:**

a. Reconstruct
b. Renounce
c. Pay for
d. Repeat

30. The welding machine *scintillated* into the dark shop.

***Scintillated* means:**

a. Emitted gases
b. Emitted light
c. Emitted fumes
d. Emitted noise

Mathematics

1. A rectangular garden has a perimeter of 600 yards. If the length of the garden is 250 yards, what is the garden's width in yards?

a. 25 yards
b. 50 yards
c. 175 yards
d. 350 yards

2. Which of these numbers is a prime number?

a. 4
b. 11
c. 12
d. 15

3. The average of six numbers is 4. If the average of two of those numbers is 2, what is the average of the other four numbers?

a. 5
b. 6
c. 7
d. 8

4. Four more than a number, x, is 2 less than $\frac{1}{3}$ of another number, y. Which of the following algebraic equations correctly represents this sentence?

a. $x + 4 = \frac{1}{3}y - 2$
b. $4x = 2 - \frac{1}{3}y$
c. $4 - x = 2 + \frac{1}{3}y$
d. $x + 4 = 2 - \frac{1}{3}y$

5. Evaluate the expression $2^3 + (4 + 1)$.

a. 9
b. 13
c. 15
d. 21

6. In a graduating high school class of 532, 15% of the students will receive As and 55% of the students will receive Bs. If 53 students receive Ds and no one failed, what approximate percentage of the students received Cs?

a. 10%
b. 20%
c. 30%
d. 40%

7. If a number, x, is subtracted from 27, the result is –5. What is the value of x?

a. 22
b. 25
c. 32
d. 35

8. 75 is 60% of what number?

a. 45
b. 125
c. 130
d. 145

9. Solve the following equation for x if $y = 2$.

$$3x - 4y = 25$$

a. $x = 10$
b. $x = 11$
c. $x = 12$
d. $x = 13$

10. If one side of an obtuse triangle equals 4 inches and the second side equals 5 inches, what does the third side equal?

a. 1 inch
b. 4.6 inches
c. 6.4 inches
d. 9 inches

11. If Nick can run 3 miles in 24 minutes, how many miles can he run in 3 hours?

a. 11.25 miles
b. 17.6 miles
c. 21.8 miles
d. 22.5 miles

12. Which of the following decimals equals 9.47%?

a. 0.000947
b. 0.00947
c. 0.0947
d. 0.9470

13. What is 0.25×0.03?

a. 75
b. 0.75
c. 0.075
d. 0.0075

14. An armoire was purchased for $340.32 at an auction, subject to a 5% tax rate. What was the additional tax charged on the armoire?

a. $15.82
b. $16.02
c. $16.39
d. $17.02

15. Jamie had $6.50 in his wallet when he left home. He spent $4.25 on drinks and $2.00 on a magazine. Later, his friend repaid him $2.50 that he had borrowed the previous day. How much money does Jamie have in his wallet now?

a. $2.75
b. $3.25
c. $12.25
d. $14.25

16. What is $8\frac{3}{4} + 6\frac{1}{2}$?

a. $14\frac{1}{2}$
b. $15\frac{1}{4}$
c. $17\frac{3}{4}$
d. 32

17. One inch is equivalent to 2.54 centimeters. How long, in centimeters, is a stick measuring 9.5 inches?

a. 241.3 centimeters
b. 24.13 centimeters
c. 12.70 centimeters
d. 3.7 centimeters

18. The ratio of 4 to 16 is equivalent to what percentage?

a. 2%
b. 4%
c. 12%
d. 25%

19. What is 20% of $\frac{12}{5}$, expressed as a percentage?

a. 48%
b. 65%
c. 72%
d. 76%

20. What is the area of a rectangle with sides 34 meters and 12 meters?

a. 408 m^2
b. 40.8 m^2
c. 22 m^2
d. 2.83 m^2

21. A woman must earn $250 in the next four days to pay a traffic ticket. How much will she have to earn each day?

a. $45.50
b. $62.50
c. $75.50
d. $100.50

22. What is $897.54 - 48.39$?

a. 813.15
b. 814.15
c. 849.15
d. 859.15

23. Factor the following expression: $x^2 + x - 12$

a. $(x - 2)(x + 6)$
b. $(x + 6)(x - 2)$
c. $(x - 4)(x + 3)$
d. $(x + 4)(x - 3)$

24. How many centimeters are in 6 meters?

a. 0.06
b. 60
c. 600
d. 6,000

25. For a cake recipe, $\frac{2}{3}$ cup of oil is needed and you have $\frac{1}{4}$ cup. How much more oil do you need?

a. $\frac{1}{2}$ cup
b. $\frac{2}{7}$ cup
c. $\frac{3}{8}$ cup
d. $\frac{5}{12}$ cup

26. A $\frac{1}{2}$ cup of skim milk is 45 calories. Approximately how many calories would $\frac{3}{4}$ cup of skim milk provide?

a. 60 calories
b. $67\frac{1}{2}$ calories
c. 68 calories
d. $76\frac{1}{2}$ calories

27. At a school carnival, three students spend an average of $10. Six other students spend an average of $4. What is the average amount of money spent by all nine students?

a. $5
b. $6
c. $7
d. $8

28. If 35% of a paycheck was deducted for taxes and 4% for insurance, what is the total percentage taken out of the paycheck?

a. 20%
b. 31%
c. 39%
d. 42%

29. The scientific notation for the diameter of a red blood cell is approximately 7.4×10^{-4} centimeters. What is that amount in standard form?

a. 0.00074
b. 0.0074
c. 740
d. 74,000

30. How many meters are equivalent to 336 millimeters?

a. 336,000
b. 33,600
c. 3.36
d. 0.336

31. Bob spends $17.90 on sodas and snacks for his study group. The expenses are to be split evenly between five people. How much is each person's share?

a. $3.45
b. $3.58
c. $3.65
d. $3.73

32. 0.10 equals which of the following fractions?

a. $\frac{1}{100}$
b. $\frac{1}{50}$
c. $\frac{1}{10}$
d. $\frac{1}{5}$

33. Which of the following is correct?

a. $\frac{4}{7} = \frac{12}{21}$
b. $\frac{3}{4} = \frac{12}{20}$
c. $\frac{5}{8} = \frac{15}{32}$
d. $\frac{7}{9} = \frac{28}{45}$

34. What is $1\frac{1}{4} \times 3\frac{2}{5} \times 1\frac{2}{3}$?

a. $5\frac{5}{6}$
b. $6\frac{7}{12}$
c. $7\frac{1}{12}$
d. $8\frac{11}{15}$

35. A recipe called for 2 ounces of cream. Lindsay didn't have a way to measure ounces, and her measuring cups were in the dishwasher, but she remembered the number of ounces and cups in a pint. The cream carton had a chart showing that a cup contains 16 tablespoons, but all she could find was her teaspoon measuring spoon. She also knew there are 3 teaspoons in a tablespoon. Which of the following shows the calculation for the number of teaspoons of cream Lindsay needs for her recipe?

a. $2 \times \frac{1}{16} \times 2 \times 16 \times 3$
b. $2 \times 16 \times \frac{1}{2} \times \frac{1}{16} \times \frac{1}{3}$
c. $\frac{1}{2} \times 16 \times 2 \times 16 \times \frac{1}{3}$
d. $\frac{2}{16} \times \frac{1}{2} \times 16 \times \frac{1}{3}$

36. A man goes to a casino with $125. He loses $30 on blackjack, then loses another $40 on roulette. How much money does he have left?

a. $35
b. $40
c. $55
d. $70

37. Four people decide to adopt a dog and take turns caring for it. Person A thinks he can take care of the dog $\frac{1}{4}$ of the time. Person B thinks she can handle $\frac{1}{8}$. Person C thinks he can take care of the dog $\frac{1}{2}$ of the time. What part is left for the fourth person to cover?

a. $\frac{1}{8}$
b. $\frac{1}{4}$
c. $\frac{1}{3}$
d. $\frac{1}{2}$

38. Sheila, Janice, and Karen, working together at the same rate, can complete a job in $3\frac{1}{3}$ days. Working at the same rate, how much of the job could Janice and Karen do in one day?

a. $\frac{1}{3}$
b. $\frac{1}{4}$
c. $\frac{1}{5}$
d. $\frac{1}{9}$

39. The table shows the cost of renting a bicycle for 1, 2, or 3 hours. Which of the following equations best represents the data, if *C* represents the cost and *h* represents the time of the rental?

Hours	1	2	3
Cost	\$3.60	\$7.20	\$10.80

a. $C = 3.60h$
b. $C = h + 3.60$
c. $C = 3.60h + 10.80$
d. $C = \frac{10.80}{h}$

40. A recipe calls for 2 cups of water for every 6 cups of flour. Josie wants to make a smaller batch using only 2 cups of flour. How much water should she use?

a. $\frac{1}{2}$ cup
b. 2 cups
c. $\frac{2}{3}$ cup
d. 12 cups

Science

1. Cardiac output is the product of what two factors?

a. Heart rate and stroke volume
b. Stroke volume and blood pressure
c. Heart rate and pulse
d. Stroke volume and oxygen consumption

2. Blood leaves the right ventricle and goes to the ____.

a. lungs
b. kidneys
c. right atrium
d. arterial circulation to the body

3. Which of the following does not help determine heart rate?

a. Body temperature
b. Physical activity
c. Concentration of ions
d. Anaerobic cellular metabolism

4. Which of the following is not considered a layer of the heart?

a. Epicardium
b. Endocardium
c. Myocardium
d. Vasocardium

5. The hormone _______ can promote increased blood volume, and increased blood pressure.

a. estrogen
b. testosterone
c. aldosterone
d. dopamine

6. Which of the following terms matches the definition: an abnormally slow heartbeat?

a. Tachycardia
b. Bradycardia
c. Fibrillation
d. Myocardial infarct

7. Blood is made of approximately __% hematocrit and ____% plasma.

a. 45, 55
b. 55, 45
c. 75, 25
d. 25, 75

8. Which of the following body systems allows a person to move?

a. integumentary system
b. digestive system
c. endocrine system
d. muscular system

9. A dihybrid cross is made between the dominant genes for brown eyes (B) and blonde hair (S), and the recessive genes for blue eyes (b) and red hair (s). What fraction of offspring would have the genotype BbSs in the F2 generation?

a. $\frac{1}{16}$
b. $\frac{3}{16}$
c. $\frac{4}{16}$
d. $\frac{9}{16}$

10. Which of the following terms matches the definition: collapse of a lung?

a. Anoxia
b. Atelectasis
c. Dyspnea
d. Hypercapnia

11. The central nervous system is composed of the _____ and the ______.

a. brain, spinal cord
b. brain, peripheral nerves
c. spinal cord, peripheral nerves
d. spinal cord, musculature system

12. The brain is made of _____ lobes.

a. 2
b. 3
c. 4
d. 5

13. ______ is a state of equilibrium within tissues.

a. Peristalsis
b. Stomatitis
c. Homeostasis
d. Synergy

14. ______ is a state of inflammation of the mouth.

a. Diverticulitis
b. Hepatitis
c. Enteritis
d. Stomatitis

15. ______ is the most important male hormone.

a. Estrogen
b. Aldosterone
c. Progesterone
d. Testosterone

16. Which of the following functions are not related to the kidneys?

a. Filtration
b. Bile production
c. Secretion
d. Re-absorption

17. Which of the following terms matches the definition: uncontrolled urination?

a. Enuresis
b. Dieuretic
c. Pyuria
d. Ureteritis

18. Auditory impulses are interpreted in the _____ lobes.

a. frontal
b. parietal
c. temporal
d. occipital

19. The outer layer of the eye is the ____.

a. cornea
b. sclera
c. retina
d. rods

20. In the marine waters, there is a beautiful, orange clown fish that lives closely with a sea anemone. This sea anemone can sting its prey with poisonous venom before devouring it; however, the clown fish is not affected by the sea anemone at all. The clown fish is only safe when hiding within the sea anemone's poisonous tentacles and protects the hiding spot from a certain type of fish who tries to eat the sea anemone. This is an example of what type of relationship?

a. Commensalism
b. Mutualism
c. Parasitism
d. None of the above

21. Which of the following elements are not halogens?

a. Chlorine
b. Bromide
c. Iodine
d. Cesium

22. The horizontal rows of the periodic table are called _____.

a. periods
b. columns
c. rows
d. families

23. Converting gas into a liquid is known as ______.

a. evaporation
b. transitioning
c. condensation
d. sublimation

24. Compounds with various structures, but the same shape are called _____.

a. polar compounds
b. isomers
c. variables
d. transient compounds

25. A gas at constant volume is cooled. Which statement about the gas must be true?

a. The kinetic energy of the gas molecules has decreased.
b. The gas has condensed to a liquid.
c. The weight of the gas has decreased.
d. The density of the gas has increased.

26. Which of the following terms matches the definition: the volume of a gas varies indirectly with temperature with pressure constant?

a. Boyle's law
b. Charles's law
c. Johnson's law
d. Avogadro's law

27. An electron moves in a uniform electric field in the same direction as the electric field from point A to point B. Which of the following statements is true?

a. The potential energy of the electron decreased
b. The potential energy of the electron increased
c. The potential energy of the electron remained constant
d. The potential energy of the electron was converted into kinetic energy

28. An acid is a substance that increases the _____ count in water.

a. chloride ion
b. hydroxide ion
c. hydrogen ion
d. oxygen

29. A scientist mixes two chemicals together, and they produce a violent reaction, generating considerable heat. Where did the thermal energy come from to heat up the chemicals?

a. The kinetic energy of the molecules in the chemicals
b. Potential energy inherent in the atomic bonds in the molecules of the chemicals
c. It was absorbed from the surrounding air
d. Nowhere; the energy was completely created by the reaction

30. Using the 2nd Law of Newton identify the formula that is applicable.

a. $F = ma$
b. $Speed = \frac{Distance}{Time}$
c. $Power = \frac{F \times D}{T}$
d. $Watts = Voltage \times Amperes$

31. In a pond, eutrophication, the pollution of water by plant nutrients, can occur, causing chemical, biological, and ecological changes to the pond. As plant material begins to decompose and carbon dioxide begins to increase, what would happen to the fish in the pond?

a. They would flourish
b. They would relocate to another area
c. They would die off
d. They would not be affected

32. The part of the human excretory system most responsible for maintaining normal body temperature is the:

a. kidney.
b. bladder.
c. liver.
d. sweat glands.

33. The main function of ______ is to reduce the number of chromosomes to half the number of parent cells?

a. mitosis
b. telophase
c. meiosis I
d. meiosis II

34. What is the name of the structure that prevents food from entering the airway?

a. Trachea
b. Esophagus
c. Diaphragm
d. Epiglottis

35. Which substance makes up the pads that provide support between the vertebrae?

a. Bone
b. Cartilage
c. Tendon
d. Fat

36. In the suburban neighborhood of Northwoods, there have been large populations of deer, and residents have complained about them eating flowers and garden plants. What would be a logical explanation for the large increase in the deer population over the last two seasons?

a. Increased quantity of food sources
b. Decreased population of a natural predator
c. Deer migration from surrounding areas
d. Increase in hunting licenses sold

Refer to the following for question 37:

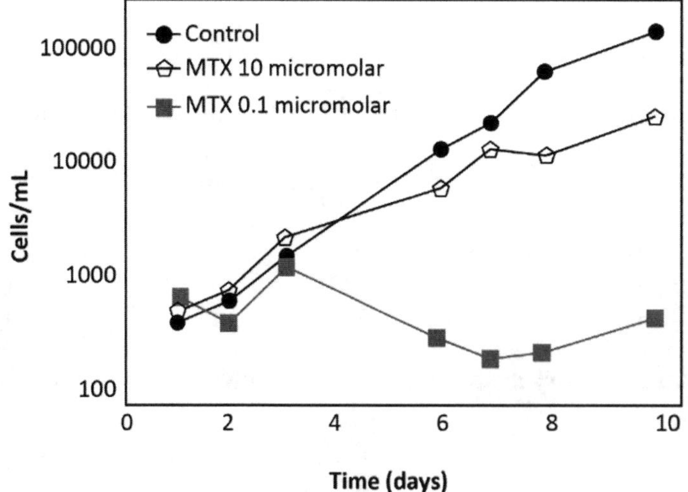

Cancer cells of the murine erythroleukemia (MEL) cell line were cultured in normal growth medium (control) and in two different concentrations of the anti-cancer drug methotrexate (MTX) for a period of ten days. Samples were removed periodically, and the number of cells per milliliter of culture was determined. Each point in the figure represents the mean of five determinations.

37. The growth of cells in the absence of drugs in this experiment can best be described as:

a. linear
b. exponential
c. derivative
d. inhibited

Refer to the following for questions 38 - 39:

1 IA	2 IIA	3 IIIB	4 IVB	5 VB	6 VIB	7 VIIB	8	9 VIIIB	10	11 IB	12 IIB	13 IIIA	14 IVA	15 VA	16 VIA	17 VIIA	18 VIIIA
1 **H** 1.01																	2 **He** 4.00
3 **Li** 6.94	4 **Be** 9.01											5 **B** 10.81	6 **C** 12.01	7 **N** 14.01	8 **O** 16.00	9 **F** 19.00	10 **Ne** 20.18
11 **Na** 22.99	12 **Mg** 24.31											13 **Al** 26.98	14 **Si** 28.09	15 **P** 30.97	16 **S** 32.07	17 **Cl** 35.45	18 **Ar** 39.95
19 **K** 39.1	20 **Ca** 40.08	21 **Sc** 44.96	22 **Ti** 47.88	23 **V** 50.94	24 **Cr** 52.00	25 **Mn** 54.94	26 **Fe** 55.85	27 **Co** 58.93	28 **Ni** 58.69	29 **Cu** 63.55	30 **Zn** 65.39	31 **Ga** 69.72	32 **Ge** 72.61	33 **As** 74.92	34 **Se** 78.96	35 **Br** 79.90	36 **Kr** 83.80
37 **Rb** 85.47	38 **Sr** 87.62	39 **Y** 88.91	40 **Zr** 91.22	41 **Nb** 92.91	42 **Mo** 95.94	43 **Tc** (98)	44 **Ru** 101.07	45 **Rh** 102.91	46 **Pd** 106.42	47 **Ag** 107.87	48 **Cd** 112.41	49 **In** 114.82	50 **Sn** 118.71	51 **Sb** 121.76	52 **Te** 127.6	53 **I** 126.9	54 **Xe** 131.29
55 **Cs** 132.9	56 **Ba** 137.3	57 **La*** 138.9	72 **Hf** 178.5	73 **Ta** 180.9	74 **W** 183.9	75 **Re** 186.2	76 **Os** 190.2	77 **Ir** 192.2	78 **Pt** 195.1	79 **Au** 197.0	80 **Hg** 200.6	81 **Tl** 204.4	82 **Pb** 207.2	83 **Bi** 209	84 **Po** (209)	85 **At** (210)	86 **Rn** (222)
87 **Fr** (223)	88 **Ra** (226)	89 **Ac^** (227)	104 **Rf** (261)	105 **Db** (262)	106 **Sg** (263)	107 **Bh** (264)	108 **Hs** (265)	109 **Mt** (268)	110 **Ds** (271)	111 **Rg** (272)							

*	58 **Ce** 140.1	59 **Pr** 140.9	60 **Nd** 144.2	61 **Pm** (145)	62 **Sm** 150.4	63 **Eu** 152.0	64 **Gd** 157.3	65 **Tb** 158.9	66 **Dy** 162.5	67 **Ho** 164.9	68 **Er** 167.3	69 **Tm** 168.9	70 **Yb** 173.0	71 **Lu** 175.0
^	90 **Th** 232.0	91 **Pa** (231)	92 **U** 238.0	93 **Np** (237)	94 **Pu** (244)	95 **Am** (243)	96 **Cm** (247)	97 **Bk** (247)	98 **Cf** (251)	99 **Es** (252)	100 **Fm** (257)	101 **Md** (258)	102 **No** (259)	103 **Lr** (260)

*Note: The row labeled with * is the lanthanide series, and the row labeled with ^ is the actinide series.*

38. On average, how many neutrons does one atom of bromine (Br) have?

a. 35
b. 44.90
c. 45
d. 79.90

39. On average, how many protons does one atom of zinc (Zn) have?

a. 30
b. 35
c. 35.39
d. 65.39

40. In your garden, you have noticed that the tomato plants on the north side of your house are growing better than those on the west side, and you have decided to figure out why. They are both planted in the same soil, and they are watered at the same time during the week. Over the course of a week, you begin to measure the amount of sunlight that hits each side of the house and determine that the north side receives more light because the sunlight is blocked on the west side by the house's shadow for much of the day. What is the name of the factor in your observations that affected the tomato plants' growth?

a. The hypothesis
b. The independent variable
c. The dependent variable
d. The conclusion

Refer to the following for question 41:

B = alleles for brown eyes; **b** = alleles for green eyes

BB	Bb
Bb	bb

41. Which word describes the allele for green eyes?

a. Dominant
b. Recessive
c. Homozygous
d. Heterozygous

42. Two species of finches are able to utilize the same food supply, but their beaks are different. They are able to coexist on an island because of:

a. Niche overlap
b. Character displacement
c. Resource partitioning
d. Realized niches

43. An electric field is pointing from south to north. If a dipole is placed in the field, how will the dipole's orientation change?

a. The positive charge will be on the northern side and the negative charge will be on the southern side.
b. The positive charge will be on the southern side and the negative charge will be on the northern side.
c. The positive charge will be on the eastern side and the negative charge will be on the western side.
d. There will be no change in the orientation.

Refer to the following for questions 44 - 45:

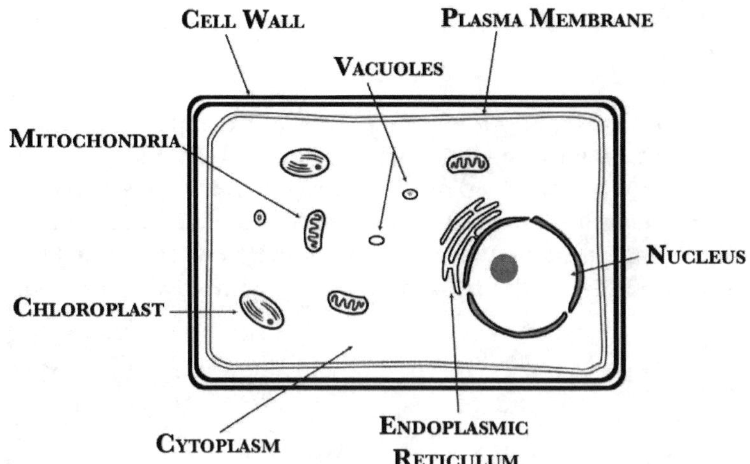

44. Which of the following structures contains DNA?

a. Cytoplasm
b. Vacuole
c. Mitochondrion
d. Nucleus

45. The mitochondria:

a. Produce energy for the cell in the form of ATP.
b. Are responsible for digesting starch.
c. Are the sites of protein synthesis.
d. Are not present in muscle cells.

Refer to the following for questions 46 - 47:

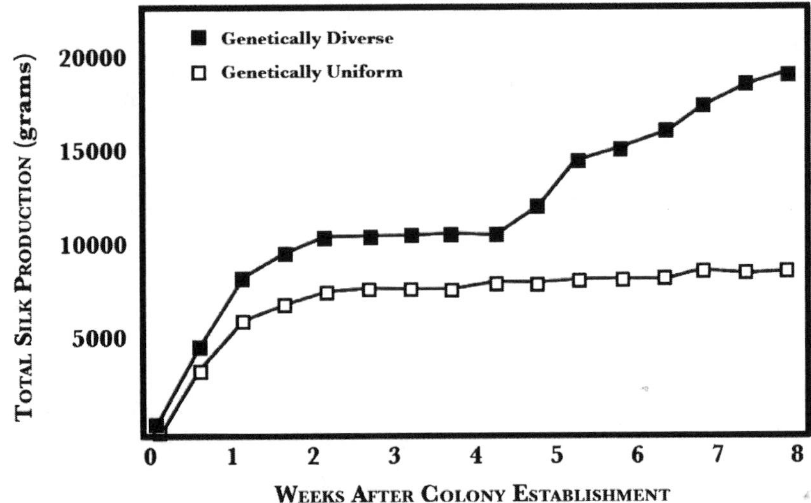

Colonies of silkworms that had the same number of genetically identical or genetically different animals were established. For several weeks after the colonies were created, silk production was estimated by removing small samples of silk from the colonies and weighing them. The results are shown in the graph. The open symbols are for the production of silk by genetically uniform worms. The closed symbols are for the production of silk by genetically diverse worms.

46. Which of the following conclusions can be drawn from the data?

a. Genetically diverse worms produce more silk than genetically uniform worms.
b. Genetically uniform worms produce more silk than genetically diverse worms.
c. Genetically diverse silkworm colonies produce more silk than genetically uniform colonies.
d. Genetically uniform silkworm colonies produce more silk than genetically diverse colonies.

47. If the generation time of a silkworm is about four weeks, which of the following hypotheses offers the best explanation for the difference in silk productivity between the two colonies?

a. Genetically diverse silkworms produce silk longer than genetically uniform worms.
b. Genetically diverse silkworms reproduce more than genetically uniform worms.
c. Genetically diverse silkworms produce heavier silk than genetically uniform worms.
d. Genetically uniform silkworms stop producing silk when they reproduce.

48. A substance is only considered acidic if it has a pH less than what?

a. 12
b. 9
c. 7
d. 4

49. Which of the following best describes a plane that divides the body into upper and lower portions?

a. Coronal
b. Transverse
c. Oblique
d. Median

50. The energy flow through an ecosystem is represented by an energy pyramid. In the energy pyramid for a terrestrial ecosystem, the producers utilize 6,000 kilocalories per square meter per year. What approximate amount of energy is transferred to the third trophic level of this ecosystem?

a. 0.6 kilocalories per square meter per year
b. 6 kilocalories per square meter per year
c. 60 kilocalories per square meter per year
d. 600 kilocalories per square meter per year

51. Which of the following quantities do *catalysts* alter to control the rate of a chemical reaction?

a. Substrate energy
b. Activation energy
c. Inhibitor energy
d. Promoter energy

52. A researcher is studying the response of bacteria to a certain chemical. In three experiments, the bacteria swim towards the chemical, and in one experiment the bacteria swim away from it. What would be the most appropriate next step for the researcher?

a. Report only the first three experiments.
b. Report all the experiments, but refrain from making any conclusions.
c. Repeat the experiment several more times and apply a statistical analysis to the data.
d. Repeat the experiment, adding a new chemical to determine its effect on the bacteria.

53. Which part of the cell is often called the cell "powerhouse" because it provides energy for cellular functions?

a. Nucleus
b. Cell membrane
c. Mitochondria
d. Cytoplasm

54. In a strenuously exercising muscle, NADH begins to accumulate in high concentration. Which of the following metabolic processes will be activated to reduce the concentration of NADH?

a. Glycolysis
b. The Krebs cycle
c. Lactic acid fermentation
d. Oxidative phosphorylation

55. What is the most likely reason that cells differentiate?

a. Cells differentiate to avoid looking like all the cells around them.
b. Cells differentiate so that simple, non-specialized cells can become highly specialized cells.
c. Cells differentiate so that multicellular organisms will remain the same size.
d. Cells differentiate for no apparent reason.

56. How is meiosis similar to mitosis?

a. Both produce daughter cells that are genetically identical.
b. Both produce daughter cells that are genetically different.
c. Both occur in humans, other animals, and plants.
d. Both occur asexually.

57. This organelle contains digestive enzymes that break down food and unneeded substances. They are also thought to be linked to the aging process. What part of a cell does this describe?

a. Lysosomes
b. Chromatin
c. Plastids
d. Golgi Apparatus

58. What type of chemical bond connects the oxygen and hydrogen atoms in a molecule of water?

a. Static bond
b. Aquatic bond
c. Ionic bond
d. Covalent bond

59. Astronauts in orbit are sometimes considered to be "weightless." Consider the three propositions about *weightlessness* and determine which ones are true.

I. Weightlessness occurs in outer space because the force of gravity becomes negligible.
II. Weightlessness occurs when a ski jumper makes a jump.
III. Weightlessness occurs when you roll a baseball on the ground.

a. I only.
b. II only.
c. I and II.
d. I, II and III.

60. When light passes between different transparent media, its speed is changed by the change in medium and it is refracted, as when a straw in a glass of water seems to break or bend at the waterline. The amount that a medium slows down the speed of light is the:

a. Normal line
b. Wavelength
c. Index of refraction
d. Angle of refraction

Answer Key and Explanations

Reading Comprehension

1. C: The passage is expository because it communicates information about the mysteries of the Bermuda Triangle and what researchers have studied and now believe. The author includes facts to inform the reader, which is the goal of expository writing. The passage does not tell a story or describe one event, so it is not a narrative. The passage also does not seek to lead the reader to take action or accept a particular conclusion, so this passage is not persuasive. The passage also does not give technical information and does not aim to help the reader understand a technical concept, so this passage is not technical.

2. D: This sentence is the best summary statement for the entire passage because it clearly describes what the author is saying about the results of studies on the Bermuda Triangle. Each paragraph in the passage includes details that support the statement that researchers have never found anything truly mysterious about the Bermuda Triangle. Choices A, B, and C are all details found in the passage, but none of these answer choices give a summary of the whole passage. Each of these answer choices support the statement in choice D, as do the rest of the details in the passage. Choice D is the best summary of these choices.

3. A: Of all the sentences provided, this is the one with which the author would most likely agree. The passage suggests that most of the "mysteries" of the Bermuda Triangle can be explained in a reasonable way. The passage mentions that some expand the Triangle to the Azores, but this is a point of fact, and the author makes no mention of whether or not this is in error. The author quotes the Navy's response to the disappearance of the planes, but there is no reason to believe the author questions this response. The author raises questions about the many myths surrounding the Triangle, but at no point does the author claim that these myths are to blame for the accidents that fall "within the expected margin of error."

4. C: The inclusion of the statement about the ships from East Asia is an opinion statement, as the author provides no support or explanation. The other statements within the answer choices offer supporting evidence and explanatory material, making them acceptable for an expository composition.

5. D: The most compelling argument from researchers stated in the passage is about the fact that the number of accidents in the Bermuda Triangle is within expected margins.

6. D: The best substitute for *discomposed* in the passage would be *disoriented*. There is no evidence given that the planes became inverted or that the pilots were forgetful. There is no way to know if the planes or pilots broke down prior to becoming lost.

7. B: The passage argues that high schools should require that students study a foreign language and gives reasons to support this argument. Choice B accurately describes the main idea of the passage. The passage does say that studying a foreign language is helpful for college acceptance and finding a job, but neither of these points are the main idea of the passage. They are both supporting details. The passage does not say that studying a foreign language will help students gain an understanding of other cultures.

8. C: The passage includes claims that studying a foreign language is helpful for participating in the global economy, being accepted into college, and being a desirable candidate for various jobs. These points are summarized in choice C, making it the best summary of the passage. The passage argues that studying a foreign language should be mandatory, but it does not claim that studying a foreign language is currently essential to high school graduation, so choice A is incorrect. Choices B and D represent claims made in the passage, but do not include all of the claims made.

9. D: Although students may find knowledge of a foreign language helpful for obtaining a job, it is clearly an exaggeration to claim that students who did not study a foreign language are unemployable. Choice A simply lists a fact that can be verified, so it cannot be an exaggeration. Choices B and C include statements that the importance of knowing a foreign language and the acceptance rates for students who have studied a foreign language have increased. These statements simply describe the direction of a trend, so while they can be incorrect, they cannot be exaggerations.

10. D: Choice D can confirm the author's claim that high school graduates who studied a foreign language are more likely to be accepted to college, so it is correct. Choices A and C would provide information regarding the opinions of students and parents, but not actual evidence regarding the influence of studying a foreign language on future success. Choice B specifies a second language taught at home, whereas the passage focuses specifically on a foreign language taught in high school.

11. B: Choice B emphasizes the passage's argument and includes a summary of the main supporting details used to defend it. This makes choice B the best conclusion. Choices A, C, and D each emphasize the passage's main argument, but each one only mentions one supporting detail. These are not effective conclusions, so they are incorrect.

12. D: The author makes their position clear that they believe learning a foreign language should be required of all students in the country, not just for those in the states that choose to have that requirement.

13. D: Only the sentence in choice D indicates an unsupported opinion on the part of the author. The author's use of phrases like "far too hasty" and "undoubtedly" make the information in this sentence subjective to the author, since it cannot be proven whether the scholars' dismissal is too hasty or whether religion's role in the situation is unable to be doubted. All other sentences in the passage offer support or an explanation that is factual and able to be confirmed.

14. C: The author actually says, "Charles's own political troubles extended beyond religion in this case, and he was beheaded in 1649." This would indicate that religion was less involved in this situation than in other situations. There is not enough information to infer that Charles II never married; the passage only notes that he had no legitimate children. (In fact, he had more than ten illegitimate children by his mistresses.) While the chance of a Catholic king frightened many in England, it is reaching beyond logical inference to assume that people were relieved when the royal children died. Finally, the author does not provide enough detail for the reader to assume that James I had no Catholic leanings. The author only says that James acknowledged the Church of England and approved a Protestant translation of the Bible.

15. A: The author notes, "In spite of a strong resemblance to the king, the young James II was generally rejected among the English and the Lowland Scots, who referred to him as "the Pretender." This indicates that there *was* a resemblance, and this increases the likelihood that the child was, in fact, that of James and Mary Beatrice. Answer choice B is too much of an opinion statement that does not have enough support in the passage. The passage essentially refutes answer choice C by pointing out that James "the Pretender" was welcomed in the Highlands. And there is little in the passage to suggest that James was unable to raise an army and mount an attack.

16. B: The passage is composed in a chronological sequence with each king introduced in order of reign, so choice B is correct. While some of the events in the passage may have a cause-and-effect relationship, the organization of the overall passage is not cause and effect. The passage also does not seek to introduce problems and solutions, so choice C is incorrect. While the people mentioned in the passage are compared and contrasted, these comparisons do not dictate the organization of the passage, so choice D is incorrect.

17. D: The passage is largely informative in focus, and the author provides extensive details about this period in English and Scottish history. There is little in the passage to suggest persuasion, and the tone of the passage has no indication of a desire to entertain. Additionally, the passage is historical, so the author avoids expressing feelings and instead focuses on factual information (with the exception of the one opinion statement).

18. D: Paragraph three states that "Charles II died without a legitimate heir, and his brother James ascended to the throne as King James II."

19. C: The author states what he believes to be the current state of the planet's environment and makes practical suggestions for making better use of its resources in the future, so choice C is correct. The author does not express expectations for improvement or regression, nor does the author condemn, complain, or make accusations in his descriptions.

20. B: As the passage states: "Locally grown food and other products manufactured within your community are the best choices. The fewer miles a product traveled to reach you, the fewer resources it required." This is summarized by choice B. The passage does not mention whether buying locally grown food supports community members, uses less packaging, or is healthier to eat, so choices A, C, and D are incorrect.

21. C: The author describes global warming and the depletion of natural resources as constant threats and makes suggestions that can slow or prevent the effects of these threats. This implies that if the author's suggestions are not followed, then these threats will continue. The author does not mention running out of resources in a specific time period, the cost of water and energy, or the possibility of hardship for local farmers.

22. D: The passage states: "You should try to be aware of your consumption of water and energy." The passage then gives examples for decreasing one's use of water and energy. The contexts of these sentences indicate that consumption means the depletion of goods. The passage instructs readers to be aware of their consumption of water and energy, but it does not suggest anything about using the greatest or least amount of water and energy. There also is no information about an illness of the lungs in the passage, so consumption does not refer to lung disease in this context.

23. C: To reduce water and energy, the author suggests that the reader turn off the water when brushing his or her teeth, limit showers to five minutes, turn off lights, and unplug appliances and chargers that are not being used. Choice C includes an item from this list, so it is correct. Choices A and B are statements related to conserving other types of resources, and choice D is a statement that applies to general conservation practices.

24. D: The author begins the third paragraph with, "You can continue to make a difference for the planet in how you use what you bought and the resources you have available." This sentence makes the connection between the second paragraph which deals with what people should buy and the third paragraph which makes suggestions for how to use what they have.

25. B: The author asserts that earning money is easy, but what often challenges people is managing money. This is the main idea of the passage. Choice B says that earning money is less difficult than managing money, so it is correct. Getting a job and the temptation to spend money are both mentioned in the passage as details. However, neither of these are the main idea, so choices A and D are both incorrect. The quote from Franklin does not advocate for working at a mill and does not summarize the main idea, so choice C is also incorrect.

26. D: The author seems to believe that there are plenty of lucrative jobs for everyone, so he or she would doubt that a person really could not find employment. This makes choice D the best choice, as *incredulous* means to struggle to believe something. *Descriptive* means describing, *conciliatory* means satisfying or appeasing, and *ingenuous* means innocent. None of these terms describe the attitude of the author, so choices A, B, and C are incorrect.

27. A: The author insists that many people who have no trouble earning money waste it through lavish spending. There are also several other statements that show the reader that the author believes managing money is more challenging than making it.

28. B: This passage is clearly intended for a non-expert adult readership.

29. D: The author suggests that many people who believe they understand economy in fact do not.

30. A: It seems clear that the author is about to describe the correct means of personal economy.

Word Knowledge

1. A: *Aberration* means a deviation from what is normal or typical. Its Latin roots are *ab-*, meaning away from, and *errare*, meaning to err or stray. Combined, these make up the Latin verb *aberrare*, to go astray (from). There are no other meanings.

2. B: To *abjure* means "to renounce." The original Latin roots are *ab-*, meaning away from, and *jurare*, meaning to swear, which is also the root of the English word jury. Hence "swearing away from" is renouncing, rejecting, or repudiating someone or something, abstaining from or avoiding something, or taking something back.

3. A: *Alchemy* refers to the hypothetical process of turning base metals into gold. While this process does not exist in reality, it was a famously popular pursuit during the Middle Ages. Today this word is also used figuratively to mean turning something common into something precious, or any mysterious transformation. The Medieval Latin *alchymia* derived from the Arabic *al-kimiya*, originating from the Late Greek word *chemeia*.

4. C: *Belligerent* means angry or hostile. Its original sense had to do with waging war. *Belligerare* in Latin means "to wage war," from *bellum*, which means war (as in the English word *antebellum*, meaning prewar), and *gerare*, which means to wage. *Hostilities* in English can refer to warfare and to anger. An English synonym of *belligerent* from the same root is *bellicose*. Both mean warlike, aggressive, combative, etc.

5. A: *Blockade* refers to preventing passage or blocking it. Its similarity to the word *block* makes it easier to define. One difference between *block* and *blockade* is that *blockade* was originally, and is still often, used to refer specifically to military maneuvers intended to block physically the transportation, trade, and communications of enemy nations. It also refers to obstruction of physiological processes and, generally, to any obstruction. It can be used as a transitive verb or a noun.

6. B: The choice closest to the meaning of *bulwark* is *obstacle*. A *bulwark* is a protective, defensive, or supportive structure that is like a wall. Synonyms include rampart, breakwater, and seawall. The (usually) plural term *bulwarks* can also refer to a ship's sides above the upper deck. It is also used abstractly, as in "Democratic ideals provide a bulwark against despotism."

7. D: The adjective *clandestine* means secretive or in secret. The Latin source word *clandestinus* derived from clam, meaning secretly. Secret, and synonyms like covert, furtive, undercover, stealthy, surreptitious, etc., represent the only meaning of this word.

8. A: *Choleric* means easily provoked. Synonyms include hot-tempered, irate, irritable, angry, etc. In ancient Greek civilization, Hippocrates and other physicians subscribed to the theory that the body contained four essential substances they called *humors*: blood, phlegm (mucus), yellow bile, and black bile, which should be balanced. The physician Galen named four temperaments resulting from unbalanced dominance of one humor: *sanguine* with blood, *phlegmatic* with mucus, *melancholic* with yellow bile, and *choleric* with black bile. This is the origin of the word and its meaning.

9. A: A *caucus* is a group with political aims. For example, the National Women's Political Caucus, the National Black Caucus, the National Caucus of Environmental Legislators, the Tea Party Caucus, etc. The origin of this word is unknown. It can mean a closed group meeting of members of a political party or faction to make policy decisions or choose candidates, or a group promoting a cause. There are no other meanings.

10. B: *Conjecture* means guessing or speculation. Synonyms include supposition, inference, and surmise. The Latin *conjectura* is the past participle of the verb *conicere*, meaning literally to throw together. The English word is a noun. It has no alternate meanings.

11. A: The closest choice is *to convey. Disseminate* means to spread or distribute, or to disperse throughout, as is done when sowing seeds. Indeed, the Latin root of this word is *semen*, which means "seed" in English and is the English biological term for male spermatic fluid, i.e., human or animal "seed."

12. B: To *dwindle* means "to decrease," usually steadily. It can be a transitive or intransitive verb, e.g., to make less or to become less. It is thought to originate from the Old English verb *dwinan*, to waste away, probably derived from the Old Norse words *dvina*, to pine away, and/or *deyja*, to die. This word has no alternate definitions.

13. D: To *bubble up* is a synonym for to *effervesce*. The related adjective is *effervescent*, meaning bubbly—literally as in bubbly liquids, or figuratively, as in bubbly personalities. The origin is the Latin verb *fervere*, meaning "to boil." The formatives *ex-* meaning out, and *fervescere*, meaning to begin to boil, combined to produce *effervescere*, meaning to effervesce or boil out, as when steam escapes.

14. D: *Evince* means "to make manifest or demonstrate." Other synonyms include: to show, display, or reveal. The Latin verb *vincere* means to conquer (e.g., Julius Caesar's "*Veni, vidi, vici*" meaning "I came, I saw, I conquered"). Derived from this is *evincere*, to vanquish or win a point.

15. C: *Disentangle* is the best choice as a synonym for *extricate*. It means to remove from entanglement, or to differentiate from something related. Its roots are the Latin *ex-*, meaning out, and *tricae*, meaning trifles or perplexities. These combine to form the verb *extricare*, whose past participle is *extricatus*.

16. C: A *filibuster* is an attempt to disrupt legislation. In United States government, it commonly takes the form of engaging in a lengthy speech on the floor of the Senate, House of Representatives, state legislature, and so on, to delay or prevent voting to pass a law or similar actions. This word's origin, the Spanish *filibustero*, meaning freebooter, is also the source of its other meaning: an irregular military adventurer, specifically an American inciting rebellion in 1850s Latin America. These are the only two definitions.

17. A: *Fortitude* refers to strength of mind or of character that enables someone to have courage in the face of adversity. Its root is the same as the words *fort* and *fortify*. *Fort* means strong in French. All these come from the Latin *fortis*, also meaning strong. (In Shakespeare's play Hamlet, the name of the supporting character Fortinbras transliterates to "strong in arm" in English.) If you chose *endurance* as the answer, this is understandable, as one can *endure* hardship; however, *endurance* refers more to lasting a long time, wearing well, etc., related to durable and duration, from Latin *durare*, to harden or last, from *durus*, or hard, rather than referring to strength. The original meaning of fortitude was simply strength, now considered obsolete, superseded by the current definition of non-physical strength.

18. B: *Genteel* means refined and comes from the French *gentil*, meaning gentle, as in *gentilhomme*, for gentleman. It can mean aristocratic, polite, elegant, or related to the gentry or upper class. Other meanings are connected with appearing or trying to appear socially superior or respectable; being falsely delicate, prudish, or affected; or being conventionally and/or ineffectually pretty, as in artistic style.

19. D: A *tirade* is the nearest synonym to a *harangue*. A *harangue* can simply mean a speech addressing a public assembly. It can also mean a lecture. A third meaning, most commonly used in contemporary English, is a spoken or written rant. While a monologue is also delivered by one person, it does not include the ranting connotations of *harangue* and *tirade*. Diatribe and philippic are other synonyms.

20. C: *Immutable* means unchangeable. The Latin verb *mutare* means to change. Its past participle is *mutates*, the root of the English verb *mutate* and noun *mutation*, as used in biology when genes or viruses mutate, or change in form or characteristics.

21. A: *Jaundice* is a yellowing condition. The French adjective *jaune* means yellow. The Latin root for the French and English words is *galbinus*, or greenish-yellow. When people or animals develop jaundice, their skin and the whites of their eyes turn yellowish. Jaundice is usually due to liver damage or dysfunction; the yellow color comes from a buildup of bile. This word is also used figuratively to mean a feeling of distaste, hostility, or being fed up, as in "a jaundiced attitude" or "a jaundiced view" of something or someone.

22. D: *Deceitfulness* is closest to *knavery* in meaning. In the Middle Ages, a roguish, rascally, mischievous, or tricky, deceitful fellow was called a *knave*. The Jack in a deck of playing cards was also formerly called the Knave. This Middle English word derived from the Old English *cnafa*.

23. C: The closest choice to *languor* is depression. *Languor* means listlessness, apathy, inertia, slowness, sluggishness, or weakness/weariness of the body or mind. The related adjective is *languid*. The root is Latin.

24. A: *Macadamize* means "to pave." The related word *macadam* refers to paving material. It originates from the name of John L. McAdam, a nineteenth-century Scottish engineer who turned road construction into a science and invented the process of *macadamization*. Over time, *macadamize* and *macadam* have evolved to refer to a variety of processes and materials for building roads.

25. B: *Necrosis* refers to tissue death. It shares roots with words like necropsy, necrophilia, and so on. The original root is the Greek *nekros*, meaning dead body. The *necro-* root is used in medical terminology and refers to death.

26. A: *Preclude* is the only synonym for *obviate* among these choices. To *obviate* means to prevent, avert, or forestall; or to render unnecessary. Both meanings incorporate the element of anticipating something in advance. The root is the Latin verb *obviare*, which meant to meet or withstand; the past participle is *obviatus*.

27. C: *Presaged* means foretold. You may recognize the Latin prefix *pre-*, meaning before. The Latin root word *sagus* means prophetic, which is also the root of the English word *seek*. *Presage* can be a verb or a noun.

28. D: *Quarantine* means isolation. *Quadraginta* is the original Latin root. *Quarantine* developed from the Latinate languages French, whose *quarante* means forty, and Italian, with its cognate *quaranta*. It was a custom in the seventeenth century to isolate ships for 40 days to prevent diseases and pests from spreading. In fact, another definition of *quarantine* is a 40-day period.

29. C: To *remunerate* means to pay for something, as in remunerating someone's services or paying someone. Synonyms include to pay, to compensate, or to recompense. In Latin, *munus* means gift. The verb for this noun is *munerare*, to give. Combined with *re-* for back, *remunerare* is to give back, and its past participle is *remuneratus*, the root of remunerate.

30. B: To *scintillate* is to emit light—literally, to sparkle. The Latin noun *scintilla* means spark. This word is also in the English vocabulary. The Latin verb "to sparkle" is *scintillare*; its past participle is *scintillatus*, the English word's root. The adjective *scintillating* is commonly used figuratively to describe a sparkling personality, conversation, or witticism.

Mathematics

1. B: The equation for perimeter of a rectangle is $P = 2l + 2w$. Substitute the perimeter and the length and solve for the width.

$$\begin{aligned} 600 &= 2(250) + 2w \\ 600 &= 500 + 2w \\ 100 &= 2w \\ 50 &= w \end{aligned}$$

Therefore, the width of the garden is 50 yards.

2. B: A prime number is any natural number that can only be divided evenly by 1 or by itself and not by any other numbers. For example, 2, 3, 5, 7, 11, 13, 17, and 19 are the first eight prime numbers in ascending order. Therefore, out of the choices given, 11 is the only prime number. 12 can be evenly divided by 2, 3, 4, and 6. 4 is evenly divisible by 2. 15 is evenly divisible by 3 and 5. Therefore, they are not prime numbers.

3. A: A set of six numbers with an average of 4 must have a collective sum of 24 because $6 \times 4 = 24$. The two numbers that average 2 will add up to 4 ($2 \times 2 = 4$), so the remaining numbers must add up to 20 ($24 - 4 = 20$). The average of these four numbers can be calculated by dividing the sum by the amount of numbers: $20 \div 4 = 5$. Therefore, the average of the other four numbers is 5.

4. A: The expression, "Four more than a number, x," can be interpreted as $x + 4$. This is equal to, "2 less than $\frac{1}{3}$ of another number, y," or $\frac{1}{3}y - 2$. Thus, the equation is $x + 4 = \frac{1}{3}y - 2$.

5. B: Evaluate following the proper order of operations, starting with the operation inside the parentheses and then the exponent. After that, perform the addition.

$$\begin{aligned} 2^3 + (4 + 1) &= 2^3 + 5 \\ &= 8 + 5 \\ &= 13 \end{aligned}$$

6. B: The students making As and Bs represent 70% of the student body ($15\% + 55\% = 70\%$). If 53 students make Ds, that is approximately 10% of the student body.

$$100\% - 70\% - 10\% = 20\%$$

That leaves 20% of the student body to make Cs.

7. C: To solve this problem, first write it as an equation: $27 - x = -5$. From here, solve using normal algebra methods.

$$\begin{aligned} 27 - x &= -5 \\ -x &= -32 \\ x &= 32 \end{aligned}$$

8. B: One simple way to figure this out is by using the fact that $60\% = \frac{6}{10}$. So, if $75 = \frac{6}{10}$, we can find out how much $\frac{1}{10}$ is by dividing 75 by 6.

$$75 \div 6 = 12.5$$

So, 12.5 is $\frac{1}{10}$ of the unknown number. To get that number, just multiply 12.5 by 10.

$$12.5 \times 10 = 125$$

Therefore, 75 is 60% of 125.

9. B: Start by substituting 2 for y.

$$3x - 4(2) = 25$$

Then, solve for x using standard algebra techniques. Start by simplifying on the left side.

$$3x - 8 = 25$$

Next, add 8 to both sides.

$$3x = 33$$

Finally, divide both sides by 3.

$$x = 11$$

10. C: An obtuse triangle has one angle greater than 90°. With a 4-inch side and a 5-inch side, the third side must be either greater than 5 inches or less than 4 inches for it to be an obtuse triangle. 1 inch is too short. The sides could not meet unless they were parallel, that is, a 180° angle. 9 inches is too long to connect with 4-inch and 5-inch sides. At the widest possible angle, the 4-inch side would still be too short to meet the others. 4.6 inches is in between 4 inches and 5 inches, so this makes an acute angle; therefore, the triangle would be acute, not obtuse. 6.4 inches is longer than the 5-inch side (the longer of the two sides given), so the angle is greater than 90° and is therefore obtuse.

11. D: If Nick runs 3 miles in 24 minutes, his rate is $\frac{24}{3} = 8$ minutes per mile. Now we need to find how many miles he can run in 3 hours, or $3 \times 60 = 180$ minutes. We can set up a ratio.

$$\frac{8\text{ min}}{1\text{ mi}} = \frac{180\text{ min}}{x\text{ mi}}$$

Now we cross-multiply.

$$8x = 180(1)$$

Dividing each side by 8 yields $x = 22.5$ miles.

12. C: When converting a percentage to a decimal number, drop the percentage sign and move the decimal point two places to the left. Therefore, 9.47% is equivalent to 0.0947.

13. D: This is multiplication with decimals. It is often easiest to perform the multiplication on the numbers without the decimals and then figure out where to put the decimal in the final result. To do this, convert the decimals to fractions and then multiply.

$$0.25 \times 0.03 = \frac{25}{100} \times \frac{3}{100} = \frac{25 \times 3}{100 \times 100} = \frac{25 \times 3}{10{,}000} \qquad \begin{array}{r} \scriptstyle 1 \\ 25 \\ \times \quad 3 \\ \hline 75 \end{array} \qquad \frac{75}{10{,}000} = 0.0075$$

14. D: To determine the tax, you must calculate 5% of \$340.32. Note that 5% = 0.05. So, you multiply 340.32 by 0.05.

$$\begin{array}{r} 340.32 \\ \times \ 0.05 \\ \hline 17.0160 \end{array}$$

Since you want cents here, the digit 6 rounds up the 1 left of it to a 2, which results in 17.02. Therefore, the additional tax charged on the armoire was \$17.02.

15. A: Jamie had \$6.50 in his wallet. To solve this problem, you subtract \$4.25 and \$2.00 from that amount: \$6.50 − \$4.25 − \$2.00 = \$0.25. So, you are left with \$0.25. Then, you add the \$2.50 that your friend had borrowed: \$0.25 + \$2.50 = \$2.75. Therefore, Jamie currently has \$2.75 in his wallet.

16. B: The common denominator for the denominators 4 and 2 is 4, so convert $\frac{1}{2}$ to a fraction with a denominator of 4.

$$\frac{1}{2}=\frac{2}{4}$$

From here, add the two fractional parts.

$$\frac{3}{4}+\frac{2}{4}=\frac{5}{4}$$

4 divides into 5 once, with $\frac{1}{4}$ left over, so $\frac{5}{4}$ is equal to $1\frac{1}{4}$ as a mixed number. Now, add the whole numbers.

$$8+6=14$$

Finally, add the two parts.

$$14+1\frac{1}{4}=15\frac{1}{4}$$

17. B: If one inch is equal to 2.54 centimeters, then we can multiply any measurement in inches by 2.54 to convert it to centimeters. To multiply decimals, we simply ignore the decimal points and multiply using the traditional algorithm. When finished, we count the total number of digits after the decimal point in each of the factors. The total number of digits after the decimal points in the factors should match the number of digits after the decimal point in the product.

```
    4 3
    2 2
    254
    ×95
 ------
    1 1
   1270
 +22860
 ------
  24130
```

Now, place the decimal 3 places from the right because there are 2 places after the decimal point in 2.54 and 1 place after the decimal point in 9.5. Therefore, the stick is 24.13 centimeters long.

18. D: Divide 4 by 16 to get 0.25. Then move the decimal two places to the right to find the percentage. 0.25 is equivalent to 25%, so the ratio 4 to 16 is equivalent to 25%.

19. A: To find 20% of $\frac{12}{5}$, multiply 20% by $\frac{12}{5}$. Since a percentage can't be multiplied by a fraction, start by converting 20% to a fraction.

$$20\% \times \frac{12}{5}=\frac{20}{100}\times\frac{12}{5}=\frac{240}{500}=\frac{12}{25}$$

Next, convert $\frac{12}{25}$ to a percentage. Do this by converting the fraction to have a denominator of 100, then the value of the numerator will be the percentage.

$$\frac{12\times 4}{25\times 4}=\frac{48}{100}$$

Therefore, 20% of $\frac{12}{5}$ is 48%.

20. A: To find the area of a rectangle, multiply the length by the width.

$$34 \text{ m} \times 12 \text{ m} = 408 \text{ m}^2$$

Therefore, the area of the rectangle is 408 m^2.

21. B: The woman has four days to earn \$250. To find the amount she must earn each day, divide the amount she must earn by 4.

$$\$250 \div 4 = \$62.50$$

Therefore, she must earn \$62.50 each day.

22. C: When subtracting numbers with a decimal point, you borrow the same way as you do when there is no decimal. Thus, the last digits subtract as 4 − 9. Borrow 1 from the 5 and change it into a 4. Then subtract 14 − 9 = 5. The next number is 4 − 3 = 1. The first digits to the left of the decimal are 7 − 8. Borrow 1 from the 9 to the left of the 7, making the 7 into 17: 17 − 8 = 9. The borrowed-from 9 becomes an 8: 8 − 4 = 4. And furthest left, 8 − 0 = 8.

```
 8 17  4 14
8 9 7. 5 4
- 4 8. 3 9
----------
8 4 9. 1 5
```

23. D: Recall that the general form of a quadratic expression is $ax^2 + bx + c$. A great way to factor quadratic expression like this, where $a = 1$ and all the answer choices are integer factors, would be to consider the factors of the last term, c. Specifically, any two factors of c that would add to b. Essentially: $f_1 \times f_2 = -12$ and $f_1 + f_2 = 1$. We can check the factors of −12.

f_1	f_2	$f_1 + f_2$
12	-1	11
6	-2	4
4	-3	1
3	-4	-1
2	-6	-4
1	-12	-11

From this the only option that works is 4 and −3, which means the expression factors as $(x + 4)(x - 3)$.

24. C: Since 1 meter equals 100 centimeters, the conversion factor is 100. Since a meter is longer than a centimeter, we multiply by the conversion factor.

$$6 \text{ m} \times \frac{100 \text{ cm}}{1 \text{ m}} = 600 \text{ cm}$$

So, there are 600 centimeters in 6 meters.

25. D: To compare these two quantities, you need to find a common denominator between 3 and 4. The simplest way to do this is to multiply the numerator and denominator of each fraction by the other denominator.

$$\frac{2}{3} = \frac{2 \times 4}{3 \times 4} = \frac{8}{12}$$

Do the same with the second fraction.

$$\frac{1}{4} = \frac{1 \times 3}{4 \times 3} = \frac{3}{12}$$

So, if you have $\frac{3}{12}$ cup of oil and you need a total of $\frac{8}{12}$ cup, you need $\frac{5}{12}$ cup more because $\frac{8}{12} - \frac{3}{12} = \frac{5}{12}$.

26. B: If $\frac{1}{2}$ cup of skim milk has 45 calories, then 1 cup has 90 calories ($45 \times 2 = 90$). So $\frac{1}{4}$ cup is equivalent to $90 \div 4 = 22.5$ calories. For $\frac{3}{4}$, multiply 22.5 calories by 3 to get 67.5 calories, which is $67\frac{1}{2}$.

27. B: The average is the total amount spent divided by the number of students. The first three students spend an average of $10, so the total amount they spend is 3 × $10 = $30. The other six students spend an average of $4, so the total amount they spend is 6 × $4 = $24. The total amount spent by all nine students is $30 + $24 = $54, and the average amount they spend is $54 ÷ 9 = $6.

28. C: To find the total percentage taken out, add the two percentages.

$$35\% + 4\% = 39\%$$

Therefore, 39% was taken out of the paycheck.

29. A: To solve, you will need to move the decimal 4 places. Since the scientific notation has a negative power of 10, move the decimal left. If the power of 10 is positive, you need to move it to the right.

$$7.4 \times 10^{-4} = 7.4 \times 0.0001 = 0.00074$$

Therefore, the standard form of the diameter of a red blood cell is 0.00074 centimeters.

30. D: Since 1 meter equals 1,000 millimeters, the conversion factor is 1,000. Since a millimeter is shorter than a meter, we divide by the conversion factor.

$$336 \text{ mm} \times \frac{1 \text{ m}}{1{,}000 \text{ mm}} = 0.336 \text{ m}$$

So, 336 millimeters is equal to 0.336 meters.

31. B: Since five people are splitting $17.90, each person's share can be calculated by dividing the total price by 5.

$$17.90 \div 5 = 3.58$$

Each person will pay $3.58.

32. C: In the decimal system, whole numbers are left of the decimal point. One decimal place to the right of the decimal point is the tenths place, two places to the right is the hundredths place, three places to the right is the thousandths place, and so on. Therefore, 0.10 represents one tenth, which is $\frac{1}{10}$ as a fraction.

33. A: To solve, test each answer. Notice that in choice A the numerator has been multiplied by 3 to get 12. The denominator has also been multiplied by 3 to get 21. In choice B, the numerator has been multiplied by 4 and the denominator has been multiplied by 5. In choice C, the numerator has been multiplied by 3 and the denominator has been multiplied by 4. In choice D, the numerator has been multiplied by 4 and the denominator has been multiplied by 5. Therefore, choice A is the only correct equation.

34. C: To multiply mixed numbers, first convert them all to improper fractions. Multiply the whole number by the denominator, then add the numerator. $1\frac{1}{4}$ becomes $\frac{5}{4}$, $3\frac{2}{5}$ becomes $\frac{17}{5}$, and $1\frac{2}{3}$ becomes $\frac{5}{3}$. Now, multiply all the numerators together and then all the denominators together.

$$\frac{5}{4} \times \frac{17}{5} \times \frac{5}{3} = \frac{5 \times 17 \times \cancel{5}}{4 \times \cancel{5} \times 3} = \frac{85}{12} = 7\frac{1}{12}$$

35. A: Lindsay used the following calculations to convert 2 ounces to teaspoons:

$$2 \text{ ounces} \times \frac{1 \text{ pint}}{16 \text{ ounces}} \times \frac{2 \text{ cups}}{1 \text{ pint}} \times \frac{16 \text{ tablespoons}}{1 \text{ cup}} \times \frac{3 \text{ teaspoons}}{1 \text{ tablespoon}} = 12 \text{ teaspoons}$$

36. C: Start by calculating how much the man lost.

$$\$40 + \$30 = \$70$$

Then, subtract that amount from the amount he had originally.

$$\$125 - \$70 = \$55$$

The man has $55 left.

37. A: There are three fractions: $\frac{1}{4}$, $\frac{1}{8}$, and $\frac{1}{2}$. To answer the question, they must be added. The common denominator is 8, so express each fraction with a denominator of 8 and then add the fractions.

$$\frac{1}{2} + \frac{1}{4} + \frac{1}{8} = \frac{4}{8} + \frac{2}{8} + \frac{1}{8} = \frac{7}{8}$$

Among just the first three people, the dog is being taken care of $\frac{7}{8}$ of the time. Therefore, to calculate the proportion of time the fourth person will have to care for the dog, subtract $\frac{7}{8}$ from 1 whole, or $\frac{8}{8}$.

$$\frac{8}{8} - \frac{7}{8} = \frac{1}{8}$$

Therefore, the fourth person will have to take care of the dog $\frac{1}{8}$ of the time.

38. C: If it takes 3 people $3\frac{1}{3}$ days to do the job, then it would take one person 10 days: $3 \times 3\frac{1}{3} = 10$. Thus, it would take 2 people 5 days, and one day of work for two people would complete $\frac{1}{5}$ of the job.

39. A: To find the slope of this equation, choose any two points to use in the slope equation. For example, (1,3.60) and (2,7.20).

$$m = \frac{y_2 - y_1}{x_2 - x_1} = \frac{7.20 - 3.60}{2 - 1} = \frac{3.60}{1} = 3.60$$

The table indicates that for each hour of rental, the cost increases by $3.60. This corresponds to the slope of the equation. Of course, if the bicycle is not rented at all (0 hours), there will be no charge ($0). If plotted on the Cartesian plane, the line would have a y-intercept of 0. Therefore, the equation of the line is $C = 3.60h$.

40. C: To start, we can write our ratio in fractional form as $\frac{2 \text{ cups of water}}{6 \text{ cups of flour}}$. We know Josie wants to lessen the flour to only 2 cups, making our proportion $\frac{2 \text{ cups of water}}{6 \text{ cups of flour}} = \frac{x \text{ cups of water}}{2 \text{ cups of flour}}$. To find the value of x, we can cross multiply the two diagonal values we know, 2 and 2, and divide their product by the remaining value, 6. $2 \times 2 = 4$, and $4 \div 6 = \frac{4}{6}$, which simplifies to $\frac{2}{3}$. This means Josie should use $\frac{2}{3}$ of a cup of water for every 2 cups of flour.

Science

1. A: Cardiac output is total volume of blood that is pumped by the heart over a certain period of time. This value is typically reported in the amount of liters per minute. Cardiac output is determined by the product of heart rate and stroke volume. Heart rate is the number of heart beats per minute and stroke volume is the amount of blood that is pumped by the left ventricle in each heart beat or contraction. A typical heart can pump approximately 5 liters of blood per minute. As the intensity of exercise increases, the cardiac output can increase as high as 40 liters per minute. An individual's heart rate will increase linearly until the maximum level is reached. Stroke volume, however, tends to increase to approximately 40-50% of the maximum and will then level off. Aerobic exercise helps to strengthen the heart, pump blood more efficiently and increase stroke volume.

2. A: Blood leaves the heart's right ventricle and goes to the lungs. The kidneys and the rest of the body receive blood from the left ventricle. The right atrium, as well as the left atrium, holds blood coming to the heart via the blood vessels; each atrium empties into the corresponding ventricle.

3. D: Anaerobic cellular metabolism refers to processes of breaking things down and converting them to other substances (metabolites) in the body's cells. Anaerobic means these processes do not use or require oxygen. Metabolic processes not involving oxygen do not affect heart rate. Increases in body temperature and physical activity increase the heart rate as the heart works harder to pump blood-supplying oxygen to the body. The concentrations of calcium, sodium, and potassium ions do affect heart rate. These ions, known as electrolytes, must stay in balance to regulate heart rate. If they are balanced, heart function is not affected, but with imbalance, cardiac function will be elevated (excess calcium) or depressed (excess potassium or sodium). Sodium deficiency causes cardiac fibrillation.

4. D: The three layers of the heart are the epicardium (outermost), myocardium (middle), and endocardium (innermost). "Vasocardium" is not a layer of the heart or even a legitimate term. The adjectives "vasocardial" or "vasocardiac" are used to refer to anything related to both blood vessels (vaso-) and heart (cardiac), as with the "vasocardial system." A related term with the order of parts reversed is "cardiovascular system."

5. C: The hormone aldosterone is secreted by the adrenal glands and regulates the levels of sodium and potassium ions (electrolytes). Aldosterone stimulates excretion of potassium and reabsorption of sodium into the bloodstream. It maintains blood pressure and body fluids. Too much aldosterone can increase the blood volume and hence the blood pressure. Estrogen is a hormone of the female reproductive system and testosterone is a hormone of the male reproductive system. Dopamine is a neurotransmitter associated with the brain's pleasure and reward circuits, and also with the regulation of motor control.

6. B: Bradycardia means a slower heartbeat than normal. The combining form *brady-* is from the Greek *bradys* meaning slow. Tachycardia means a faster heartbeat than normal. (*Tachy-* from Greek *tachos* means speed, as also in "tachometer.") Fibrillation means uncoordinated, ineffectual heart movements. A myocardial infarct is a type of heart attack.

7. A: Hematocrit is the red blood cell portion of the blood. Plasma is mainly water, plus some plasma proteins, blood glucose, and so on. Normal levels of hematocrit are around 36% to 45% for women, and about 40% to 50% for men. Thus, an approximate normal level is around 45%. A hematocrit >50% can cause blood clots and heart attacks with exertion. If a hematocrit is 45%, it follows that the remaining plasma portion of the blood would be 55%.

8. D: The muscular system includes muscles, which allow a person's body to move. The integumentary system (A) includes organs such as the skin. While injuries to the skin can limit a person's range of movement, it does not enable movement. The digestive system (B) allows a person to eat and digest food, but does not allow a person to move. The endocrine system (C) is related to hormones, not a person's ability to move.

9. C: The fraction of offspring that that have the genotype BbSs is $\frac{4}{16}$. A dihybrid cross considers two traits at a time, in this case, eye color and hair color. In the parent (P) generation, a parent with the genotype BBSS would be crossed with a parent with the genotype bbss. The offspring are considered the F1 generation and all would have the genotype BbSs. This question asks about the F2 generation, which is the offspring between a cross of the F1 generation. Therefore, the parent genotypes in this question would be BbSs. To solve, develop a Punnet square of 16 cells. Each parent will produce the following gametes: BS, Bs, bS, bs. Place these across the top and the side. After completing the square, the resulting offspring show that four would have the genotype BbSs.

P → F1

	BS
bs	BbSs

F1 → F2

	BS	**Bs**	**bS**	**bs**
BS	BBSS	BBSs	BbSS	BbSs
Bs	BBSs	BBss	BbSs	Bbss
bS	BbSS	BbSs	bbSS	bbSs
bs	BbSs	Bbss	bbSs	bbss

10. B: Atelectasis is the medical term for collapse of a lung. Its Greek roots are *ateles*, incomplete or defective, and *ektasis*, extension or stretching out, as a collapsed lung cannot inflate and expand properly. Anoxia literally means no oxygen. It commonly refers to a lack of oxygen to the brain, especially in a fetus before or during childbirth. Dyspnea means difficulty breathing. Hypercapnia means too much carbon dioxide (a waste product of aerobic respiration) in the blood.

11. A: The central nervous system is another term for the brain and the spinal cord. It does not include the peripheral nerves (peripheral is the opposite of central) or the muscular system. Choices omitting the brain are necessarily incorrect.

12. C: The brain is composed of four lobes: the frontal lobe, the parietal lobe in the midbrain, the temporal lobe at the bottom, and the occipital lobe at the back. Some people also refer specifically to the left and right of each lobe. This is because the brain has two hemispheres (left and right), so each lobe also has two hemispheres. Each lobe has different functions.

13. C: Homeostasis is a state of equilibrium, or balance, within the body. The natural tendency is to maintain or restore homeostasis. Peristalsis is the wavelike muscular contractions of the digestive system to process food. Stomatitis is an inflammation of the mouth's mucosa.

14. D: Stomatitis is a state of oral inflammation, usually caused by viral or bacterial infection. Diverticulitis is inflammation of a diverticulum, or an abnormal pouch, in the wall of the large intestine. Hepatitis is inflammation of the liver. Enteritis is inflammation of the small intestine.

15. D: The most important male hormone is testosterone. Estrogen is the most important female hormone. Aldosterone is a hormone that regulates blood volume and pressure in both sexes. Progesterone is the second most important female hormone.

16. B: Bile production is a function of the liver, not of the kidneys. The kidneys filter the blood to clean it, removing waste products like urea and ammonium, excreting them in urine. They secrete hormones such as renin, calcitriol, and erythropoietin. The kidneys also reabsorb water, glucose, and amino acids.

17. A: Enuresis is the medical term for uncontrolled urination. A diuretic is an agent (a drug or substance) that stimulates urination. (Diuretics are not the same as enuresis but can cause it.) Pyuria means pus in the urine. Ureteritis means an inflammation of the ureter(s), muscular tubes that send urine from the kidneys into the bladder.

18. C: Auditory impulses, meaning sounds received through the ears, are interpreted in the brain's temporal lobes. Acoustic impulses travel through the external ear canal, are amplified and transmitted by the middle ear mechanism, converted into electrical energy in the inner ear's cochlea, and sent via the auditory nerve to the primary auditory cortex in the temporal lobe for analysis.

19. B: The eye's outer layer is the sclera, or the white of the eye. The cornea is the clear, protuberant, main refractive surface at the eye's front. The retina is a layered sensory tissue lining the eye's inner surface that is sensitive to light that creates images of what the eye sees. The retina contains two kinds of photoreceptors: rods and cones. Cones are responsible for color vision and high visual acuity. Rods are responsible for peripheral vision, night vision/low-light vision, and detecting motion.

20. B: The relationship between the clown fish and the sea anemone is an example of mutualism - because both organisms are benefitting from the relationship. The Clown fish gains the protection from the anemone while offering protection to the anemone from being eaten by a certain type of fish.

21. D: Halogens are nonmetallic chemical elements. There are five halogens: fluorine, chlorine, bromine, iodine, and astatine. At room temperature, iodine and astatine are solids, bromine is a liquid, and fluorine and chlorine are gases. Cesium is not a halogen; it is a metal element.

22. A: In the periodic table of the chemical elements, the numbers of the periods 1, 2, 3, and so forth, are listed vertically in a column on the left, and each period runs horizontally across the table. The groups 1, 2, 3, et cetera, are listed horizontally, and each group runs vertically down the table.

23. C: Condensation is the process whereby gas is converted to liquid. For example, when water vapor (a gas) in the air is cooled, it becomes liquid. This is how condensation forms on the outside of a glass containing cold liquid. Evaporation is the opposite: the process of a liquid becoming a gas, as when water evaporates into the air. Sublimation is the process of a solid becoming a gas, as with dry ice.

24. B: Isomers are compounds with the same shapes even if their structures vary. Polar compounds are molecules with polar covalent bonds; electromagnetically, their electrons are not equally shared in chemical bonds. Variables in the sciences are any entities or factors that can change. Experimenters manipulate variables to determine their effects on other variables. In research, a variable can be a logical set of attributes. A transient compound is one that disappears rapidly in the body.

25. A: The kinetic energy of the gas molecules is directly proportional to the temperature. If the temperature decreases, so does the molecular motion. A decrease in temperature will not necessarily mean a gas condenses to a liquid. Neither the mass nor the density is impacted, as no material was added or removed, and the volume remained the same.

26. B: Charles' Law is also known as the law of volumes. It describes how gases expand when heated. Boyle's law states that for a given mass at a constant temperature, the product of pressure times volume is a constant. Johnson's Law, attributed to California Senator Hiram Johnson (1918), states that "the first casualty when war comes is truth." Dr. Samuel Johnson (1730) had stated the same principle in much wordier terms. Avogadro's Law states that when a gas is at a constant temperature and pressure, its volume is in direct proportion to the number of moles of gas. These are all gas laws except Johnson's.

27. B: The direction of the electric field is the same as the direction of the force on a positive test charge. Moving a negative charge in the direction of the electric field requires an external force to oppose the electric field. This would increase the electron's potential energy.

28. C: Acids increase the number of hydrogen ions in water. The pH scale measures how acidic or basic a liquid is. Hydrogen ions and hydroxide ions are the focus of pH. The strongest acids have low pH values: 0–4. High pH values (10–14) are found in the strongest bases or alkali, the opposites of acids. Sodium hydroxide is a base or alkaline compound. When dissolved in water, acids break down to hydrogen (H^+) ions and another compound, while bases break down to hydroxide (OH^-) ions and another compound.

29. B: If the chemicals heat up, their temperatures increase, and their kinetic energies therefore increase, so energy could not have been obtained from kinetic energy. Chemical reactions also do not typically involve absorption of heat from the environment. Instead, chemical bonds contain some amount of potential energy, which may be released in certain chemical reactions.

30. A: Newton's Second law of motion states that when all existing forces are not balanced, the acceleration of an object depends on the net force acting on the object and the object's mass. When net force is represented as F_{net} and mass as m, and acceleration as a, net force is the product of mass times acceleration, or $F_{net} = ma$. $Speed = \frac{Distance}{Time}$ is the equation of the basic formula for calculating velocity. $Power = \frac{F \times D}{T}$ is the basic power equation: work done, that is, force times distance, divided by time. The formula of voltage times amperes is for calculating watts, or units of power, in the measurement of electrical energy.

31. C: In a pond, plants produce oxygen as a byproduct of photosynthesis. During eutrophication, plants die and decompose, causing increased levels of carbon dioxide. Fish cannot relocate from the pond, and they cannot live without oxygen, so they would die.

32. D: Blood is cooled as it passes through capillaries surrounding the sweat glands. Heat is absorbed along with excess salt and water and transferred to the glands as sweat. Droplets of sweat then evaporate from the skin surface to dissipate heat and cool the body. The kidney, bladder, and liver are not involved in regulating body temperature.

33. C: In humans, diploid cells are those that contain 46 chromosomes. There are 23 pairs of chromosomes each made up of one chromosome from the father and one from the mother. In meiosis I, each chromosome replicates itself and lines up, or synapses, with its homologous chromosome, and each of the daughter cells ends up with one copy of each of the chromosomes. The two daughter cells at the end of meiosis I are haploid because they contain half of the chromosomes of the parent cell. In humans, this would be 23 chromosomes. However, each of these chromosomes are made of two sister chromatids. In meiosis II, the sister chromatids in the daughter cells separate and result in the production of the gametes. These are also haploid cells because they contain one copy of half of the genetic material of the parent cell. Four haploid cells result from meiosis. Choice A, mitosis, can be eliminated as it refers to the process of cell division where each daughter cell contains exactly the same genetic material as the parent cell. Choice B, telophase, refers to phases of both mitosis and meiosis, during which chromosomes move toward the opposite ends of the cell.

34. D: The epiglottis covers the trachea during swallowing, thus preventing food from entering the airway. The trachea, also known as the windpipe, is a cylindrical portion of the respiratory tract that joins the larynx with the lungs. The esophagus connects the throat and the stomach. When a person swallows, the esophagus contracts to force the food down into the stomach. Like many other structures in the digestive and respiratory systems, the esophagus secretes mucus for lubrication.

35. B: The pads that support the vertebrae are made up of cartilage. Cartilage, a strong form of connective tissue, cushions and supports the joints. Cartilage also makes up the larynx and the outer ear. Bone is a form of connective tissue that makes up the majority of the skeleton. It includes both organic and inorganic substances. Tendons connect the muscles to other structures of the body, typically bones. Tendons can increase and decrease in length as the bones move. Fat is a combination of lipids; in humans, fat forms a layer beneath the skin and on the outside of the internal organs.

36. B: A decrease in a natural predator, such as a wolves, coyotes, bobcat, or wild dogs, would allow the population to become out of control. In a population of deer that has increased, there would be a natural decrease in a food source for the nutritional needs for the animals. Although deer have been known to share a human's developed habitat, it is often forced by reduced territory and food sources. An increase in hunting licenses would be used by local officials to try to control the population, helping to decrease the number of adults of breeding age.

37. B: The vertical axis of this graph is an exponential scale, with each regularly-spaced tick mark corresponding to a ten-fold increase in the quantity being measured. The curve corresponding to the control cells, those grown in the absence of the drug, shows a cell concentration of approximately 500 cells/mL at the start, 5000 cells/mL after 4 days, and 50,000 cells per mL after 8 days, indicating an exponential growth pattern in which the number of cells increases by a factor of ten every four days.

38. B: To determine the average number of neutrons in one atom of an element, subtract the atomic number from the average atomic mass. For bromine (Br), subtract its atomic number (35) from its average atomic mass (79.9) to acquire the average number of neutrons, 44.9.

39. A: The number of protons is the same for every atom of a given element and is the element's atomic number: in this case, 30 for zinc (Zn).

40. B: The conclusion was that the amount of sunlight received by the plants was affecting their growth. The independent variable was the amount of light that was given to the plants and could have been manipulated by the experimenter by moving the plants or adding equal parts of light. No hypothesis was clearly stated in this experiment.

41. B: Recessive alleles are represented by lowercase letters, while dominant alleles are represented by uppercase letters. Organisms that are *homozygous* for a trait have two identical alleles (BB or bb), while those that are *heterozygous* for a trait have two different alleles (Bb).

42. D: Species may theoretically be able to inhabit a particular area, called its fundamental niche. But the presence of competing species may mean that it only occupies part of its niche, called a realized niche.

43. A: Since like charges repel and opposite charges attract, putting a dipole in an electric field would cause the dipole to orient so that its negative side will point towards the electric field's positive side. Since electric fields flow from positive towards negative, an electric field pointing from south to north could be caused by positive charges in the south and negative charges in the north. Consequently, the dipole will line up opposite to this, with the positive charge on the north side. Answer B is not correct because such an orientation would be unstable. The least disturbance would cause the dipole to flip 180°.

44. D: The nucleus is the home for the chromosomes. These chromosomes are made of DNA and a protein component. The chromosomes have the genetic code in a certain sequence of bases that make up the DNA chain.

45. A: Mitochondria give chemical energy for the cell in the form of ATP (i.e., adenosine triphosphate). They give energy by converting nutritional energy sources (e.g., glucose) through a complex series of chemical reactions. These reactions take place on the extensive membrane system located in the mitochondria's outer membranes.

46. C: The data indicates that up until about 4 weeks, the silk production from both colonies was similar. This suggests that the worms from each colony produced the same amount of silk, and that choices A and B are incorrect. The data does indicate that, over the long term, the silk produced by the entire colony of genetically diverse worms was greater than the silk produced by the entire colony of genetically uniform worms. This might be because the worms produce for a longer time, or because of some other mechanism. The experiment does not indicate what that mechanism might be.

47. B: The increase in productivity from the diverse culture occurs at about 4 weeks, coinciding with the time at which new worms are hatched and begin to produce silk.

48. C: The number of 7 is the "breaking point" between basic and acidic. Above 7 solutions are considered basic; below 7 solutions are considered acidic. For instance, milk, with a pH of 6.5, is actually considered acidic. Bleach, with a pH of 12.5, is considered basic.

49. B: The transverse plane separates the body into upper and lower portions. The oblique plane is when a cylindrical organ is sectioned with an angular cut across the organ. The midsagittal or medial plane refers to a lengthwise cut that divides the body into equal right and left portions. The frontal or coronal plane refers to a cut that divides the body into anterior and posterior sections.

50. C: Producers always form the base of an energy pyramid as the first trophic level. Each successive level receives about 10% of the energy from the previous level. In this energy pyramid, the second trophic level receives 10% of 6,000 or 600 kilocalories per square meter per year. The third trophic level receives 10% of 600, or 60 kilocalories per square meter per year.

51. B: Catalysts alter the activation energy during a chemical reaction and therefore control the rate of the reaction. The substrate is the actual surface that enzymes use during a chemical reaction (and there is no such term as *substrate energy*). Inhibitors and promoters participate in the chemical reaction, but it is the activation energy that catalysts alter to control the overall rate as the reaction occurs.

52. C: By repeating the experiment, the researcher could determine whether the instance of the bacteria swimming away from the chemical was simply due to chance. Observing the same results would allow the researcher to make conclusions with more certainty, and statistical analysis would help determine the significance of the data. Researchers must report all data (A), and reaching a conclusion is a vital part of any experiment (B). Adding a new chemical would completely change the experiment, so it would not be helpful (D).

53. C: Mitochondria are often called the power house of the cell because they provide energy for the cell to function. The nucleus is the control center for the cell. The cell membrane surrounds the cell and separates the cell from its environment. Cytoplasm is the thick fluid within the cell membrane that surrounds the nucleus and contains organelles.

54. C: Lactic acid fermentation converts pyruvate into lactate using high-energy electrons from NADH. This process allows ATP production to continue in anaerobic conditions by providing NAD^+ so that ATP can be made in glycolysis.

55. B: Cells differentiate so that simple, less specialized cells can become highly specialized cells. For example, humans are multicellular organisms who undergo cell differentiation numerous times. Cells begin as simple zygotes after fertilization and then differentiate to form a myriad of complex tissues and systems before birth.

56. C: Both meiosis and mitosis occur in humans, other animals, and plants. Mitosis produces cells that are genetically identical, and meiosis produces cells that are genetically different. Only mitosis occurs asexually.

57. A: A lysosome is an organelle that is thought to be linked to the aging process and contains digestive enzymes that break down food and unneeded substances. Chromatin is the structure created by DNA and various proteins in the cell nucleus during interphase and condenses to form chromosomes. Plastids are found in plants and algae. They often contain pigments and usually help make chemical compounds for the plant. The Golgi apparatus prepares macromolecules like proteins and lipids for transport.

58. D: A covalent bond is one in which atoms share valence electrons. Within a water molecule, one oxygen atom and two hydrogen atoms share valence electrons to yield the H_2O structure.

59. B: The phenomenon known as weightlessness is caused by an object being in free fall. An object in space still experiences a gravitational force due to the earth, but if that object is in orbit, it's effectively free falling around the earth, which causes it to experience weightlessness. Here, proposition I is wrong because you have to be pretty far away from a star for gravity to become negligible. In fact, objects only stay in orbit because the earth's gravity pulls on them and causes them to change direction. This means the usual experience of weight is lost, as you can see by the floating objects and people inside an orbiting spaceship. The same thing happens to a ski jumper, who is in free fall after he or she jumps. If the jumper is carrying a rock, for example, that rock will feel weightless while the jumper is in the air. A rolled baseball is not in freefall and does not experience weightlessness.

60. C: The amount that a transparent medium slows down the speed of light through it is called the index of refraction. The normal line (A) is an imaginary line that runs at a right angle to the surface of a medium; in the example given, it would be the waterline in the glass of water. The wavelength (B) of the light becomes shorter in proportion to how much the speed of light is slowed by the medium (but the medium does not change the frequency of the light wave, which is a property of the light source). The angle of refraction (D) is the degree to which the light wave is bent by the medium. As an example of refraction indices, diamonds trap light and slow its speed more than water because they are much denser and harder than water; thus, they sparkle more than water does and have a higher index of refraction than water.

Image Credits

LICENSED UNDER CC BY 4.0 (CREATIVECOMMONS.ORG/LICENSES/BY/4.0/)

Meiosis: "Meiosis Overview New" by Wikimedia user Rdbickel (https://commons.wikimedia.org/wiki/File:Meiosis_Overview_new.svg)

LICENSED UNDER CC BY 3.0 (CREATIVECOMMONS.ORG/LICENSES/BY/3.0/)

Biomagnification Mercury: "Mercury Food Chain" by Bretwood Higman (https://commons.wikimedia.org/wiki/File:MercuryFoodChain.svg)

Energy Flow: "Trophic Web" by Wikimedia user Thompsma (https://en.wikipedia.org/wiki/File:TrophicWeb.jpg)

LICENSED UNDER CC BY-SA 3.0 (CREATIVECOMMONS.ORG/LICENSES/BY-SA/3.0/DEED.EN)

Secondary Succession: "Secondary Succession" by Wikimedia user Katelyn Murphy (https://commons.wikimedia.org/wiki/File:Secondary_Succession.png)

PAX Practice Tests #2 and #3

To take these additional PAX practice tests, visit our bonus page:
mometrix.com/bonus948/pax

How to Overcome Test Anxiety

Just the thought of taking a test is enough to make most people a little nervous. A test is an important event that can have a long-term impact on your future, so it's important to take it seriously and it's natural to feel anxious about performing well. But just because anxiety is normal, that doesn't mean that it's helpful in test taking, or that you should simply accept it as part of your life. Anxiety can have a variety of effects. These effects can be mild, like making you feel slightly nervous, or severe, like blocking your ability to focus or remember even a simple detail.

If you experience test anxiety—whether severe or mild—it's important to know how to beat it. To discover this, first you need to understand what causes test anxiety.

Causes of Test Anxiety

While we often think of anxiety as an uncontrollable emotional state, it can actually be caused by simple, practical things. One of the most common causes of test anxiety is that a person does not feel adequately prepared for their test. This feeling can be the result of many different issues such as poor study habits or lack of organization, but the most common culprit is time management. Starting to study too late, failing to organize your study time to cover all of the material, or being distracted while you study will mean that you're not well prepared for the test. This may lead to cramming the night before, which will cause you to be physically and mentally exhausted for the test. Poor time management also contributes to feelings of stress, fear, and hopelessness as you realize you are not well prepared but don't know what to do about it.

Other times, test anxiety is not related to your preparation for the test but comes from unresolved fear. This may be a past failure on a test, or poor performance on tests in general. It may come from comparing yourself to others who seem to be performing better or from the stress of living up to expectations. Anxiety may be driven by fears of the future—how failure on this test would affect your educational and career goals. These fears are often completely irrational, but they can still negatively impact your test performance.

Elements of Test Anxiety

As mentioned earlier, test anxiety is considered to be an emotional state, but it has physical and mental components as well. Sometimes you may not even realize that you are suffering from test anxiety until you notice the physical symptoms. These can include trembling hands, rapid heartbeat, sweating, nausea, and tense muscles. Extreme anxiety may lead to fainting or vomiting. Obviously, any of these symptoms can have a negative impact on testing. It is important to recognize them as soon as they begin to occur so that you can address the problem before it damages your performance.

The mental components of test anxiety include trouble focusing and inability to remember learned information. During a test, your mind is on high alert, which can help you recall information and stay focused for an extended period of time. However, anxiety interferes with your mind's natural processes, causing you to blank out, even on the questions you know well. The strain of testing during anxiety makes it difficult to stay focused, especially on a test that may take several hours. Extreme anxiety can take a huge mental toll, making it difficult not only to recall test information but even to understand the test questions or pull your thoughts together.

Effects of Test Anxiety

Test anxiety is like a disease—if left untreated, it will get progressively worse. Anxiety leads to poor performance, and this reinforces the feelings of fear and failure, which in turn lead to poor performances on subsequent tests. It can grow from a mild nervousness to a crippling condition. If allowed to progress, test anxiety can have a big impact on your schooling, and consequently on your future.

Test anxiety can spread to other parts of your life. Anxiety on tests can become anxiety in any stressful situation, and blanking on a test can turn into panicking in a job situation. But fortunately, you don't have to let anxiety rule your testing and determine your grades. There are a number of relatively simple steps you can take to move past anxiety and function normally on a test and in the rest of life.

Physical Steps for Beating Test Anxiety

While test anxiety is a serious problem, the good news is that it can be overcome. It doesn't have to control your ability to think and remember information. While it may take time, you can begin taking steps today to beat anxiety.

Just as your first hint that you may be struggling with anxiety comes from the physical symptoms, the first step to treating it is also physical. Rest is crucial for having a clear, strong mind. If you are tired, it is much easier to give in to anxiety. But if you establish good sleep habits, your body and mind will be ready to perform optimally, without the strain of exhaustion. Additionally, sleeping well helps you to retain information better, so you're more likely to recall the answers when you see the test questions.

Getting good sleep means more than going to bed on time. It's important to allow your brain time to relax. Take study breaks from time to time so it doesn't get overworked, and don't study right before bed. Take time to rest your mind before trying to rest your body, or you may find it difficult to fall asleep.

Along with sleep, other aspects of physical health are important in preparing for a test. Good nutrition is vital for good brain function. Sugary foods and drinks may give a burst of energy but this burst is followed by a crash, both physically and emotionally. Instead, fuel your body with protein and vitamin-rich foods.

Also, drink plenty of water. Dehydration can lead to headaches and exhaustion, especially if your brain is already under stress from the rigors of the test. Particularly if your test is a long one, drink water during the breaks. And if possible, take an energy-boosting snack to eat between sections.

Along with sleep and diet, a third important part of physical health is exercise. Maintaining a steady workout schedule is helpful, but even taking 5-minute study breaks to walk can help get your blood pumping faster and clear your head. Exercise also releases endorphins, which contribute to a positive feeling and can help combat test anxiety.

When you nurture your physical health, you are also contributing to your mental health. If your body is healthy, your mind is much more likely to be healthy as well. So take time to rest, nourish your body with healthy food and water, and get moving as much as possible. Taking these physical steps will make you stronger and more able to take the mental steps necessary to overcome test anxiety.

Mental Steps for Beating Test Anxiety

Working on the mental side of test anxiety can be more challenging, but as with the physical side, there are clear steps you can take to overcome it. As mentioned earlier, test anxiety often stems from lack of preparation, so the obvious solution is to prepare for the test. Effective studying may be the most important weapon you have for beating test anxiety, but you can and should employ several other mental tools to combat fear.

First, boost your confidence by reminding yourself of past success—tests or projects that you aced. If you're putting as much effort into preparing for this test as you did for those, there's no reason you should expect to fail here. Work hard to prepare; then trust your preparation.

Second, surround yourself with encouraging people. It can be helpful to find a study group, but be sure that the people you're around will encourage a positive attitude. If you spend time with others who are anxious or cynical, this will only contribute to your own anxiety. Look for others who are motivated to study hard from a desire to succeed, not from a fear of failure.

Third, reward yourself. A test is physically and mentally tiring, even without anxiety, and it can be helpful to have something to look forward to. Plan an activity following the test, regardless of the outcome, such as going to a movie or getting ice cream.

When you are taking the test, if you find yourself beginning to feel anxious, remind yourself that you know the material. Visualize successfully completing the test. Then take a few deep, relaxing breaths and return to it. Work through the questions carefully but with confidence, knowing that you are capable of succeeding.

Developing a healthy mental approach to test taking will also aid in other areas of life. Test anxiety affects more than just the actual test—it can be damaging to your mental health and even contribute to depression. It's important to beat test anxiety before it becomes a problem for more than testing.

Study Strategy

Being prepared for the test is necessary to combat anxiety, but what does being prepared look like? You may study for hours on end and still not feel prepared. What you need is a strategy for test prep. The next few pages outline our recommended steps to help you plan out and conquer the challenge of preparation.

Step 1: Scope Out the Test

Learn everything you can about the format (multiple choice, essay, etc.) and what will be on the test. Gather any study materials, course outlines, or sample exams that may be available. Not only will this help you to prepare, but knowing what to expect can help to alleviate test anxiety.

Step 2: Map Out the Material

Look through the textbook or study guide and make note of how many chapters or sections it has. Then divide these over the time you have. For example, if a book has 15 chapters and you have five days to study, you need to cover three chapters each day. Even better, if you have the time, leave an extra day at the end for overall review after you have gone through the material in depth.

If time is limited, you may need to prioritize the material. Look through it and make note of which sections you think you already have a good grasp on, and which need review. While you are studying, skim quickly through the familiar sections and take more time on the challenging parts. Write out your plan so you don't get lost as you go. Having a written plan also helps you feel more in control of the study, so anxiety is less likely to arise from feeling overwhelmed at the amount to cover.

Step 3: Gather Your Tools

Decide what study method works best for you. Do you prefer to highlight in the book as you study and then go back over the highlighted portions? Or do you type out notes of the important information? Or is it helpful to make flashcards that you can carry with you? Assemble the pens, index cards, highlighters, post-it notes, and any other materials you may need so you won't be distracted by getting up to find things while you study.

If you're having a hard time retaining the information or organizing your notes, experiment with different methods. For example, try color-coding by subject with colored pens, highlighters, or post-it notes. If you learn better by hearing, try recording yourself reading your notes so you can listen while in the car, working out, or simply sitting at your desk. Ask a friend to quiz you from your flashcards, or try teaching someone the material to solidify it in your mind.

Step 4: Create Your Environment

It's important to avoid distractions while you study. This includes both the obvious distractions like visitors and the subtle distractions like an uncomfortable chair (or a too-comfortable couch that makes you want to fall asleep). Set up the best study environment possible: good lighting and a comfortable work area. If background music helps you focus, you may want to turn it on, but otherwise keep the room quiet. If you are using a computer to take notes, be sure you don't have any other windows open, especially applications like social media, games, or anything else that could distract you. Silence your phone and turn off notifications. Be sure to keep water close by so you stay hydrated while you study (but avoid unhealthy drinks and snacks).

Also, take into account the best time of day to study. Are you freshest first thing in the morning? Try to set aside some time then to work through the material. Is your mind clearer in the afternoon or evening? Schedule your study session then. Another method is to study at the same time of day that you will take the test, so that your brain gets used to working on the material at that time and will be ready to focus at test time.

Step 5: Study!

Once you have done all the study preparation, it's time to settle into the actual studying. Sit down, take a few moments to settle your mind so you can focus, and begin to follow your study plan. Don't give in to distractions or let yourself procrastinate. This is your time to prepare so you'll be ready to fearlessly approach the test. Make the most of the time and stay focused.

Of course, you don't want to burn out. If you study too long you may find that you're not retaining the information very well. Take regular study breaks. For example, taking five minutes out of every hour to walk briskly, breathing deeply and swinging your arms, can help your mind stay fresh.

As you get to the end of each chapter or section, it's a good idea to do a quick review. Remind yourself of what you learned and work on any difficult parts. When you feel that you've mastered the material, move on to the next part. At the end of your study session, briefly skim through your notes again.

But while review is helpful, cramming last minute is NOT. If at all possible, work ahead so that you won't need to fit all your study into the last day. Cramming overloads your brain with more information than it can process and retain, and your tired mind may struggle to recall even previously learned information when it is overwhelmed with last-minute study. Also, the urgent nature of cramming and the stress placed on your brain contribute to anxiety. You'll be more likely to go to the test feeling unprepared and having trouble thinking clearly.

So don't cram, and don't stay up late before the test, even just to review your notes at a leisurely pace. Your brain needs rest more than it needs to go over the information again. In fact, plan to finish your studies by noon or early afternoon the day before the test. Give your brain the rest of the day to relax or focus on other things, and get a good night's sleep. Then you will be fresh for the test and better able to recall what you've studied.

Step 6: Take a Practice Test

Many courses offer sample tests, either online or in the study materials. This is an excellent resource to check whether you have mastered the material, as well as to prepare for the test format and environment.

Check the test format ahead of time: the number of questions, the type (multiple choice, free response, etc.), and the time limit. Then create a plan for working through them. For example, if you have 30 minutes to take a 60-question test, your limit is 30 seconds per question. Spend less time on the questions you know well so that you can take more time on the difficult ones.

If you have time to take several practice tests, take the first one open book, with no time limit. Work through the questions at your own pace and make sure you fully understand them. Gradually work up to taking a test under test conditions: sit at a desk with all study materials put away and set a timer. Pace yourself to make sure you finish the test with time to spare and go back to check your answers if you have time.

After each test, check your answers. On the questions you missed, be sure you understand why you missed them. Did you misread the question (tests can use tricky wording)? Did you forget the information? Or was it something you hadn't learned? Go back and study any shaky areas that the practice tests reveal.

Taking these tests not only helps with your grade, but also aids in combating test anxiety. If you're already used to the test conditions, you're less likely to worry about it, and working through tests until you're scoring well gives you a confidence boost. Go through the practice tests until you feel comfortable, and then you can go into the test knowing that you're ready for it.

Test Tips

On test day, you should be confident, knowing that you've prepared well and are ready to answer the questions. But aside from preparation, there are several test day strategies you can employ to maximize your performance.

First, as stated before, get a good night's sleep the night before the test (and for several nights before that, if possible). Go into the test with a fresh, alert mind rather than staying up late to study.

Try not to change too much about your normal routine on the day of the test. It's important to eat a nutritious breakfast, but if you normally don't eat breakfast at all, consider eating just a protein bar. If you're a coffee drinker, go ahead and have your normal coffee. Just make sure you time it so that the caffeine doesn't wear off right in the middle of your test. Avoid sugary beverages, and drink enough water to stay hydrated but not so much that you need a restroom break 10 minutes into the test. If your test isn't first thing in the morning, consider going for a walk or doing a light workout before the test to get your blood flowing.

Allow yourself enough time to get ready, and leave for the test with plenty of time to spare so you won't have the anxiety of scrambling to arrive in time. Another reason to be early is to select a good seat. It's helpful to sit away from doors and windows, which can be distracting. Find a good seat, get out your supplies, and settle your mind before the test begins.

When the test begins, start by going over the instructions carefully, even if you already know what to expect. Make sure you avoid any careless mistakes by following the directions.

Then begin working through the questions, pacing yourself as you've practiced. If you're not sure on an answer, don't spend too much time on it, and don't let it shake your confidence. Either skip it and come back later, or eliminate as many wrong answers as possible and guess among the remaining ones. Don't dwell on these questions as you continue—put them out of your mind and focus on what lies ahead.

Be sure to read all of the answer choices, even if you're sure the first one is the right answer. Sometimes you'll find a better one if you keep reading. But don't second-guess yourself if you do immediately know the answer. Your gut instinct is usually right. Don't let test anxiety rob you of the information you know.

If you have time at the end of the test (and if the test format allows), go back and review your answers. Be cautious about changing any, since your first instinct tends to be correct, but make sure you didn't misread any of the questions or accidentally mark the wrong answer choice. Look over any you skipped and make an educated guess.

At the end, leave the test feeling confident. You've done your best, so don't waste time worrying about your performance or wishing you could change anything. Instead, celebrate the successful completion of this test. And finally, use this test to learn how to deal with anxiety even better next time.

Review Video: Test Anxiety
Visit mometrix.com/academy and enter code: 100340

Important Qualification

Not all anxiety is created equal. If your test anxiety is causing major issues in your life beyond the classroom or testing center, or if you are experiencing troubling physical symptoms related to your anxiety, it may be a sign of a serious physiological or psychological condition. If this sounds like your situation, we strongly encourage you to seek professional help.

Additional Bonus Material

Due to our efforts to try to keep this book to a manageable length, we've created a link that will give you access to all of your additional bonus material:

mometrix.com/bonus948/pax